Thyroid Cancer

Giorgio Grani • David S. Cooper
Cosimo Durante
Editors

Thyroid Cancer

A Case-Based Approach

Second Edition

Springer

Editors
Giorgio Grani
Department of Translational and Precision Medicine
Sapienza University of Rome
Rome
Italy

Cosimo Durante
Department of Translational and Precision Medicine
Sapienza University of Rome
Rome
Italy

David S. Cooper
Division of Endocrinology, Diabetes, and Metabolism
The Johns Hopkins University School of Medicine
Baltimore, MD
USA

ISBN 978-3-030-61918-3 ISBN 978-3-030-61919-0 (eBook)
https://doi.org/10.1007/978-3-030-61919-0

This Springer imprint is published by the registered company Springer Nature Switzerland AG
The registered company address is: Gewerbestrasse 11, 6330 Cham, Switzerland

Preface to the Second Edition

There have been few instances in the field of thyroidology as startling and dramatic as the epidemic of differentiated thyroid cancer in virtually all developed and developing countries around the world. Whether this is due, as many suspect, to increases in radiologic procedures and screening, or to environmental factors, such as radiation, or both, continues to be a matter of intense debate. However, for the clinicians caring for the large number of new and prevalent thyroid cancer patients, there is no debate about the need for current, practical, and evidence-based information on management. This is especially the case for our patients with low-risk papillary thyroid cancer, who represent the vast majority of thyroid cancer patients in the twenty-first century. In this group, we are learning that "less is more" in terms of the traditional treatments of surgery, radioiodine, and thyroxine suppressive therapy. Also, the need for immediate biopsy (and surgery) in the case of small, subcentimeter, low-risk suspected papillary thyroid cancer is questioned. On the other end of the spectrum, patients with more advanced disease are benefitting from new targeted therapies with a host of new pharmaceutical agents, as well as local treatments directed at individual metastatic lesions. In addition, new approaches to less common forms of thyroid malignancy, including medullary thyroid cancer and anaplastic cancer, are also being developed.

There are textbooks of thyroid disease in general and of thyroid cancer specifically; they provide the reader with a vast amount of important information related to etiology, epidemiology, diagnosis, and management. We also know that there are extensive data available electronically that provide helpful guidance with the click of a mouse. The object of this text, however, is to provide the practitioner with clinically relevant information in the context of the classical medical learning tool, the case history.

These illustrative thyroid cancer cases have been selected to cover the almost innumerable clinical issues encountered in the care of thyroid cancer patients. The textbook begins with cases highlighting the initial management of differentiated thyroid cancer. Part I includes diagnostic difficulties in patients with indeterminate thyroid nodules and encompasses a host of examples of the initial management of differentiated thyroid cancer of varying degrees of complexity. Part II provides case histories of patients who are undergoing postoperative follow-up with surveillance of varying degrees of intensity, including those who have undergone lobectomy as well as patients discovered to have metastatic disease. Part III presents special issues in thyroid cancer, including the management of thyroid cancer in pregnant patients, the elderly, and in those who have had postsurgical complications such as hypoparathyroidism and recurrent laryngeal nerve damage. Part IV comprises case histories of high-risk patients with local or distant metastatic disease, including children and the elderly. Part V presents a series of patients with locally invasive and/or widely metastatic disease who have become radioiodine refractory. This section includes detailed discussions of "targeted therapies," their indications, adverse effects, and expected therapeutic outcomes. Finally, we have included individual sections devoted to the care of patients with medullary thyroid cancer and anaplastic thyroid cancer. For this second edition, we have invited Giorgio Grani, M.D., Ph.D., from the University of Rome to edit the volume with us, and we have asked all contributors to update their cases to reflect current evidence-based practice. Some chapters were removed, and others added, to reflect the changing picture of thyroid cancer care over the last five years.

All the case histories are written by an international group of authorities in the field of thyroid cancer, and all recommendations are based on evidence-based clinical practice guidelines and data from the recent published literature. We wish to thank all the contributors to the book. They have done what we asked: to ensure that their case reports were brief, succinct, and current, and to provide guidance in areas of controversy. We also wish to thank our partners at Springer for their superb assistance and support in the production of the book. We hope this novel text will provide guidance to all those who seek to increase their understanding of thyroid cancer management.

Rome, Italy Giorgio Grani, MD, PhD
Baltimore, MD, USA David S. Cooper, MD
Rome, Italy Cosimo Durante, MD, PhD

Contents

Contributors

Monica L. Arango, MD, FAAP Division of Pediatric Endocrinology, McGovern Medical School, UTHealth, Houston, TX, USA

Douglas W. Ball, MD Division of Endocrinology, Diabetes, and Metabolism, and Department of Oncology, Johns Hopkins University School of Medicine, Baltimore, MD, USA

Keith C. Bible, MD, PhD Division of Medical Oncology, Mayo Clinic, Rochester, MN, USA

Valeria Bottici, MD Endocrine Unit, Department of Clinical and Experimental Medicine, University Hospital of Pisa, Pisa, Italy

Sarah J. Bottomley, DNP, APRN, CPNP Department of Endocrine Neoplasia & Hormonal Disorders, University of Texas MD Anderson Cancer Center, Houston, TX, USA

Laura Boucai, MD Division of Endocrinology, Diabetes, and Metabolism, Memorial Sloan-Kettering Cancer Center, Weill Cornell Medical College, New York, NY, USA

Ingrid Breuskin, MD, PhD Department of Head and Neck Oncology, Thyroid Surgery Unit, Gustave Roussy and Paris-Sud University, Villejuif, France

James Brierley, MB Department of Radiation Oncology, University of Toronto, Toronto, Canada

Department of Radiation Oncology, Princess Margaret Cancer Centre, Toronto, Canada

Lucia Brilli, MD Policlinico Santa Maria alle Scotte, Siena, Italy

Maria E. Cabanillas, MD Department of Endocrine Neoplasia and Hormonal Disorders, The University of Texas MD Anderson Cancer Center, Houston, TX, USA

Virginia Cappagli, MD Endocrine Unit, Department of Clinical and Experimental Medicine, University Hospital of Pisa, Pisa, Italy

David Carruthers, MD Department of Endocrinology, Diabetes, and Metabolism, New York University, New York, NY, USA

Maria Grazia Castagna, MD, PhD Policlinico Santa Maria alle Scotte, Siena, Italy

Department of Medical, Surgical and Neurological Sciences, University of Siena, Siena, Italy

Ashish V. Chintakuntlawar, MBBS, PhD Division of Medical Oncology, Mayo Clinic, Rochester, MN, USA

Marcela Vaisberg Cohen, MD Department of Endocrinology, Universidade Federal do Rio de Janeiro- Medical School, Rio de Janeiro, RJ, Brazil

David S. Cooper, MD Division of Endocrinology, Diabetes, and Metabolism, The Johns Hopkins University School of Medicine, Baltimore, MD, USA

Giuseppe Costante, MD Endocrinology Clinic, Medicine Department, Institut Jules Bordet, Comprehensive Cancer Center – Université Libre de Bruxelles, Brussels, Belgium

Ramona Dadu, MD Department of Endocrine Neoplasia and Hormonal Disorders, The University of Texas MD Anderson Cancer Center, Houston, TX, USA

Désirée Deandreis, MD Division of Nuclear Medicine, Department of Medical Sciences, University of Turin, AOU Città della Salute e della Scienza, Turin, Italy

Dimpi Desai, MD Division of Endocrinology, Diabetes and Metabolism, Baylor College of Medicine, Houston, TX, USA

Gerard M. Doherty, MD Department of Surgery, Brigham and Women's Hospital/ Harvard Medical School, Boston, MA, USA

Henning Dralle, MD FRCS, FACS, FEBS Department of General, Visceral and Transplantation Surgery, Section of Endocrine Surgery, University Hospital, Essen, Germany

Medical Faculty, University of Duisburg-Essen, Essen, Germany

Cosimo Durante, MD, PhD Department of Translational and Precision Medicine, Sapienza University of Rome, Rome, Italy

Rossella Elisei, MD Endocrine Unit, Department of Clinical and Experimental Medicine, University Hospital of Pisa, Pisa, Italy

Rosa Falcone, MD Department of Translational and Precision Medicine, Sapienza University of Rome, Rome, Italy

Sebastiano Filetti, MD Department of Translational and Precision Medicine, Sapienza University of Rome, Rome, Italy

Monica Finessi, MD Division of Nuclear Medicine, Department of Medical Sciences, University of Turin, AOU Città della Salute e della Scienza, Turin, Italy

Carlotta Giani, MD Endocrine Unit, Department of Clinical and Experimental Medicine, University Hospital of Pisa, Pisa, Italy

Meredith Giuliani, MB Department of Radiation Oncology, University of Toronto, Toronto, Canada

Department of Radiation Oncology, Princess Margaret Cancer Centre, Toronto, Canada

Alyse S. Goldberg, MD Division of Endocrinology, Department of Medicine, Sunnybrook Health Sciences Centre, Toronto, Ontario, Canada

Adam D. Goodale, MD The Christ Hospital Physicians – Ear, Nose & Throat, Liberty Township, OH, USA

Giorgio Grani, MD, PhD Department of Translational and Precision Medicine, Sapienza University of Rome, Rome, Italy

Joanne Guerlain, MD Department of Head and Neck Oncology, Thyroid Surgery Unit, Gustave Roussy and Paris-Sud University, Villejuif, France

Dana M. Hartl, MD, PhD Department of Head and Neck Oncology, Thyroid Surgery Unit, Gustave Roussy and Paris-Sud University, Villejuif, France

Steven P. Hodak, MD Department of Endocrinology, Diabetes, and Metabolism, New York University, New York, NY, USA

Michael E. Hopkins, MBchB, BSC, MRCS(ENT) Department of Otolaryngology, Head and Neck Surgery, NHS Lothian, Edinburgh, UK

Mimi I. Hu, MD Department of Endocrine Neoplasia and Hormonal Disorders, The University of Texas MD Anderson Cancer Center, Houston, TX, USA

Yasuhiro Ito, MD, PhD Department of Clinical Trial Management, Kuma Hospital, Center for Excellence in Thyroid Care, Kobe, Japan

Department of Surgery, Kuma Hospital, Center for Excellence in Thyroid Care, Kobe, Japan

Ana P. Kiess, MD, PhD Department of Radiation Oncology, Johns Hopkins School of Medicine, Baltimore, MD, USA

Jina Kim, MD Department of Surgery, University of California San Francisco, San Francisco, CA, USA

Carmen Kut, MD, PhD Department of Radiation Oncology, Johns Hopkins School of Medicine, Baltimore, MD, USA

Angela Liang, B.A. Johns Hopkins School of Medicine, Baltimore, MD, USA

Virginia Liberini, MD Division of Nuclear Medicine, Department of Medical Sciences, University of Turin, AOU Città della Salute e della Scienza, Turin, Italy

Andreas Machens, MD Department of Visceral, Vascular and Endocrine Surgery, University Hospital, Halle (Saale), Germany

Medical Faculty, University of Halle-Wittenberg, Halle (Saale), Germany

Susan J. Mandel, MD, MPH Division of Endocrinology, Diabetes and Metabolism, Perelman School of Medicine University of Pennsylvania, Philadelphia, PA, USA

Antonio Matrone, MD Endocrine Unit, Department of Clinical and Experimental Medicine, University Hospital of Pisa, Pisa, Italy

Donald S. A. McLeod, MBBS (Hon I), FRACP, MPH, PhD Department of Endocrinology & Diabetes, Royal Brisbane & Women's Hospital, Herston, QLD, Australia

Department of Population Health, QIMR Berghofer Medical Research Institute, Herston, QLD, Australia

Salvatore Minisola, MD Department of Clinical, Internal, Anesthesiological and Cardiovascular Sciences, "Sapienza" University of Rome, Rome, Italy

Akira Miyauchi, MD, PhD Department of Surgery, Kuma Hospital, Center for Excellence in Thyroid Care, Kobe, Japan

Iain J. Nixon, MBChB, FRCS (ORL-HNS), PhD Department of Otolaryngology, Head and Neck Surgery, NHS Lothian, Edinburgh, UK

Furio Pacini, MD Department of Medical, Surgical and Neurological Sciences, University of Siena, Siena, Italy

Jessica Pepe, MD, PhD Department of Clinical, Internal, Anesthesiological and Cardiovascular Sciences, "Sapienza" University of Rome, Rome, Italy

Tania Pilli, MD Policlinico Santa Maria alle Scotte, Siena, Italy

Valeria Ramundo, MD Department of Translational and Precision Medicine, Sapienza University of Rome, Rome, Italy

Lorne E. Rotstein, MD Department of Surgery, University Health Network and University of Toronto, Toronto, Ontario, Canada

Anna M. Sawka, MD, PhD Division of Endocrinology, University Health Network and University of Toronto, Toronto, Ontario, Canada

Wen T. Shen, MD, MA Department of Surgery, University of California San Francisco, San Francisco, CA, USA

Steven I. Sherman, MD University of Texas M.D. Anderson Cancer Center, Houston, TX, USA

Zachary Simons, MD Division of Endocrinology, Diabetes, and Metabolism, The Johns Hopkins University School of Medicine, Baltimore, MD, USA

Robert C. Smallridge, MD Division of Endocrinology, Mayo Clinic, Jacksonville, FL, USA

Julie Ann Sosa, MD, MA Department of Surgery, University of California San Francisco, San Francisco, CA, USA

David L. Steward, MD Department of Otolaryngology – Head & Neck Surgery, University of Cincinnati College of Medicine, Cincinnati, OH, USA

Fernanda Vaisman, MD, PhD Department of Endocrinology, National cancer Institute- INCa, Universidade Federal do Rio de Janeiro- Medical School, Rio de Janeiro, RJ, Brazil

Steven G. Waguespack, MD, FACE Department of Endocrine Neoplasia and Hormonal Disorders, The University of Texas MD Anderson Cancer Center, Houston, TX, USA

Jennifer R. Wang, MD, ScM Department of Head and Neck Surgery, The University of Texas MD Anderson Cancer Center, Houston, TX, USA

Leonard Wartofsky, MD MedStar Health Research Institute, MedStar Washington Hospital Center, Washington, DC, USA

Georgetown University School of Medicine, Washington, DC, USA

Swaytha Yalamanchi, MD Division of Endocrinology, Diabetes, and Metabolism, Palo Alto Medical Foundation, Palo Alto, CA, USA

Part I
Differentiated Thyroid Cancer: Initial Management

Chapter 1
A Patient with a Single Thyroid Nodule Suspicious for Follicular Neoplasm According to the Bethesda System for Reporting Thyroid Cytopathology: Molecular Evaluation

Dimpi Desai and Susan J. Mandel

Abbreviation

ACR TI-RADS	American College of Radiology Thyroid Imaging Reporting and Data System
ATA	American Thyroid Association
EFVPTC	Encapsulated follicular variant papillary thyroid cancer
FN	Follicular neoplasm
FNA	Fine-needle aspiration
GC	Genomic Classifier
GEC	Gene Expression Classifier
GSC	Gene Sequencing Classifier
NIFTP	Noninvasive follicular thyroid neoplasm with papillary-like nuclear features
NPV	Negative predictive value
PPV	Positive predictive value
TBSRTC	The Bethesda System for Reporting Thyroid Cytopathology

D. Desai
Division of Endocrinology, Diabetes and Metabolism, Baylor College of Medicine, Houston, TX, USA

S. J. Mandel (✉)
Division of Endocrinology, Diabetes and Metabolism, Perelman School of Medicine University of Pennsylvania, Philadelphia, PA, USA
e-mail: Susan.Mandel@pennmedicine.upenn.edu

G. Grani et al. (eds.), *Thyroid Cancer*,
https://doi.org/10.1007/978-3-030-61919-0_1

Case Presentation

A 76-year-old woman presents for the evaluation of a thyroid nodule that was found incidentally on carotid ultrasound. She denies a family history of thyroid cancer or exposure to external beam radiation as a child. Her serum TSH level is 2.3 mIU/L. On physical exam, there is a 2.5 cm palpable right thyroid nodule. A diagnostic ultrasound reveals a 27 × 29 × 38 mm solid, isoechoic nodule with smooth margins and without any microcalcifications; cervical lymph nodes appear normal (Fig. 1.1). A fine-needle aspiration (FNA) with ultrasound guidance yields a cytologic diagnosis of "suspicious for follicular neoplasm" (Bethesda IV).

Assessment and Literature Review

Once a clinician is confronted with a patient with a cytologic diagnosis of follicular neoplasm, now classified as Bethesda IV in The Bethesda System for Reporting Thyroid Cytopathology (TBSRTC) [1], the relevant clinical question is that patient's likelihood of having thyroid cancer. The malignancy risk for a nodule with a cytologic diagnosis of "suspicious for follicular neoplasm"/"follicular neoplasm" (henceforth referred to as a FN nodule) is approximately 25–40%, and this decreases by up to 40% if tumors now classified as noninvasive follicular thyroid neoplasm with papillary-like nuclear features (NIFTPs) are removed from the calculation [1].

Recent studies have shown that the sonographic pattern of a FN nodule, if either likely benign or highly suspicious, may modify malignancy risk and lead directly to recommendations to either surveillance or surgery, respectively [2, 3]. However, for 80–85% of FN nodules, the sonographic pattern does not alter the FN cytology associated with malignancy risk; for these nodules, molecular testing may be indicated.

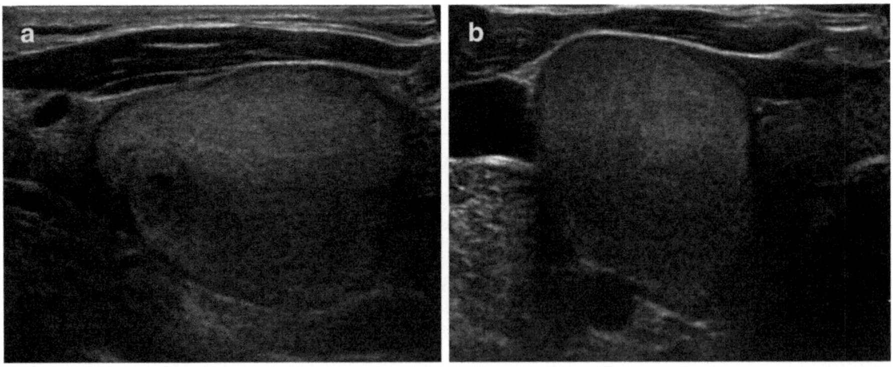

Fig. 1.1 Longitudinal (**a**) and transverse (**b**) grayscale sonographic appearance of a 27 × 29 × 38 mm solid, isoechoic, noncalcified nodule with regular margins (ATA low suspicion, TR3)

The application of molecular diagnostic tools to FN nodules is predicated upon the assumption that results can further refine malignancy risk in these patients where cytology is not definitive. If molecular testing techniques were 100% sensitive and specific for the diagnosis of all thyroid cancer histologies, this technology could replace cytologic analysis. Perhaps future testing strategies will achieve this goal, but current commercially available molecular diagnostics do not. Therefore, to interpret the results of these molecular tests for an individual patient, the clinician must understand the reported negative and positive predictive values and their derivation from recently published studies.

A high negative predictive value (NPV) signifies that the false negative rate is very low when the test result is negative, e.g., NPV of 97% is associated with a cancer risk of only 3%. On the other hand, a high positive predictive value (PPV) indicates that the likelihood of malignancy is high when the test is positive, e.g., PPV of 90% means that cancer is present in 90% of patients with this result. The point estimates for NPV and PPV for a given test vary based upon the prevalence of disease (thyroid cancer) in the tested population. For example, when the cancer risk is low, e.g., 10%, even a test with a sensitivity of 60% will be associated with an NPV of over 95%. Here, because there are so few cancers in the population, the absolute number of cases where the test fails to accurately diagnose cancer is very low, and this does not significantly decrease the NPV. But, as the cancer rate rises, this same test with 60% sensitivity will miss more diagnoses leading to a higher false-negative rate and lowering the NPV. On the other hand, the PPV rises as the population disease risk increases because false-positive results decrease when there are fewer patients without thyroid cancer.

Therefore, for a given patient, the interpretation of results from currently available molecular diagnostics depends upon the patient's baseline malignancy risk after cytologic diagnosis, i.e., the "pretest probability." Certain factors may modify the risk of malignancy associated with a FN cytologic result and could potentially alter the interpretation of subsequent molecular diagnostic results. Prior to the discussion of the recent publications about the application of molecular testing, we will review the literature on patient demographics and nodule sonographic imaging that may alter the malignancy risk associated with a FN nodule.

Part I: Risk of Malignancy

Limitations of Cytologic and Histologic Interpretations

Using TBSRTC, the diagnosis of Bethesda IV ("suspicious for follicular neoplasm"/"follicular neoplasm") is rendered on average in 10–15% of FNAs, but center-specific rates may vary from 1.2% to 25.3% [4]. Of the three indeterminate cytology classifications defined by TBSRTC [1], follicular neoplasm is the most reliably reproducible. Interobserver diagnostic agreement is considered fair (kappa 0.5), based on Fleiss' criteria for interpreting kappa values [5].

Prior to the widespread adoption of molecular testing, the standard of care for patients with this cytologic diagnosis had been diagnostic lobectomy, eventually followed by completion thyroidectomy if histology was malignant. In large studies predating molecular testing, about 60–70% of patients with FN nodules have been observed to undergo surgery [4, 6]. Approximately 25% of these FN nodules were malignant on histology [4, 7], with center-specific rates ranging from 14% to 49% [7]. Of these cancers, 27% were follicular carcinomas, but most (68%) were papillary thyroid cancers, with the low-risk follicular variant as the most common subtype [6].

However, this observed risk of malignancy for a FN nodule predates the 2016 reclassification of the encapsulated follicular variant papillary thyroid cancer (EFVPTC) as a noncancerous lesion termed "noninvasive follicular thyroid neoplasm with papillary-like nuclear features (NIFTP)," a name more accurately describing its behavior [8]. The diagnosis of NIFTP is applied to tumors previously called EFVPTC when no capsular invasion is identified after sampling the entire tumor capsule. The NIFTP reclassification was done because of its extremely low recurrence risk, hence mandating de-escalation of clinical management to prevent overtreatment [8].

In contemporary practice, if NIFTP tumors are no longer considered malignant, the risk of malignancy for FN cytology nodules decreases by 20–40% and may vary depending upon institutional prevalence of EFVPTC [9, 10]. Overall, TBSRTC estimates the range for the cancer risk of Bethesda IV cytology as 25–40% if NIFTP is considered malignant and as 10–40% if it is not [1]. Nevertheless, the diagnosis of NIFTP requires surgical removal to be confirmed by documentation of the lack of tumor capsular invasion. Patients with these tumors require the same surveillance as a very low-risk malignancy.

Demographic and Sonographic Features Predictive of Malignancy

Once a nodule has a cytologic diagnosis of FN, some studies have reported that certain clinical features, including male gender, age, and the presence of a solitary nodule, are predictive of malignancy, but these findings have not been consistent [11–15]. Large nodule size, in contrast, may be a reliable predictor of follicular thyroid carcinoma [12, 14]. Nodule size greater than or equal to 2.8 cm has been associated with an 11-fold increased risk of follicular thyroid carcinoma, but not with an increased risk of papillary thyroid carcinoma, which is typically smaller [14]. For example, in one study [12], nodule size only achieved statistical significance as a predictor of malignancy in FN nodules after papillary carcinoma was excluded from the analysis. Consistent with these findings, nodule size was not predictive in three studies when the malignant histologic diagnoses were predominately papillary [15–17]. Only a single study with predominately follicular cancers failed to show nodule size as a significant predictor [18].

Ultrasound examination of the thyroid is the initial diagnostic test of choice when an abnormal thyroid is palpated or an "incidental" thyroid nodule is discovered on another radiologic study. Several professional societies have created tiered risk-stratification systems (RSS) to classify thyroid nodules into categories based on combinations of sonographic features associated with cancer. Each class is associated with a size cut-off for FNA recommendations. The two systems most commonly used in the United States are the American Thyroid Association (ATA) sonographic pattern classification [19] and the American College of Radiology Thyroid Imaging Reporting and Data System (ACR TI-RADS) [20].

The ATA system is based on the identification of sonographic patterns derived from nodule composition, echogenicity, margins, and shape, in addition to the presence/absence of microcalcifications and abnormal cervical lymph nodes. Based upon combinations of these characteristics, it stratifies thyroid nodules into five levels of suspicion with respective risks of malignancy: benign, 1%; very low suspicion, <3%; low suspicion, 5–10%; intermediate suspicion, 10–20%; and high suspicion, >70–90% [19]. On the other hand, the ACR TI-RADS system is a scoring system where 0–3 points are assigned to the characteristics of five ultrasound features: composition, echogenicity, shape, margins, and echogenic foci. A sum of these assigned points stratifies the risk of malignancy into five levels (TR1 to TR5) classified respectively as benign, not suspicious, minimally suspicious, moderately suspicious, or highly suspicious for malignancy [20]. The recommended nodule size thresholds are slightly different between these classification systems (Table 1.1).

Table 1.1 Comparison of ATA classification system of thyroid nodules and ACR TI-RADS system

ATA (2015)	ACR TI-RADS (2017)
Benign *Risk of malignancy < 1%* *FNA is not indicated* Purely cystic nodules (no solid component)	**TR1 benign** *Risk of malignancy 2%* *FNA is not indicated* Spongiform Pure cyst **TR2 not suspicious** *Risk of malignancy 2%* *FNA is not indicated* Mixed cystic or solid noncalcified nodules with smooth margins and oval shape
Very low suspicion *Risk of malignancy <3%* *FNA ≥20 mm or observation* Spongiform or partially cystic nodules without any of the US features defining low-, intermediate-, or high-suspicion patterns	**TR3 mildly suspicious** *Risk of malignancy 3%* *FNA ≥ 25 mm* Isoechoic solid or hypoechoic cystic noncalcified nodules with smooth margins and oval shape
Low suspicion *Risk of malignancy 5–10%* *FNA ≥15 mm* Isoechoic or hyperechoic solid nodule or partially cystic nodule with eccentric solid area without: microcalcifications, irregular margin, extrathyroidal extension, taller-than-wide shape	

(continued)

Table 1.1 (continued)

ATA (2015)	ACR TI-RADS (2017)
Intermediate suspicion *Risk of malignancy 10–20%* *FNA ≥10 mm* Hypoechoic solid nodule with smooth margins without: microcalcifications, extrathyroidal extension, or taller-than-wide shape	**TR4 moderately suspicious** *Risk of malignancy 5–20%* *FNA >15 mm* Hypoechoic solid noncalcified nodules with oval shape and either smooth or irregular or lobulated margins Isoechoic solid or mixed noncalcified nodules with either nonparallel orientation (taller than wide) or punctate echogenic foci
High suspicion *Risk of malignancy >70–90%* *FNA ≥10 mm* Solid hypoechoic nodule or solid hypoechoic component of partially cystic nodule with ≥1 of the following: Irregular margins (infiltrative, microlobulated) Microcalcifications Taller-than-wide shape Rim calcifications with small extrusive soft tissue Extrathyroidal extension	**TR5 suspicious** *Risk of malignancy "at least 20%"* *FNA >10 mm* Hypoechoic solid nodule with any of the following: Nonparallel orientation (taller than wide) Extrathyroidal extension Punctate echogenic foci Isoechoic solid nodule with irregular or lobulated margins and either peripheral rim calcifications or punctate echogenic foci

Adapted from [28]

Recent studies have evaluated whether the sonographic appearance of a FN nodule may better refine the cancer risk (including NIFTP) within the range reported by TBSRTC [2, 3]. For the sonographically low suspicious nodules (ATA very low suspicion and TR1 and TR2), there were no cases of malignancy. Hence for these nodules, clinical observation may be offered without further testing. For the sonographically high suspicious nodules (ATA high suspicion and TR5), the risk of malignancy was observed to be 50–60%. Hence, surgical intervention should be considered as molecular testing may not offer any additional benefit. However, most (~80%) FN nodules have imaging features that fall into low to intermediate suspicion categories (ATA low and intermediate suspicion, TR3, and TR4), and for these, the cancer risk remains at 15–35%, the range for which molecular testing is generally considered. Hence, molecular testing has become an important diagnostic tool for nodules with indeterminate cytology [21].

Part II: Molecular Evaluation

The appropriate application of diagnostic molecular testing is based upon three principles: analytical validation, clinical validation, and clinical usefulness. Analytical validation refers to test precision and reproducibility, even across different processing and storage methods. As determined by Congress, all molecular tests should be performed in Clinical Laboratory Improvements Amendments-certified laboratory. Clinical validation is the ability of the test to detect either thyroid nodule benignity or malignancy when applied in prospective blinded clinical studies. This includes the determination of test sensitivity and specificity, and the calculation of NPV and PPV. While NPV and PPV are dependent on the disease prevalence in a population, the sensitivity and specificity are independent of the same and intrinsic features of the method. The third principle of clinical usefulness signifies the socioeconomic consequences of molecular testing in real clinical practice and the overall health outcome while considering the broader needs of an individual, family, and society [21, 22].

Commercial molecular diagnostic testing for thyroid nodules may include analysis for DNA point mutations and fusions, mRNA expression, and miRNA changes. Earlier generation molecular tests had either more limited specificity, e.g., Afirma Gene Expression Classifier (GEC), or sensitivity, e.g., ThyroSeq v2. However, the two most commonly used current molecular diagnostics have improved performance.

The Afirma Gene Sequencing Classifier (GSC) is a RNA-sequencing-based test that includes 12 classifiers composed of 10,196 genes (1115 core genes) plus 7 additional components to identify parathyroid lesions, MTC, *BRAF* V600 E mutations, *RET/PTC1* or *RET/PTC3* fusions, and Hürthle cell lesions. A blinded clinical validation study, using the same cohort of the original GEC study, assessed the performance of GSC in 191 indeterminate nodules (Bethesda III and IV) from 49 sites, and the test revealed a high sensitivity of 90% and improved specificity of 64% compared to the GEC (38%) for Bethesda IV. With a baseline 47% cancer prevalence for Bethesda IV, the NPV was 97% and the PPV was 47% [23].

The ThyroSeq v3 Genomic Classifier (GC) adopts next-generation sequencing technology to analyze 112 genes using 5 classes of genetic alterations, including point mutations, insertions/deletions, gene fusions, copy number alterations, and abnormal gene expression. Then based upon algorithmic analysis, the result is classified as either negative or positive. A small number of ThyroSeq results (~5%) are classified as "currently negative" because of the presence of a low-risk mutation at a low allelic frequency. The reported cancer risk for such nodules is 5–10% [24]. A recent prospective, double-blinded, multicenter validation study reported 97% sensitivity and 75% specificity for cases diagnosed as Bethesda IV. Given a baseline cancer prevalence of 35%, the NPV and PPV estimates were 97% and 66%, respectively [25]. Publications discussing real-world application of both tests report consistent findings.

If resected, FN nodules with a positive Afirma GSC or ThyroSeq v3 GC results are generally low-risk follicular-patterned cancers [26]. In our institution, for the FN nodules that were ThyroSeq v3 GC positive, the most common mutations observed were *RAS* mutations corresponding to low-risk carcinomas. It is unusual for mutational analysis of a FN nodule to reveal the high-risk combination of both *BRAF* V600E and *TERT* mutations [25] for which more aggressive surgery is indicated.

Part III: Surgical Management

The most recent ATA recommendations state that lobectomy suffices for low-risk papillary and follicular cancers, defined by tumor size less than 4 cm and without vascular invasion, extrathyroidal extension, or metastatic lymph node involvement [19]. Hence, for a FN nodule with positive result from either Afirma GSC or ThyroSeq v3 GC, lobectomy should be considered after sonographic evaluation of cervical lymph nodes. Other considerations may influence the extent of surgery: the presence of contralateral nodules, concomitant hypothyroidism or hyperparathyroidism, as well as patient preference and comorbidities. Patients with preoperative serum TSH levels <1.7 mIU/L are more likely to remain euthyroid after lobectomy alone than those with higher levels [27].

Management of the Case

This patient has a follicular neoplasm cytologic diagnosis (Bethesda IV) without any known risk factor for thyroid cancer. On ultrasound, the nodule is 27 × 29 × 38 mm in size, solid, isoechoic, with regular margin, and without any microcalcifications. The sonographic appearance is consistent with ATA low suspicion or TR3. Hence, the pretest risk of malignancy associated with this nodule is ~15–35%. The patient elected to proceed with molecular testing with the ThyroSeq v3 GC for risk stratification. Her result was "negative," associated with an NPV of ~97%. A repeat ultrasound 18 months later documented stability in size and sonographic appearance.

Clinical Pearls

- The risk of malignancy for a FN nodule is approximately 25–40% (and decreases to 10–40% if NIFTP is considered benign).
- The sonographic appearance of a FN nodule using an ultrasound risk stratification system (ATA or ACR TI-RADS) may refine the nodule's malignancy risk. While an ATA very low suspicion or TR1 or TR2 nodule can be observed, an ATA high suspicion or TR5 nodule should be directly referred to surgery. For ATA low or intermediate suspicion or TR3 or TR4 nodules, molecular testing should be considered.
- ThyroSeq v3 GC and Afirma GSC are the most common molecular tests in current practice and have improved performance compared to earlier versions. The application of these tests is predicated upon understanding that as the baseline risk of cancer (i.e., the "pretest probability") increases, the negative predictive value decreases and the positive predictive value increases.
- If FN nodules that test positive on molecular testing are malignant, these are generally low-risk tumors, and, often, lobectomy suffices.

References

1. Cibas ES, Ali SZ. The 2017 Bethesda system for reporting thyroid cytopathology. Thyroid. 2017;27(11):1341–6.
2. Ahmadi S, Herbst R, Oyekunle T, Jiang X, Strickland K, Roman S, et al. Using the Ata and Acr Ti-Rads sonographic classifications as adjunctive predictors of malignancy for indeterminate thyroid nodules. Endocr Pract. 2019;25(9):908–17.
3. Valderrabano P, McGettigan MJ, Lam CA, Khazai L, Thompson ZJ, Chung CH, et al. Thyroid nodules with indeterminate cytology: utility of the American Thyroid Association Sonographic patterns for cancer risk stratification. Thyroid. 2018;28(8):1004–12.
4. Bongiovanni M, Spitale A, Faquin WC, Mazzucchelli L, Baloch ZW. The Bethesda system for reporting thyroid cytopathology: a meta-analysis. Acta Cytol. 2012;56(4):333–9.
5. Walts AE, Bose S, Fan X, Frishberg D, Scharre K, de Peralta-Venturina M, et al. A simplified Bethesda system for reporting thyroid cytopathology using only four categories improves intra- and inter-observer diagnostic agreement and provides non-overlapping estimates of malignancy risks. Diagn Cytopathol. 2012;40 Suppl 1:E62–8.
6. Yang J, Schnadig V, Logrono R, Wasserman PG. Fine-needle aspiration of thyroid nodules: a study of 4703 patients with histologic and clinical correlations. Cancer. 2007;111(5):306–15.
7. Wang CC, Friedman L, Kennedy GC, Wang H, Kebebew E, Steward DL, et al. A large multicenter correlation study of thyroid nodule cytopathology and histopathology. Thyroid. 2011;21(3):243–51.
8. Nikiforov YE, Seethala RR, Tallini G, Baloch ZW, Basolo F, Thompson LD, et al. Nomenclature revision for encapsulated follicular variant of papillary thyroid carcinoma: a paradigm shift to reduce overtreatment of indolent tumors. JAMA Oncol. 2016;2(8):1023–9.
9. Faquin WC, Wong LQ, Afrogheh AH, Ali SZ, Bishop JA, Bongiovanni M, et al. Impact of reclassifying noninvasive follicular variant of papillary thyroid carcinoma on the risk of malignancy in The Bethesda System for Reporting Thyroid Cytopathology. Cancer Cytopathol. 2016;124(3):181–7.
10. Strickland KC, Howitt BE, Marqusee E, Alexander EK, Cibas ES, Krane JF, et al. The impact of noninvasive follicular variant of papillary thyroid carcinoma on rates of malignancy for fine-needle aspiration diagnostic categories. Thyroid. 2015;25(9):987–92.
11. Tuttle RM, Lemar H, Burch HB. Clinical features associated with an increased risk of thyroid malignancy in patients with follicular neoplasia by fine-needle aspiration. Thyroid. 1998;8(5):377–83.
12. Lubitz CC, Faquin WC, Yang J, Mekel M, Gaz RD, Parangi S, et al. Clinical and cytological features predictive of malignancy in thyroid follicular neoplasms. Thyroid. 2010;20(1):25–31.
13. Schlinkert RT, van Heerden JA, Goellner JR, Gharib H, Smith SL, Rosales RF, et al. Factors that predict malignant thyroid lesions when fine-needle aspiration is "suspicious for follicular neoplasm.". Mayo Clin Proc. 1997;72(10):913–6.
14. Lee SH, Baek JS, Lee JY, Lim JA, Cho SY, Lee TH, et al. Predictive factors of malignancy in thyroid nodules with a cytological diagnosis of follicular neoplasm. Endocr Pathol. 2013;24(4):177–83.
15. Raber W, Kaserer K, Niederle B, Vierhapper H. Risk factors for malignancy of thyroid nodules initially identified as follicular neoplasia by fine-needle aspiration: results of a prospective study of one hundred twenty patients. Thyroid. 2000;10(8):709–12.
16. Gulcelik NE, Gulcelik MA, Kuru B. Risk of malignancy in patients with follicular neoplasm: predictive value of clinical and ultrasonographic features. Arch Otolaryngol Head Neck Surg. 2008;134(12):1312–5.
17. Rago T, Di Coscio G, Basolo F, Scutari M, Elisei R, Berti P, et al. Combined clinical, thyroid ultrasound and cytological features help to predict thyroid malignancy in follicular and Hupsilonrthle cell thyroid lesions: results from a series of 505 consecutive patients. Clin Endocrinol. 2007;66(1):13–20.

18. Choi YJ, Yun JS, Kim DH. Clinical and ultrasound features of cytology diagnosed follicular neoplasm. Endocr J. 2009;56(3):383–9.
19. Haugen BR, Alexander EK, Bible KC, Doherty GM, Mandel SJ, Nikiforov YE, et al. 2015 American Thyroid Association management guidelines for adult patients with thyroid nodules and differentiated thyroid cancer: the American Thyroid Association guidelines task force on thyroid nodules and differentiated thyroid cancer. Thyroid. 2016;26(1):1–133.
20. Tessler FN, Middleton WD, Grant EG, Hoang JK, Berland LL, Teefey SA, et al. ACR thyroid imaging, reporting and data system (TI-RADS): white paper of the ACR TI-RADS Committee. J Am Coll Radiol. 2017;14(5):587–95.
21. Mayson SE, Haugen BR. Molecular diagnostic evaluation of thyroid nodules. Endocrinol Metab Clin N Am. 2019;48(1):85–97.
22. Teutsch SM, Bradley LA, Palomaki GE, Haddow JE, Piper M, Calonge N, et al. The evaluation of genomic applications in practice and prevention (EGAPP) initiative: methods of the EGAPP Working Group. Genet Med. 2009;11(1):3–14.
23. Patel KN, Angell TE, Babiarz J, Barth NM, Blevins T, Duh QY, et al. Performance of a genomic sequencing classifier for the preoperative diagnosis of cytologically indeterminate thyroid nodules. JAMA Surg. 2018;153(9):817–24.
24. Nikiforova MN, Mercurio S, Wald AI, Barbi de Moura M, Callenberg K, Santana-Santos L, et al. Analytical performance of the ThyroSeq v3 genomic classifier for cancer diagnosis in thyroid nodules. Cancer. 2018;124(8):1682–90.
25. Steward DL, Carty SE, Sippel RS, Yang SP, Sosa JA, Sipos JA, et al. Performance of a multigene genomic classifier in thyroid nodules with indeterminate cytology: a prospective blinded multicenter study. JAMA Oncol. 2019;5(2):204–12.
26. Endo M, Nabhan F, Porter K, Roll K, Shirley LA, Azaryan I, et al. Afirma gene sequencing classifier compared with gene expression classifier in indeterminate thyroid nodules. Thyroid. 2019;29(8):1115–24.
27. Park S, Jeon MJ, Song E, Oh HS, Kim M, Kwon H, et al. Clinical features of early and late postoperative hypothyroidism after lobectomy. J Clin Endocrinol Metab. 2017;102(4):1317–24.
28. Durante C, Grani G, Lamartina L, Filetti S, Mandel SJ, Cooper DS. The diagnosis and management of thyroid nodules: a review. JAMA. 2018;319(9):914–24.

Chapter 2
A Young Patient with Intrathyroidal Papillary Thyroid Cancer and Family History of Differentiated Thyroid Cancer

Giorgio Grani, Valeria Ramundo, and Cosimo Durante

Case Presentation

A general practitioner referred an asymptomatic 39-year-old man to our center for thyroid ultrasonography. The patient had no evidence of thyroid disease, and his past medical history was unremarkable. However, his mother and his uncle had both been diagnosed with papillary thyroid cancer (PTC). Both had been treated with thyroidectomy followed by radioactive iodine (RAI) remnant ablation (RRA), and the uncle also had had multiple RAI therapies for RAI-avid lung metastases. At the time of the patient's referral, they had been disease-free for 5 and 1.5 years, respectively. There was no documentable history of radiation exposure.

The patient's physical examination was negative, but thyroid and neck ultrasonography revealed multiple solid hypoechoic nodules in both lobes of the thyroid. The largest one, which was located in the left lobe, measured 10 mm and exhibited intranodular punctate hyperechoic foci. There was no clinical or sonographic evidence of lymph node involvement. The patient was euthyroid (serum TSH: 1.4 mIU/L). The dominant nodule, being classified as high suspicion by the 2015 American Thyroid Association (ATA) guidelines [1] (and other sonographic risk-stratification systems) [2], was subjected to fine-needle aspiration biopsy (FNAB), and the cytology findings were consistent with PTC (Bethesda class VI) [3]. A total thyroidectomy was performed. The pathology showed multifocal, bilateral, classic variant PTC (lesion diameters: left lobe, 9 and 2 mm; isthmus, 4 mm; right lobe, 5 mm). There was no evidence of extrathyroidal extension or vascular invasion

G. Grani · V. Ramundo · C. Durante (✉)
Department of Translational and Precision Medicine, Sapienza University of Rome, Rome, Italy
e-mail: cosimo.durante@uniroma1.it

G. Grani et al. (eds.), *Thyroid Cancer*,
https://doi.org/10.1007/978-3-030-61919-0_2

(pT1am, N0b—Stage 1, AJCC/TNM VIII Edition) [4, 5] . Based on the 2009 ATA Initial Risk Stratification System [6], and its update [1], the patient's disease was considered at low risk for recurrence. Because the case met the current criteria for familial nonmedullary thyroid cancer (FNMTC), however, the possibilities that the patient might actually be at higher risk than he seemed to be and that other members of his family might be genetically predisposed to thyroid cancer had to be considered.

Literature Review

Approximately 3–10% of all NMTCs appear to be familial [7]. Excluding those tumors linked to syndromes (e.g., familial adenomatous polyposis, Gardner's syndrome, PTEN hamartoma tumor syndrome, Werner's syndrome, or Carney's complex), most of these cases have not been linked to specific genetic causes. Some candidate loci (MNG1, TCO, fPTC/PRN, NMTC1, FTEN) and genes (*FOXE1*, telomere telomerase complex, *TITF-1/NKX2·1*, and *SRGAP1*) have been proposed, but a specific genetic testing approach is not available [7, 8]. Therefore, the diagnosis is generally made when NMTC has been found in two or more first-degree relatives. When cases are defined in this manner, the probability that affected family members actually have sporadic tumors has been estimated at about 30–40%, but when three of more members of a kindred are affected, the probability of hereditary disease climbs to over 96% [9].

Management of patients with FNMTC should be based for the most part on the ATA risk class of the individual patient, although a positive family history is considered to be a potential risk modifier. In terms of surgery, for example, the 2015 ATA guidelines list familial disease as one of the *possible* indications for choosing thyroidectomy over lobectomy (others being age >45 years, the presence of nodules in the contralateral lobe, or a personal history of radiation therapy to the head and neck). The issue of RRA in this context is even more of a gray area. Our patient had multiple foci of PTC, each with a maximum diameter of less than 1 cm, and his risk for recurrence was thus classified as low. There is an appreciable difference between the risks of recurrence associated with unifocal and multifocal papillary microcarcinomas (1–2% vs. 4–6%, respectively), especially when the sum of the diameters of the tumor foci exceeds 1 cm (as it did in our patient) [10, 11]. Nonetheless, the risk remains low in both cases, and there is no evidence that RRA improves the disease-specific or disease-free survival in either case—unless there are other high-risk features [1].

Does the fact that the multifocal disease is familial rather than sporadic constitute an additional high-risk feature that could tip the scales in favor of RRA? Conflicting data have been published on the clinical behavior of FNMTCs. Some studies suggest that they are indeed more aggressive than their sporadic counterparts, as reflected by higher rates of extrathyroidal invasion, lymph node metastases, and postoperative recurrence and significantly lower rates of disease-free survival [12–14]. Others studies, however, have found that the prognosis for FNMTC (even in kindreds with three or more affected members) is not significantly different from that of similarly treated sporadic NMTCs, even though the familial cases were associated with higher rates of multifocal involvement in index cases and a possibly greater tendency to spread outside the thyroid [15]. The discrepancies between these findings have been attributed to the possible polygenetic etiology of FNMTC suggested by the wide variation in penetrance documented in many large pedigrees [7]. It has also been suggested that closer surveillance of the relatives of patients who have FNMTCs leads to earlier diagnosis and treatment of familial forms of the disease, thereby improving the prognosis and attenuating evidence of their increased aggressiveness relative to sporadic NMTCs [7].

The actual value of screening thyroid ultrasonography for unaffected family members is also uncertain. Formal cost-benefit studies have yet to be undertaken, but the results will in any case reflect features of the local health-care system. In general, screening of apparently healthy individuals believed to be at increased risk for cancer is recommended when five criteria proposed by the World Health Organization are satisfied. To implement an early detection program, (1) the candidate cancers should be frequent; (2) a high rate of patients should present in advanced stages; (3) cost-effective, early detection methods should be available and easily accessible for the candidate group; (4) diagnosis, treatment, follow-up, and quality assurance procedures can be implemented; and (5) the benefits of early detection should outweigh the risks, in terms of complications and negative effects. Thyroid ultrasonography with FNAB confirmation is available and easily accessible, as well as treatment and follow-up protocols. However, there is no conclusive evidence that FNMTCs are more aggressive than their sporadic counterparts or that an early detection may improve patient outcomes [16]. For this reason, ultrasound-based screening is discouraged in asymptomatic adults by the US Preventive Services Task Force [17, 18]. The 2015 ATA guidelines acknowledge that ultrasound-based screening may lead to earlier diagnosis of thyroid cancer in these cases, but the panel refrains from recommending for or against this practice since evidence is lacking that it would diminish morbidity or mortality [1].

Back to the Patient

In kindreds with only two members having DTCs, the possibility that the cancers may actually be sporadic is substantial. Our patient, however, was the third member of his family to develop PTC, so the likelihood of true familial disease was much higher. We discussed the fact that his own cancer had all the earmarks of being low risk for recurrence, and we reviewed the pros and cons of RRA, including data showing lack of benefit from radioiodine therapy in patients with multifocal microPTC [19, 20]. Nevertheless, the patient opted for ablation, noting that both his mother and uncle had received the same treatment and “they seem to be doing pretty well.” He was also strongly in favor of sonographic screening for his siblings and his children. Following the diagnosis of her brother’s thyroid cancer, he said his mother had had a thyroid scan (it was not clear who had ordered the test) and that “as a result of that precaution,” she had experienced far less morbidity than her brother.

The patient underwent RRA (administered activity: 30 mCi), and at the 1-year follow-up visit, the cervical ultrasound examination revealed no macroscopic evidence of residual thyroid tissue and no findings suggestive of lymph node involvement. The recombinant human TSH-stimulated thyroglobulin level was 0.8 ng/mL (normal: <1), and the thyroglobulin antibody assay was negative. His sister (age 41) and his two brothers (51 and 48 years old) have all undergone screening sonography in our center. The sister's examination revealed a 12-mm nodule in the right lobe, with suspicious sonographic and cytologic features (Bethesda class V) [1]. She is scheduled for surgery in the near future and promises to become the fourth member of the family with thyroid cancer. The patient's two children, currently 2 and 3 years old, will be screened after puberty.

Clinical Pearls

- At present, there is no convincing evidence that the treatment strategies indicated by the initial ATA risk classification of NMTC should be substantially modified solely because the disease seems to be familial rather than sporadic.
- Likewise, there is no evidence that sonographic screening of unaffected family members in these kindreds will have any significant impact on morbidity or mortality.
- Treatment planning with patients who have been diagnosed with familial neoplastic disease can be "complicated" by psychological factors that are absent in cases of sporadic cancer, e.g., the patient's recall of loved ones who have had the disease and anxiety over the prospect of other cases in the family.

References

1. Haugen BR, Alexander EK, Bible KC, Doherty GM, Mandel SJ, Nikiforov YE, et al. 2015 American Thyroid Association management guidelines for adult patients with thyroid nodules and differentiated thyroid cancer: the American Thyroid Association guidelines task force on thyroid nodules and differentiated thyroid cancer. Thyroid. 2016;26(1):1–133.
2. Durante C, Grani G, Lamartina L, Filetti S, Mandel SJ, Cooper DS. The diagnosis and management of thyroid nodules a review. JAMA. 2018;319(9):914–24.
3. Cibas ES, Ali SZ. The 2017 Bethesda system for reporting thyroid cytopathology. Thyroid. 2017;27(11):1341–6.
4. Tuttle M, Morris LF, Haugen B, Shah J, Sosa JA, Rohren E, et al. Thyroid-differentiated and anaplastic carcinoma. In: Amin MB, Cancer. AJCo, American Cancer Society, editors. AJCC cancer staging manual. Chicago: American Joint Committee on Cancer, Springer; 2017. p. 873–90.
5. Wittekind C, Brierley JD, Lee A, van Eycken E. Optional proposals for testing new subcategories of TNM. In: Sobin LH, editor. TNM Online. p. 209–17.
6. Cooper DS, Doherty GM, Haugen BR, Hauger BR, Kloos RT, Lee SL, et al. Revised American Thyroid Association management guidelines for patients with thyroid nodules and differentiated thyroid cancer. Thyroid. 2009;19(11):1167–214.

7. Mazeh H, Sippel RS. Familial nonmedullary thyroid carcinoma. Thyroid. 2013;23(9):1049–56.
8. Peiling Yang S, Ngeow J. Familial non-medullary thyroid cancer: unraveling the genetic maze. Endocr Relat Cancer. 2016;23(12):R577–r95.
9. Charkes ND. On the prevalence of familial nonmedullary thyroid cancer in multiply affected kindreds. Thyroid. 2006;16(2):181–6.
10. Tam AA, Ozdemir D, Cuhaci N, Baser H, Aydin C, Yazgan AK, et al. Association of multifocality, tumor number, and total tumor diameter with clinicopathological features in papillary thyroid cancer. Endocrine. 2016;53(3):774–83.
11. Tam AA, Ozdemir D, Ogmen BE, Faki S, Dumlu EG, Yazgan AK, et al. Should multifocal papillary thyroid carcinomas classified as t1a with a tumor diameter sum of 1 to 2 centimeters be reclassified as T1B? Endocr Pract. 2017;23(5):526–35.
12. Wang X, Cheng W, Li J, Su A, Wei T, Liu F, et al. Endocrine tumours: familial nonmedullary thyroid carcinoma is a more aggressive disease: a systematic review and meta-analysis. Eur J Endocrinol. 2015;172(6):R253–62.
13. Uchino S, Noguchi S, Kawamoto H, Yamashita H, Watanabe S, Shuto S. Familial nonmedullary thyroid carcinoma characterized by multifocality and a high recurrence rate in a large study population. World J Surg. 2002;26(8):897–902.
14. El Lakis M, Giannakou A, Nockel PJ, Wiseman D, Gara SK, Patel D, et al. Do patients with familial nonmedullary thyroid cancer present with more aggressive disease? Implications for initial surgical treatment. Surgery. 2019;165(1):50–7.
15. Pinto AE, Silva GL, Henrique R, Menezes FD, Teixeira MR, Leite V, et al. Familial vs sporadic papillary thyroid carcinoma: a matched-case comparative study showing similar clinical/prognostic behaviour. Eur J Endocrinol. 2014;170(2):321–7.
16. Lamartina L, Grani G, Durante C, Filetti S, Cooper DS. Screening for differentiated thyroid cancer in selected populations. Lancet Diabetes Endocrinol. 2020;8(1):81–8.
17. Bibbins-Domingo K, Grossman DC, Curry SJ, Barry MJ, Davidson KW, Doubeni CA, et al. Screening for thyroid cancer: US preventive services task force recommendation statement. JAMA. 2017;317(18):1882–7.
18. Lin JS, Bowles EJA, Williams SB, Morrison CC. Screening for thyroid cancer: updated evidence report and systematic review for the US preventive services task force. JAMA. 2017;317(18):1888–903.
19. Hay ID, Hutchinson ME, Gonzalez-Losada T, McIver B, Reinalda ME, Grant CS, et al. Papillary thyroid microcarcinoma: a study of 900 cases observed in a 60-year period. Surgery. 2008;144(6):980–7; discussion 7–8.
20. Ross DS, Litofsky D, Ain KB, Bigos T, Brierley JD, Cooper DS, et al. Recurrence after treatment of micropapillary thyroid cancer. Thyroid. 2009;19(10):1043–8.

Chapter 3
A Case of a Small (1–2 cm) Papillary Thyroid Cancer in a Young Patient: Lobectomy Versus Total Thyroidectomy

Gerard M. Doherty

Case Presentation

A 35-year-old woman was referred to a thyroid clinic due to a newly identified palpable nodule in the left thyroid lobe. She had no history of neck surgery, voice changes, prior thyroid nodules, significant radiation exposure, or family history of thyroid disease. Physical examination included a palpable firm left thyroid nodule, a normal voice, and no cervical adenopathy. Thyroid ultrasound confirmed that the palpable nodule was a solitary hypoechoic 18 mm left thyroid nodule with irregular borders and scattered microcalcifications (classified as "high suspicion" according to the 2015 American Thyroid Association (ATA) guidelines). A formal ultrasound nodal survey showed no abnormal lymph nodes, and fine-needle aspiration cytology of the dominant nodule revealed papillary thyroid cancer (Bethesda VI). After discussion, the patient elected a strategy of left thyroid lobectomy with intraoperative node assessment, including a planned intraoperative switch to total thyroidectomy and level 6 node dissection only if there were higher-risk features detected during the procedure, such as gross lymph node metastases. The operation was an uncomplicated left thyroid lobectomy under local anesthesia with sedation done as an ambulatory procedure. At 8-week follow-up, her TSH without exogenous thyroid hormone was 1.1 mU/L, and thyroglobulin was 1.8 ng/mL without antithyroglobulin antibodies.

G. M. Doherty (✉)
Department of Surgery, Brigham and Women's Hospital/Harvard Medical School, Boston, MA, USA
e-mail: gmdoherty@bwh.harvard.edu

G. Grani et al. (eds.), *Thyroid Cancer*,
https://doi.org/10.1007/978-3-030-61919-0_3

Assessment and Literature Review

Small papillary thyroid carcinomas are very common and rarely threaten long-term survival, especially in young people, unless associated with some poor prognostic features. The management strategy for this common tumor requires coordination of the plan prior to operation, in order to ensure that the procedure performed supports the intended adjuvant therapies and follow-up surveillance.

Prognostic Features

The 2015 version of the ATA thyroid cancer guidelines includes a three-tiered *recurrence risk* stratification system that classified patients as low, intermediate, or high risk [1]. The pathological features that increase the risk of recurrence include vascular invasion by the tumor, invasion of tumor into tissues outside of the thyroid capsule, clinically apparent lymph node metastases, or aggressive histologic features. The presence of *BRAF* or *TERT* mutations, if known, increases the risk of recurrence [2, 3]. The findings during treatment that increase the patient's risk of recurrence include the presence of local or distant metastases on postoperative radioiodine scan or other imaging modalities and a persistently elevated serum thyroglobulin. High-risk pathological features include gross extrathyroidal extension or incomplete tumor resection; distant metastases, thyroglobulin levels that suggest distant metastases, large node metastases (>3 cm), and extranodal extension are other high-risk findings. These features have been shown to predict recurrence risk and can therefore be used to inform patients and clinicians who are choosing treatment and follow-up plans, rather than basing those plans solely on predictions of survival, which is typically unaffected in low-risk patients [4].

The ATA initial risk stratification also predicts the type of persistent or recurrent disease pattern observed; most persistent disease in low-risk patients is solely an abnormal serum thyroglobulin level without structurally identifiable disease which is unlikely to lead to disease-related morbidity. Greater proportions of intermediate- and high-risk patients who have persistent or recurrent disease have clinically or radiologically identifiable structural disease and have a greater likelihood of disease-related morbidity or mortality.

Management Strategies

The operation for thyroid cancer is the initial step in the treatment strategy and follow-up plan established by the managing team. In the past, total thyroidectomy has been promoted as the optimal option for papillary thyroid cancers greater than 1 cm. There are data showing that total thyroidectomy leads to decreased recurrence rates and improved survival [5], as well as optimally positioning the patient for subsequent follow-up using serum thyroglobulin measurements. However, there are also data to support more limited thyroid resection as an equivalent strategy for patients with low-risk disease [6]. As a selective approach to RAI ablation has become more favored in low-risk patients, the utilization of total thyroidectomy specifically as preparation for the use of RAI in treatment or follow-up has become a less important rationale. If a patient population can be identified that has equivalent long-term disease outcomes with thyroid lobectomy, without radioiodine therapy or TSH suppression, then they would best be served by limiting the aggressiveness of treatment, minimizing adverse events, and maximizing quality of life. This is a very important clinical issue, since patients with very low-risk thyroid cancer comprise a very large proportion of the thyroid cancer population [7].

A bilateral thyroidectomy (total or near-total) is preferred if the treatment strategy is to include RAI scanning or therapy postoperatively. This is most clearly applicable to the high-risk groups. For patients at intermediate risk, either a bilateral or unilateral thyroidectomy may serve as the surgical platform for an overall treatment plan. Features that place the patient at increased risk of recurrent disease or of concomitant contralateral disease, such as age >45 years, contralateral thyroid nodules, known multifocal cancer in the lobe to be operated upon, a personal history of radiation therapy to the head and neck, or a family history of differentiated thyroid cancer, may inform the decision to employ a bilateral procedure to preserve the option of RAI scanning or therapy or to resolve questions of bilateral disease. It is clearly in the patient's best interest to work with a treatment team that can discuss and coordinate this decision-making prior to the initial operation, to avoid awkward planning compromises at later points in the treatment course [8].

Complications of Total Thyroidectomy

Though both are quite safe operations, total thyroidectomy carries a significantly greater risk of complications than thyroid lobectomy. A 2013 meta-analysis showed a relative risk (RR) that was greater for total thyroidectomy for all significant complications [9]. These included permanent recurrent laryngeal nerve injury ($RR = 1.9$), permanent hypocalcemia ($RR = 3.2$), and hemorrhage/hematoma ($RR = 2.6$). Most importantly, thyroid lobectomy has a negligible risk of permanent hypoparathyroidism because the parathyroid glands near the contralateral lobe are not dissected, making it impossible to cause permanent hypoparathyroidism. Thyroid lobectomy may also obviate the need for levothyroxine treatment in 50–80% of patients.

There is a relationship between surgeon volume and patient outcomes for thyroid surgery that may inform the choice of approach in some instances. Differences have been identified in studies evaluating data at the state and national levels in the USA and in other countries [10, 11]. These studies have consistently shown that patients operated on by low-volume surgeons (as variably defined) have more complications than those operated on by intermediate- or high-volume surgeons. Furthermore, the majority of thyroid surgery is performed by low-volume surgeons. These data suggest that patients should ideally receive care from high-volume thyroid surgeons where, overall, they are more likely to have good results. However, the distribution and limited number of high-volume surgeons make this impractical in the USA. The ATA guidelines do support a policy of sending patients with more extensive disease and concern for grossly invasive disease to high-volume centers that have experience in the management of advanced thyroid cancer.

For an individual patient, the decision regarding the extent of surgery should depend upon the clinical status, preoperative risk assessment, and treatment team plans for adjuvant therapy and follow-up. Since even high-volume surgeons have a higher risk of complications with bilateral procedures, the decision is more dependent upon the clinical scenario than upon the available surgeon.

Indications for Adjuvant Radioiodine Therapy

The patient risk category as informed by the preoperative, intraoperative, and postoperative findings can be used to determine the utility of thyroid remnant ablation or adjuvant radioiodine therapy for papillary thyroid cancer. The use of postoperative administration of radioactive iodine after total thyroidectomy is to further some combination of these goals:

- Remnant ablation is intended to destroy the remaining normal thyroid tissue in order to enable detection of persistent and recurrent disease by RAI scan and thyroglobulin measurement.
- Adjuvant therapy is intended to affect disease-free survival by destroying microscopic undetected metastatic disease in lymph nodes or distant sites.
- Radioiodine therapy is intended to improve disease-specific and disease-free survival by treating known persistent disease.

The use of radioiodine in any of these contexts (ablation, adjuvant therapy, or RAI therapy) can also be accompanied by scanning that can provide diagnostic information regarding the presence or absence of RAI-avid persistent disease.

For patients with low-risk papillary thyroid cancer, follow-up without RAI ablation, using neck ultrasound and thyroglobulin, is reasonable [1]. Because of the low risk of disease recurrence and the feasibility of follow-up without the use of radioiodine scans, radioiodine ablation or adjuvant therapy is not generally recommended for patients in the ATA low-risk category. However, practices vary widely, with great variation in the use of radioiodine for low-risk patients in the USA [12, 13], and there is still a significant overtreatment in many parts of the world [14, 15].

Management of the Case

In this case, the patient's clinical features are all low risk. She is <45 years of age, with papillary thyroid cancer confined to the thyroid. There are no features (contralateral nodules, radiation exposure history, family history) to suggest a significant current or future risk of contralateral disease. Her formal node survey done with ultrasound does not show evidence of clinically significant metastases in the central or lateral neck.

Her preoperative discussion focused on the likelihood that in her clinical scenario she would not benefit from adjuvant therapy with radioiodine. The main risk factor that could be discovered at operation without being evident preoperatively is small but grossly identifiable central neck (level 6) lymphadenopathy. With her preoperative assent, the plan for intraoperative decision-making could have led to a bilateral thyroid procedure to facilitate postoperative radioiodine treatment and scanning if there were confirmed central neck metastases (clinical N1 disease). This would have placed her into the intermediate-risk group, where the benefit of this strategy is still somewhat uncertain, but was recommended and agreed upon by the patient and treatment team. Whether RAI therapy in this setting is done for remnant ablation to make follow-up easier or as adjuvant therapy is a matter of clinical viewpoint, but in any case was not indicated for her management. Finally, her postoperative TSH level without exogenous hormone therapy falls within the target range for low-risk thyroid cancer (0.5–2.0 mU/mL), and so no additional therapy is indicated [1].

Clinical Pearls/Pitfalls

- The treatment should be based upon the defined risk category of the patient.
- The "doses" of therapy, including surgery, radioiodine administration, and TSH suppression, can each be altered in response to the risk of the disease and the therapy for that individual patient.
- The current trend in the management of low-risk differentiated thyroid cancer is toward more conservative therapy (lower doses of surgery and radioiodine in particular) based upon patient risk group.

References

1. Haugen BR, Alexander EK, Bible KC, Doherty GM, Mandel SJ, Nikiforov YE, Pacini F, Randolph GW, Sawka AM, Schlumberger M, et al. 2015 American Thyroid Association management guidelines for adult patients with thyroid nodules and differentiated thyroid cancer: the American Thyroid Association guidelines task force on thyroid nodules and differentiated thyroid cancer. Thyroid. 2016;26:1):1–133.
2. Xing M, Liu R, Liu X, Murugan AK, Zhu G, Zeiger MA, Pai S, Bishop J. BRAF V600E and TERT promoter mutations cooperatively identify the most aggressive papillary thyroid cancer with highest recurrence. J Clin Oncol. 2014;32(25):2718–26.
3. Huang Y, Qu S, Zhu G, Wang F, Liu R, Shen X, Viola D, Elisei R, Puxeddu E, Fugazzola L, et al. BRAF V600E mutation-assisted risk stratification of solitary intrathyroidal papillary thyroid cancer for precision treatment. J Natl Cancer Inst. 2018;110(4):362–70.
4. Tuttle RM, Alzahrani AS. Risk stratification in differentiated thyroid cancer: from detection to final follow-up. J Clin Endocrinol Metab. 2019;104(9):4087–100.
5. Bilimoria KY, Bentrem DJ, Ko CY, Stewart AK, Winchester DP, Talamonti MS, Sturgeon C. Extent of surgery affects survival for papillary thyroid cancer. [see comment]. Ann Surg. 2007;246(3):375–81; discussion 381-374.

6. Matsuzu K, Sugino K, Masudo K, Nagahama M, Kitagawa W, Shibuya H, Ohkuwa K, Uruno T, Suzuki A, Magoshi S, et al. Thyroid lobectomy for papillary thyroid cancer: long-term follow-up study of 1,088 cases. World J Surg. 2014;38(1):68–79.
7. Welch HG, Doherty GM. Saving thyroids - overtreatment of small papillary cancers. N Engl J Med. 2018;379(4):310–2.
8. Carty SE, Doherty GM, Inabnet WB 3rd, Pasieka JL, Randolph GW, Shaha AR, Terris DJ, Tufano RP, Tuttle RM. Surgical Affairs Committee of the American Thyroid A: American Thyroid Association statement on the essential elements of interdisciplinary communication of perioperative information for patients undergoing thyroid cancer surgery. Thyroid. 2012;22(4):395–9.
9. Kandil E, Krishnan B, Noureldine SI, Yao L, Tufano RP. Hemithyroidectomy: a meta-analysis of postoperative need for hormone replacement and complications. ORL J Otorhinolaryngol Relat Spec. 2013;75(1):6–17.
10. Sosa JA, Bowman HM, Tielsch JM, Powe NR, Gordon TA, Udelsman R. The importance of surgeon experience for clinical and economic outcomes from thyroidectomy. Ann Surg. 1998;228(3):320–30.
11. Dralle H, Sekulla C, Lorenz K, Brauckhoff M, Machens A, German ISG. Intraoperative monitoring of the recurrent laryngeal nerve in thyroid surgery. World J Surg. 2008;32(7):1358–66.
12. Haymart MR, Banerjee M, Yang D, Stewart AK, Sisson JC, Koenig RJ, Doherty GM, Griggs JJ. Variation in the management of thyroid cancer. J Clin Endocrinol Metab. 2013;98(5):2001–8.
13. Wallner LP, Reyes-Gastelum D, Hamilton AS, Ward KC, Hawley ST, Haymart MR. Patient-perceived lack of choice in receipt of radioactive iodine for treatment of differentiated thyroid cancer. J Clin Oncol. 2019;37(24):2152–61.
14. Lamartina L, Durante C, Lucisano G, Grani G, Bellantone R, Lombardi CP, Pontecorvi A, Arvat E, Felicetti F, Zatelli MC, et al. Are evidence-based guidelines reflected in clinical practice? An analysis of prospectively collected data of the Italian thyroid cancer observatory. Thyroid. 2017;27(12):1490–7.
15. Sastre Marcos J, Aznar S, Álvarez V, Torres B, Delgado M, González J, Quiroga I. Follow-up and results in patients with differentiated thyroid carcinoma in Castilla-La Mancha (2001-2015). The CADIT-CAM study. Endocrinol Diabetes Nutr. 2019;66(3):164–72.

Chapter 4
A Patient with Papillary Microcarcinoma Undergoing Active Surveillance

Laura Boucai

Case Presentation

A 63-year-old female was referred for recommendations on management of a biopsy-proven microcarcinoma of the thyroid. She initially consulted with her neurologist for headaches and neck pain. A cervical magnetic resonance image incidentally detected the presence of a 1.2 cm right thyroid nodule. A thyroid ultrasound with lymph node mapping was recommended for better characterization of this finding which revealed a solid, hypoechoic, hypovascular nodule, with well-defined margins, measuring 1.2 × 1.1 × 1.0 cm, located in the right thyroid lobe and extending into the isthmus (Fig. 4.1). There was normal thyroid tissue surrounding this nodule, no nodules in the left thyroid lobe, and no cervical lymphadenopathy. The patient denied masses in her neck, hoarseness, dysphagia, or dyspnea. Her TSH was normal at 1.8 mIU/L. She denied any history of head or neck irradiation or family history of thyroid carcinoma. The right thyroid nodule was classified as "intermediate suspicion" according to the 2015 American Thyroid Association (ATA) guidelines; a fine-needle aspiration (FNA) of it was positive for papillary thyroid carcinoma (Bethesda VI), and she sought endocrinologic consultation for discussion of treatment options.

L. Boucai (✉)
Division of Endocrinology, Diabetes, and Metabolism, Memorial Sloan-Kettering Cancer Center, Weill Cornell Medical College, New York, NY, USA
e-mail: boucail@mskcc.org

G. Grani et al. (eds.), *Thyroid Cancer*,
https://doi.org/10.1007/978-3-030-61919-0_4

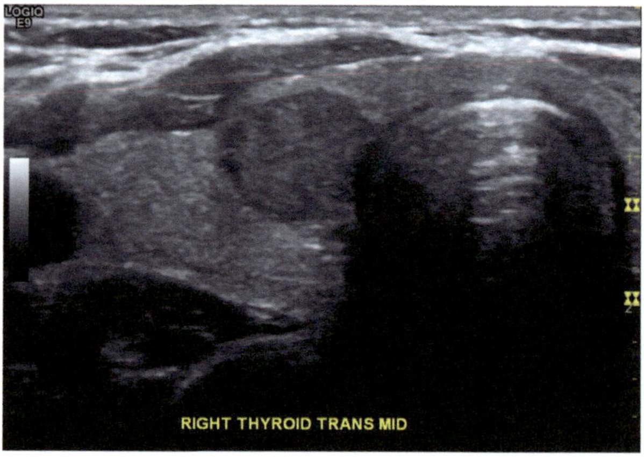

Fig. 4.1 Ultrasound transverse view of right mid thyroid lobe. Hypoechoic, hypovascular nodule measuring 1.2 × 1.1 × 1.0 cm located in the right thyroid lobe and extending into the isthmus

Literature Review

With the widespread use of screening and diagnostic imaging studies, there has been a logarithmic rise in the discovery of incidental papillary thyroid carcinomas (PTCs). This phenomenon is not unique to the United States [1, 2]. South Korea [3], France [4], and Canada [5], among others [6], have witnessed an epidemic of thyroid microcarcinoma, mainly due to the increased detection of asymptomatic, subcentimeter, low-risk PTCs [7, 8]. The traditional approach to thyroid carcinomas has been total thyroidectomy followed by radioactive iodine ablation and levothyroxine suppressive therapy [9, 10], even though the vast majority of these subclinical tumors progress either slowly or not at all [11–13]. The favorable prognosis of papillary microcarcinomas (PMCs) detected incidentally on cross-sectional imaging studies has been documented by Ito et al. in a 10-year cohort study of patients undergoing total thyroidectomy: the lymph node recurrence-free survival rate, distant recurrence-free survival rate, and cause-specific survival rate were 99%, 100%, and 100%, respectively [14]. Moreover, thyroid surgery can result in significant morbidity including hoarseness due to injury of the recurrent laryngeal nerve and pitch changes due to injury to the external branch of the superior laryngeal nerve, tracheostomy in the case of bilateral recurrent laryngeal nerve injury, hypoparathyroidism, formation of hematomas, and infections, particularly when the surgery is performed by low-volume surgeons [15]. Consequently, more conservative approaches to PMCs that include thyroid lobectomy or enrollment in an active surveillance program have been proposed and are slowly being adopted [16]. Defined as a conservative observational management strategy, active surveillance for papillary microcarcinomas was first conceived at Kuma Hospital in Japan, when patients with biopsy-proven PMC under observation demonstrated the same risk of locoregional spread, distant metastasis, and disease-specific mortality as patients undergoing immediate surgery [11, 12]. Ito et al. followed 340 patients and found that only

15.9% of them had tumor enlargement of 3 mm or more and only 3.45% of the cohort developed cervical metastases after 10 years of follow-up [11]. Sugitani et al. followed 230 patients and similarly found that 7% of tumors enlarged and only 1% metastasized to cervical lymph nodes after 11 years of follow-up [12]. In the United States, Tuttle et al. followed 291 patients with biopsy-proven PMC of the thyroid for a median of 2 years and found that 3.8% of these grew by 3 mm or more in 2 years with a cumulative incidence of 12.1% in 5 years [13]. Factors associated with disease progression were age at the time of diagnosis and pregnancy during surveillance. Young patients (<40 years) were more likely to experience tumor enlargement and spread to cervical lymph nodes compared to older patients (>60 years) [17]. Also, 44% of pregnant patients showed enlargement of PMCs compared to 11% of age-matched non-pregnant controls, possibly due to the thyroid-stimulating activity of human chorionic gonadotropin [18]. Importantly, even patients who demonstrated disease progression while under active surveillance were effectively treated with thyroid surgery, indicating that a delayed surgical management approach in properly selected patients had no impact on disease-specific survival [11, 12]. In a recent study by Oda et al. [19] comparing unfavorable outcomes of surgery for microcarcinomas of the thyroid, the incidence of transient vocal cord paralysis, transient hypoparathyroidism, and permanent hypoparathyroidism was higher in the immediate-surgery group compared to the active-surveillance group (4.1% vs 0.6%, $p < 0.001$; 16.7% vs 2.8%, $p < 0.001$; 1.6% vs 0.08%, $p < 0.001$, respectively).

Therefore, in light of the very low disease-specific mortality, low rates of recurrence, and the potential for complications from surgery, the traditional management approach of immediate thyroid surgery for PMC is being reconsidered. The 2015 ATA thyroid cancer management guidelines state that while surgery is generally recommended for biopsy-proven thyroid cancer, an active surveillance management approach "can be considered" as an alternative to immediate surgery in patients with very low-risk tumors (e.g., PMCs without clinically evident metastases or local invasion and no convincing cytology or molecular evidence of aggressive disease) [16]. Furthermore, the guidelines strongly discourage biopsy of asymptomatic subcentimeter nodules, even if sonographically highly suspicious. On the whole, they advocate for a reduction of the diagnostic and therapeutic burden of low-risk thyroid cancer patients.

Tailoring the Management Approach

While this conservative management approach is endorsed, the guidelines do not specifically discuss the factors that may make tumors and patients ideal candidates for an observational approach. Brito et al. [20] published a clinical framework to facilitate risk stratification when considering an active surveillance alternative to immediate surgery for papillary microcarcinomas. The authors describe tumor

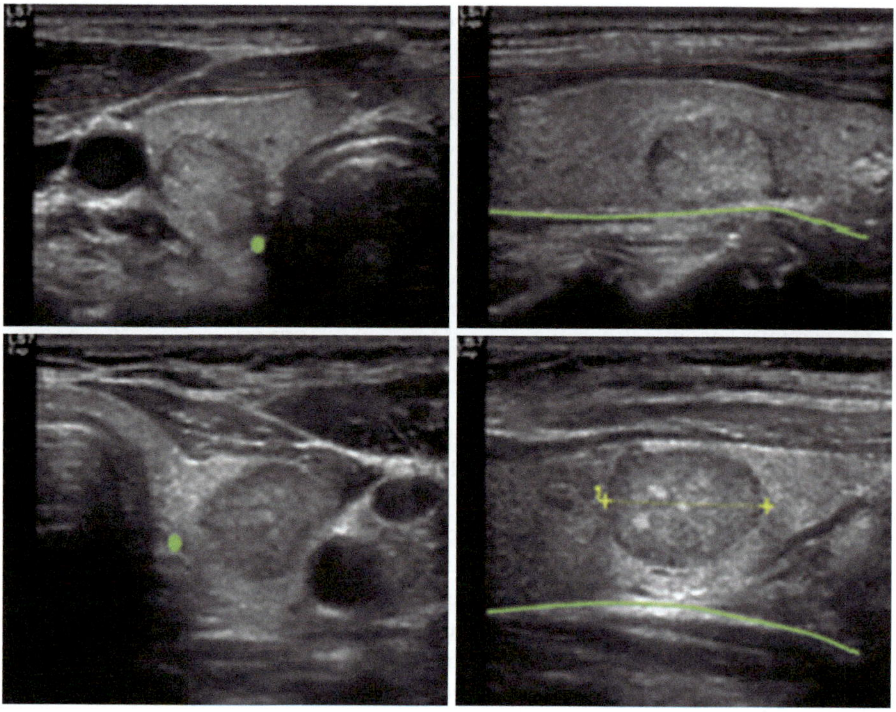

Fig. 4.2 Anatomical pathway of the recurrent laryngeal nerve (green). The top panel shows a thyroid nodule in the right lobe with a closer proximity to the recurrent laryngeal nerve than the nodule in the left thyroid lobe (bottom panel)

characteristics, patient characteristics, and medical team characteristics that make PMCs ideal, appropriate, and inappropriate for active surveillance. Ideal tumors would be solitary thyroid nodules, with well-defined margins, surrounded by ≥2 mm normal thyroid parenchyma, without evidence of extrathyroidal extension, without clinical cervical or distant metastases, and with a previous ultrasound documenting stability. Inappropriate tumors to observe or, conversely, appropriate tumors to excise would be those with aggressive cytology on FNA (e.g., tall-cell, columnar, and hobnail variants and poorly differentiated features), those with subcapsular locations adjacent to the recurrent laryngeal nerve (RLN) (Fig. 4.2), evidence of extrathyroidal extension, clinical symptoms/signs suspicious for invasion into the RLN or trachea (such as vocal cord paralysis, hemoptysis), proof of cervical or distant metastases on initial evaluation or during follow-up, or a documented increase in size ≥3 mm during surveillance. Also, isthmic tumors are generally considered appropriate for surgery because of their proximity to the trachea and strap muscles.

Evaluation of the patient and the medical team characteristics are as important when weighing the decision to proceed with active surveillance. An older patient expected to comply with follow-ups, with life-threatening comorbidities, with a supportive social environment, and followed by an experienced multidisciplinary management team constitutes an ideal candidate for surveillance. On the contrary, young patients (<18 years), unlikely to be compliant with follow-up plans, not willing to accept an observational approach for the fear of living with cancer or for other reasons, followed by teams with little experience in thyroid cancer management and without reliable neck ultrasonography are examples of inappropriate candidates for surveillance that should be referred for immediate surgery. Modalities of follow-up include clinical exam, ultrasound, and occasionally CT with contrast for better definition of tumors located posteriorly or near the trachea. The time interval between examinations is still unclear, but it is prudent to envision biannual follow-ups initially to establish stability or progression of disease and yearly examinations thereafter if disease is stable, also based on location and patient choice.

Molecular Markers

The role of molecular markers as predictors of PMC progression has received considerable attention in an attempt to refine the methodology through which patients are selected for an active surveillance approach. Identifying a gene or group of genes that confer an aggressive potential to PMC would be the ideal way of distinguishing patients likely to benefit from immediate surgery as opposed to an observational approach. The $BRAF^{V600E}$ mutation, which constitutes ~60% of all driver mutations found in papillary thyroid cancer, has received particular attention since it has been associated with the presence of distant metastases, more advanced clinical stage, and higher mortality [21, 22], but much uncertainty exists around the prognostic and predictive power of BRAF alone since, by itself, it has not proven to be independently associated with worse outcomes [22–25]. Other clinicopathological unfavorable characteristics in combination with BRAF confer the worse prognosis [26, 27]. Telomerase reverse transcriptase (TERT) promoter mutations in thyroid cancer were first reported in 2013 [28, 29], and their coexistence with BRAF has been shown to be associated with particularly aggressive thyroid cancer behavior and poor clinical outcomes, including tumor recurrence and cancer-specific mortality [30, 31]. More recently, Tuttle et al. compared the genomic landscape of 40 PMC patients with N1b disease to that of 71 PMC patients with N0 disease and found that TERT promoter mutations (3%) and TP53 mutations (1%) were exclusively present in patients with N1b disease and that there was a differential expression of 43 selected genes between PMC patients with N1b and N0 disease [32]. The latter study provides the basis for a molecular classifier that may offer risk stratification in PMCs.

Long-Term Planning and Communication with the Patients

Once the patient has elected to pursue active surveillance, the parameters for the decision to exit an active surveillance program and proceed to surgery must be clearly defined. Sugitani et al. provided the option of conventional surgical therapy to all asymptomatic patients with PMC [12]. In both Japanese active surveillance studies [11, 12], the patients were advised to undergo surgery if they met the following criteria during active surveillance: (1) a change in the patient's desire to remain under active surveillance; (2) tumor enlargement (of 3 mm or more); (3) the appearance of clinically evident lymph node metastases; and (4) tumor growth towards the dorsal surface of the thyroid gland or adjacent structures. The Ito and Sugitani trials differed slightly in that Ito et al. [11] also recommended surgery for patients who were diagnosed as having familial carcinoma, young age, suspicion of multicentricity, or the coexistence of other thyroid diseases (e.g., enlargement of associated benign nodules). Additional criteria may be considered: (1) suspicion of invasion of the recurrent laryngeal nerve (RLN) (such as the development of hoarseness or dysphagia); (2) the development of any other cancer-related symptoms; and (3) a new biopsy diagnosis that indicates higher-grade malignancy. In future studies these criteria may change or be refined, particularly with ongoing research on molecular markers, which may help identify tumors that are likely to grow or spread.

Back to the Patient

A detailed discussion with the endocrinologist informed the patient of the minimal risks of growth and spread of her papillary microcarcinoma. Among the treatment options, total thyroidectomy, right thyroid lobectomy, and active surveillance were discussed. The patient was living in a rural area 2 hours away from a tertiary center that would be optimal to follow her microcarcinoma with updated sonographic equipment and radiologic and medical expertise. After careful consideration of multiple strategies, she decided she would travel twice a year to follow her nodule to avoid removing her thyroid. Her initial sonogram at 6 months demonstrated no growth of her PTC and no cervical lymphadenopathy. Eighteen months after her initial visit, her tumor had enlarged by 2 mm. At this point she was advised that this increase falls within the measurement error of different studies, but she was offered to rebiopsy her PMC to measure key genetic markers. She declined given the lack of insurance coverage of this test. The patient is currently 69 years of age, and she has completed 6 years of active surveillance every 6–12 months, without evidence of growth or spread of her biopsy-proven microcarcinoma of the thyroid and without need for levothyroxine replacement therapy.

Clinical Pearls/Pitfalls

- An active surveillance program for biopsy-confirmed papillary microcarcinomas of the thyroid is feasible and is slowly being adopted as an alternative to immediate thyroid surgery.
- Tumor characteristics including solitary thyroid nodules, with well-defined margins, surrounded by ≥2 mm normal thyroid parenchyma, without evidence of extrathyroidal extension, without clinical cervical or distant metastases; patient characteristics including age, comorbidities, ability to comply with follow-ups, and supportive social environment; and medical team factors including quality of sonographic equipment, expertise of the treating team, and ability to collaborate with patient's doctors should all be integrated to define appropriate, adequate, and inappropriate candidates for an active surveillance approach.
- The role of molecular markers as predictors of progression of PMCs is becoming important among the factors used to recommend an active surveillance approach. The presence of TERT promoter mutations and TP53 mutations has been recently found to be only present in PMC with N1b disease, and a panel of 43 genes were differentially expressed among N1b and N0 patients. Future studies are directed at validating these genetic associations with prognosis of PMCs.
- Once an active surveillance approach has been elected, a clear definition of the parameters that will favor a surgical intervention including tumor growth, spread to cervical lymph nodes, extension outside the thyroid capsule, and signs of clinical aggressiveness ought to be discussed with the patient.

References

1. Davies L, Welch HG. Increasing incidence of thyroid cancer in the United States, 1973-2002. JAMA. 2006;295(18):2164–7.
2. Vaccarella S, Franceschi S, Bray F, Wild CP, Plummer M, Dal Maso L. Worldwide thyroid-cancer epidemic? The increasing impact of overdiagnosis. N Engl J Med. 2016;375(7):614–7.
3. Ahn HS, Kim HJ, Welch HG. Korea's thyroid-cancer "epidemic" – screening and overdiagnosis. N Engl J Med. 2014;371(19):1765–7.
4. Leenhardt L, Grosclaude P, Cherie-Challine L, Thyroid Cancer C. Increased incidence of thyroid carcinoma in France: a true epidemic or thyroid nodule management effects? Report from the French Thyroid Cancer Committee. Thyroid. 2004;14(12):1056–60.
5. Liu S, Semenciw R, Ugnat AM, Mao Y. Increasing thyroid cancer incidence in Canada, 1970-1996: time trends and age-period-cohort effects. Br J Cancer. 2001;85(9):1335–9.
6. Reynolds RM, Weir J, Stockton DL, Brewster DH, Sandeep TC, Strachan MW. Changing trends in incidence and mortality of thyroid cancer in Scotland. Clin Endocrinol. 2005;62(2):156–62.
7. Davies L, Welch HG. Current thyroid cancer trends in the United States. JAMA Otolaryngol Head Neck Surg. 2014;140(4):317–22.

8. Brito JP, Morris JC, Montori VM. Thyroid cancer: zealous imaging has increased detection and treatment of low risk tumours. BMJ. 2013;347:f4706.
9. American Thyroid Association Guidelines Taskforce on Thyroid N, Differentiated Thyroid C, Cooper DS, Doherty GM, Haugen BR, Kloos RT, et al. Revised American Thyroid Association management guidelines for patients with thyroid nodules and differentiated thyroid cancer. Thyroid. 2009;19(11):1167–214.
10. Pacini F, Schlumberger M, Dralle H, Elisei R, Smit JW, Wiersinga W, et al. European consensus for the management of patients with differentiated thyroid carcinoma of the follicular epithelium. Eur J Endocrinol. 2006;154(6):787–803.
11. Ito Y, Miyauchi A, Inoue H, Fukushima M, Kihara M, Higashiyama T, et al. An observational trial for papillary thyroid microcarcinoma in Japanese patients. World J Surg. 2010;34(1):28–35.
12. Sugitani I, Toda K, Yamada K, Yamamoto N, Ikenaga M, Fujimoto Y. Three distinctly different kinds of papillary thyroid microcarcinoma should be recognized: our treatment strategies and outcomes. World J Surg. 2010;34(6):1222–31.
13. Tuttle RM, Fagin JA, Minkowitz G, Wong RJ, Roman B, Patel S, et al. Natural history and tumor volume kinetics of papillary thyroid cancers during active surveillance. JAMA Otolaryngol Head Neck Surg. 2017;143(10):1015–20.
14. Ito Y, Fukushima M, Kihara M, Takamura Y, Kobayashi K, Miya A, et al. Investigation of the prognosis of patients with papillary thyroid carcinoma by tumor size. Endocr J. 2012;59(6):457–64.
15. Hauch A, Al-Qurayshi Z, Randolph G, Kandil E. Total thyroidectomy is associated with increased risk of complications for low- and high-volume surgeons. Ann Surg Oncol. 2014;21(12):3844–52.
16. Haugen BR, Alexander EK, Bible KC, Doherty GM, Mandel SJ, Nikiforov YE, et al. 2015 American Thyroid Association management guidelines for adult patients with thyroid nodules and differentiated thyroid cancer: the American Thyroid Association guidelines task force on thyroid nodules and differentiated thyroid cancer. Thyroid. 2016;26:1):1–133.
17. Ito Y, Miyauchi A, Kobayashi K, Miya A. Prognosis and growth activity depend on patient age in clinical and subclinical papillary thyroid carcinoma. Endocr J. 2014;61(3):205–13.
18. Shindo H, Amino N, Ito Y, Kihara M, Kobayashi K, Miya A, et al. Papillary thyroid microcarcinoma might progress during pregnancy. Thyroid. 2014;24(5):840–4.
19. Oda H, Miyauchi A, Ito Y, Yoshioka K, Nakayama A, Sasai H, et al. Incidences of unfavorable events in the management of low-risk papillary microcarcinoma of the thyroid by active surveillance versus immediate surgery. Thyroid. 2016;26(1):150–5.
20. Brito JP, Ito Y, Miyauchi A, Tuttle RM. A clinical framework to facilitate risk stratification when considering an active surveillance alternative to immediate biopsy and surgery in papillary microcarcinoma. Thyroid. 2016;26(1):144–9.
21. Namba H, Nakashima M, Hayashi T, Hayashida N, Maeda S, Rogounovitch TI, et al. Clinical implication of hot spot BRAF mutation, V599E, in papillary thyroid cancers. J Clin Endocrinol Metab. 2003;88(9):4393–7.
22. Xing M, Alzahrani AS, Carson KA, Viola D, Elisei R, Bendlova B, et al. Association between BRAF V600E mutation and mortality in patients with papillary thyroid cancer. JAMA. 2013;309(14):1493–501.
23. Gouveia C, Can NT, Bostrom A, Grenert JP, van Zante A, Orloff LA. Lack of association of BRAF mutation with negative prognostic indicators in papillary thyroid carcinoma: the University of California, San Francisco, experience. JAMA Otolaryngol Head Neck Surg. 2013;139(11):1164–70.
24. Kim TH, Park YJ, Lim JA, Ahn HY, Lee EK, Lee YJ, et al. The association of the BRAF(V600E) mutation with prognostic factors and poor clinical outcome in papillary thyroid cancer: a meta-analysis. Cancer. 2012;118(7):1764–73.

25. Li C, Lee KC, Schneider EB, Zeiger MA. BRAF V600E mutation and its association with clinicopathological features of papillary thyroid cancer: a meta-analysis. J Clin Endocrinol Metab. 2012;97(12):4559–70.
26. Roti E, degli Uberti EC, Bondanelli M, Braverman LE. Thyroid papillary microcarcinoma: a descriptive and meta-analysis study. Eur J Endocrinol. 2008;159(6):659–73.
27. Niemeier LA, Kuffner Akatsu H, Song C, Carty SE, Hodak SP, Yip L, et al. A combined molecular-pathologic score improves risk stratification of thyroid papillary microcarcinoma. Cancer. 2012;118(8):2069–77.
28. Liu X, Bishop J, Shan Y, Pai S, Liu D, Murugan AK, et al. Highly prevalent TERT promoter mutations in aggressive thyroid cancers. Endocr Relat Cancer. 2013;20(4):603–10.
29. Landa I, Ganly I, Chan TA, Mitsutake N, Matsuse M, Ibrahimpasic T, et al. Frequent somatic TERT promoter mutations in thyroid cancer: higher prevalence in advanced forms of the disease. J Clin Endocrinol Metab. 2013;98(9):E1562–6.
30. Liu X, Qu S, Liu R, Sheng C, Shi X, Zhu G, et al. TERT promoter mutations and their association with BRAF V600E mutation and aggressive clinicopathological characteristics of thyroid cancer. J Clin Endocrinol Metab. 2014;99(6):E1130–6.
31. Melo M, da Rocha AG, Vinagre J, Batista R, Peixoto J, Tavares C, et al. TERT promoter mutations are a major indicator of poor outcome in differentiated thyroid carcinomas. J Clin Endocrinol Metab. 2014;99(5):E754–65.
32. Perera D, Ghossein R, Camacho N, Senbabaoglu Y, Seshan V, Li J, et al. Genomic and transcriptomic characterization of papillary microcarcinomas with lateral neck lymph node metastases. J Clin Endocrinol Metab. 2019;104(10):4889–99.

Chapter 5
Completion Thyroidectomy in a Patient with Low-Risk Papillary Cancer

David S. Cooper

The Case

The patient is a 25-year-old woman who was found to have a 2 cm right thyroid nodule on routine physical examination by her gynecologist. Thyroid function was normal, with serum TSH 2.6 mU/L. Thyroid ultrasound revealed a 2 cm nodule that was mildly hypoechoic with a sonolucent rim and internal vascularity (an "intermediate suspicion" nodule according to the American Thyroid Association [ATA] guidelines, thus a candidate for fine-needle aspiration biopsy). The contralateral lobe looked normal sonographically. FNA showed a "follicular lesion of undetermined significance" (Bethesda class III). Molecular testing using a gene expression classifier was "suspicious." After discussing the pros and cons of lobectomy versus total thyroidectomy, she underwent a right hemithyroidectomy. The final pathology revealed a 1.5 cm unifocal follicular variant papillary cancer with no extrathyroidal extension, negative margins, and no evidence of venous or lymphatic invasion. Lymphocytic thyroiditis was noted in the specimen. No lymph nodes were removed at the time of surgery. Her surgeon recommended a completion thyroidectomy in the near future, and she comes to discuss whether this is really necessary.

Assessment and Literature Review

Many patients undergo thyroid lobectomy because of indeterminate thyroid nodules. Even with molecular testing, only about 50% of these patients prove to have thyroid cancer [1–3], and the question of completion thyroidectomy is often raised.

D. S. Cooper (✉)
Division of Endocrinology, Diabetes, and Metabolism, The Johns Hopkins University School of Medicine, Baltimore, MD, USA
e-mail: dscooper@jhmi.edu

G. Grani et al. (eds.), *Thyroid Cancer*,
https://doi.org/10.1007/978-3-030-61919-0_5

But, it remains unsettled whether completion thyroidectomy is necessary in patients who are found to have low-risk papillary cancer in the operated lobe. Theoretically, there are two reasons to consider completion thyroidectomy: the contralateral lobe may harbor occult disease which could be the source of recurrence in the future, and, in order to enable the patient to receive radioiodine ablative therapy, a total thyroidectomy is generally required. A third, less compelling reason may be that follow-up with thyroglobulin measurements may be less ambiguous in patients who have been thyroidectomized. After lobectomy, serum thyroglobulin monitoring is probably not useful [4].

With regard to the first potential indication, numerous studies have shown that there is 30–80% prevalence of contralateral thyroid cancer [5]. This is typically micropapillary thyroid cancer (foci <10 mm), with a higher frequency in patients who have multifocal disease in the removed lobe and possibly also in patients who are older or who have larger primary tumors (e.g., [5]). However, despite this high frequency of residual malignant foci, the clinical recurrence rates in the contralateral lobe are very low, in the 1–4% range, consistent with the concept that these small thyroid cancer foci are relatively innocuous [6]. This observation is similar to what is known about small subclinical central lymph node metastases that are found after a prophylactic central neck dissection, which have a similar prevalence (30–80%), but which also have a very low rate of clinical recurrence, in the 1–2% range [7].

In the 2009 American Thyroid Association guidelines for the management of thyroid cancer, completion thyroidectomy was recommended for patients with primary tumors ≥1 cm in diameter [8]. This recommendation was based on two studies. The first was an older study by Hay et al. showing that while completion thyroidectomy did not improve cause-specific mortality, it did decrease the risk of locoregional recurrence [19% nodal metastasis rate at 20 years for lobectomy versus 6% recurrence rate for "bilateral lobar resection" ($P = 0.0001$)] [9]. However, it was the large study by Bilimoria et al. [10] which used data from the National Cancer Data Base that included over 52,000 patients that was the main driver of the 2009 ATA recommendation. These authors found that recurrence rates were higher [hazard ratio 1.24 (95% confidence interval 1.01–1.54, $P = 0.04$)] and overall survival was lower [hazard ratio 1.49 (95% CI 1.02–2.17, $P = 0.04$)] when patients underwent less than a total thyroidectomy for tumors 1–2 cm in diameter, compared to no difference in outcomes in patients with tumors <1 cm in diameter. However, this study has been faulted because only "overall survival" and not "disease-specific survival" was reported [11]. Since the mortality rates for differential thyroid cancer are extremely low, disease-specific survival is a much more important indicator of treatment efficacy. Also, information on extrathyroidal extension and completeness of tumor removal was not available, and if lobectomy was performed in some patients because of other comorbid conditions, or because of a compromised contralateral recurrent nerve, then these factors may have biased the results. Furthermore, the paper reported that 18% of patients who underwent lobectomy received radioiodine therapy postoperatively, suggesting the possibility that some of the patients were misclassified and actually had undergone completion thyroidectomy.

In addition to the study cited above [6], there have now been other studies also showing no advantage of total thyroidectomy over lobectomy. For example, in a paper using data extracted from the Surveillance, Epidemiology, and End Results (SEER) database involving almost 23,000 patients, of whom almost 6000 patients underwent lobectomy, there were no differences in disease-specific survival between patients who underwent total thyroidectomy versus lobectomy in multivariate analyses, and this was true for all tumor sizes up to 4 cm [12]. Similarly, in another study from Memorial Sloan Kettering Cancer Center involving a retrospective analysis of almost 900 patients with low-risk papillary thyroid cancer followed for an average of 10 years, there were no differences in disease-specific survival and in recurrence-free survival between patients who received a total thyroidectomy versus lobectomy (10-year disease-specific survival was 100% for the lobectomy group versus 98.5% for the total thyroidectomy group) [13]. Similarly, local recurrence rates were 0% for both groups, and regional recurrence rates were 0% versus 0.8% in the lobectomy versus total thyroidectomy groups, respectively. In multivariate analyses, only age >45 years and male gender were predictors of worse outcome, whereas the T stage and type of surgery were not predictive [13]. Finally, a study of over 61,000 patients from the National Cancer Database [14] found no survival advantage of total thyroidectomy versus lobectomy for thyroid cancers up to 4 cm in size. Thus, data showing better outcomes after total thyroidectomy (or completion thyroidectomy) has been questioned in more recent studies and is the basis of the 2015 American Thyroid Association guideline stating: "For patients with thyroid cancer >1 cm and <4 cm without extrathyroidal extension and without clinical evidence of any lymph node metastases (cN0) the initial surgical procedure can be either a bilateral procedure (near-total or total thyroidectomy) or a unilateral procedure (lobectomy)" [15]. And while completion thyroidectomy does not have greater morbidity than an initial total thyroidectomy, the morbidity of a total thyroidectomy is higher than that of a lobectomy even in the hands of high-volume surgeons [16].

The need for radioiodine remnant ablation is the second major reason to recommend completion thyroidectomy in some patients in whom the diagnosis of thyroid cancer is not known preoperatively. In this scenario, the decision to recommend completion thyroidectomy would depend on whether postoperative radioiodine therapy was deemed to be appropriate for the patient's risk of recurrence and death. Since the indications for remnant ablation have been made more stringent [15], and are now typically reserved for patients considered to be at intermediate risk rather than at low risk for recurrence, many patients would not be considered for postoperative radioactive iodine therapy, even if they had undergone a total thyroidectomy at the first surgery.

Based on these newer data, the 2015 American Thyroid Association guidelines state that "Completion thyroidectomy should be offered to those patients for whom a bilateral thyroidectomy would have been recommended had the diagnosis been available before the initial surgery" [15]. This decision would be based on the size of the tumor, the presence of clinical nodal metastases, or other high-risk histologic features that may have been known about preoperatively. Indeed, in a recent report, completion thyroidectomy was performed more frequently in patients with higher-risk tumors (T3) or other higher-risk features [17]. In the future, the presence of certain high-risk mutations, e.g., BRAF and TERT mutations, may also dictate a more aggressive approach [18]. These clinical, radiologic, and pathologic features would also likely inform the decision to administer radioiodine postoperatively. Thus, in those patients who are not known to have thyroid cancer preoperatively, it makes sense to do a lobectomy in those patients in whom a total thyroidectomy would not have been done, even if the diagnosis of thyroid cancer had been known preoperatively [15]. One might anticipate that the question of completion thyroidectomy will continue to be raised if lobectomy becomes a more common primary surgical treatment in the future, given the new ATA guideline recommendations. Patient preference is another factor which will always need to be considered.

Back to the Patient

It was explained to the patient that her cancer was very low risk and that, as a stage 1 patient, her risk of cancer-related mortality was 0%. Furthermore, the rate of recurrence was also extremely low, even without additional surgery or radioiodine therapy. Since serum thyroglobulin measurement is less helpful after lobectomy [4], we recommended annual neck ultrasound for the next 3–5 years with maintenance of serum TSH in the low normal range. Following surgery, her serum TSH was in the 3–4 mU/L range, so she was started on 50 μg of levothyroxine per day. The presence of positive TPO antibodies and/or preoperative serum TSH > ~2.5 mU/L has been shown to be predictors of the need for levothyroxine therapy after a lobectomy [19, 20]. She has now been followed for 5 years without any evidence of recurrent disease.

Clinical Pearls

1. In patients with indeterminate thyroid nodules, lobectomy is reasonable since the risk of cancer is only ~50% even with molecular testing. Lobectomy should be offered to those patients in whom lobectomy would have been reasonable even if the diagnosis of thyroid cancer had been known preoperatively.
2. Recent studies suggest that patients with low-risk thyroid cancer do not benefit from completion thyroidectomy.
3. Similarly, since total thyroidectomy is often recommended for patients with more advanced disease, with postoperative radioiodine remnant ablation in mind, the typical patient for whom lobectomy would be recommended would not be a candidate for radioiodine, even if thyroid cancer was discovered on final pathology.
4. Patients with low-risk thyroid cancer who have undergone thyroid lobectomy can be followed with neck ultrasound, since serum thyroglobulin monitoring is not useful.

References

1. Bongiovanni M, Spitale A, Faquin WC, Mazzucchelli L, Baloch ZW. The Bethesda system for reporting thyroid cytopathology: a meta-analysis. Acta Cytol. 2012;56:333–9.
2. Patel KN, Angell TE, Babiarz J, et al. Performance of a genomic sequencing classifier for the preoperative diagnosis of cytologically indeterminate thyroid nodules. JAMA Surg. 2018;153:817–24.
3. Steward DL, Carty SE, Sippel RS, et al. Performance of a multigene genomic classifier in thyroid nodules with indeterminate cytology: a prospective blinded multicenter study. JAMA Oncol. 2019;5:204–12.
4. Park S, Jeon MJ, Oh HS, et al. Changes in serum thyroglobulin levels after lobectomy in patients with low-risk papillary thyroid cancer. Thyroid. 2018;28:997–1003.
5. Kim ES, Kim TY, Koh JM, Kim YI, Hong SJ, Kim WB, Shong YK. Completion thyroidectomy in patients with thyroid cancer who initially underwent unilateral operation. Clin Endocrinol. 2004;61:145–8.
6. Vaisman F, Shaha A, Fish S, Tuttle RM. Initial therapy with either thyroid lobectomy or total thyroidectomy without radioactive iodine remnant ablation is associated with very low rates of structural disease recurrence in properly selected patients with differentiated thyroid cancer. Clin Endocrinol. 2011;75:112–9.
7. Randolph GW, Duh QY, Heller KS, LiVolsi VA, Mandel SJ, Steward DL, Tufano RP, Tuttle RM, American Thyroid Association Surgical Affairs Committee's Taskforce on Thyroid Cancer Nodal Surgery. The prognostic significance of nodal metastases from papillary thyroid carcinoma can be stratified based on the size and number of metastatic lymph nodes, as well as the presence of extranodal extension. Thyroid. 2012;22:1144–52.
8. Cooper DS, Doherty GM, Haugen BR, Kloos RT, Lee SL, Mandel SJ, Mazzaferri EL, McIver B, Pacini F, Schlumberger M, Sherman SI, Steward DL, Tuttle RM. Revised American Thyroid Association management guidelines for patients with thyroid nodules and differentiated thyroid cancer. Thyroid. 2009;19:1167–214.
9. Hay ID, Grant CS, Bergstralh EJ, Thompson GB, van Heerden JA, Goellner JR. Unilateral total lobectomy: is it sufficient surgical treatment for patients with AMES low-risk papillary thyroid carcinoma? Surgery. 1998;124:958–64.
10. Bilimoria KY, Bentrem DJ, Ko CY, Stewart AK, Winchester DP, Talamonti MS, Sturgeon C. Extent of surgery affects survival for papillary thyroid cancer. Ann Surg. 2007;246:375–81.
11. Shaha AR. Extent of surgery for papillary thyroid carcinoma: the debate continues: comment on "surgery for papillary thyroid carcinoma". Arch Otolaryngol Head Neck Surg. 2010;136:1061–3.
12. Mendelsohn AH, Elashoff DA, Abemayor E, St John MA. Surgery for papillary thyroid carcinoma: is lobectomy enough? Arch Otolaryngol Head Neck Surg. 2010;136:1055–61.
13. Nixon IJ, Ganly I, Patel SG, Palmer FL, Whitcher MM, Tuttle RM, Shaha A, Shah JP. Thyroid lobectomy for treatment of well differentiated intrathyroid malignancy. Surgery. 2012;151:571–9.
14. Adam MA, Pura J, Gu L, et al. Extent of surgery for papillary thyroid cancer is not associated with survival: an analysis of 61,775 patients. Ann Surg. 2014;260:601–7.
15. Haugen BR, Alexander EK, Bible KC, et al. 2015 American Thyroid Association management guidelines for adult patients with thyroid nodules and differentiated thyroid cancer: the American Thyroid Association guidelines task force on thyroid nodules and differentiated thyroid cancer. Thyroid. 2016;26:1–133.
16. Hauch A, Al-Qurayshi Z, Randolph G, Kandil E. Total thyroidectomy is associated with increased risk of complications for low- and high-volume surgeons. Ann Surg Oncol. 2014;21:3844–52.
17. Untch BR, Palmer FL, Ganly I, Patel SG, Tuttle RM, Shah JP, Shaha AA. Oncologic outcomes after completion thyroidectomy for patients with well-differentiated thyroid carcinoma. Ann Surg Oncol. 2014;21:1374–8.

18. Nikiforov YE. Role of molecular markers in thyroid nodule management: then and now. Endocr Pract. 2017;23:979–88.
19. Lee DY, Seok J, Jeong WJ, Ahn SH. Prediction of thyroid hormone supplementation after thyroid lobectomy. J Surg Res. 2015;193:273–8.
20. Zatelli MC, Lamartina L, Meringolo D, et al. Thyroid nodule recurrence following lobo-isthmectomy: incidence, patient's characteristics, and risk factors. J Endocrinol Investig. 2018;41:1469–75.

Chapter 6
Papillary Thyroid Cancer with Microscopic Extra-thyroidal Extension

Donald S. A. McLeod

Case Presentation

A 33-year-old woman with no past medical history presented with a right thyroid nodule. Fine needle aspiration was nondiagnostic (Bethesda system I), but on the basis of suspicious ultrasound features, diagnostic right lobectomy was performed. Histopathology revealed a classical 1.9 cm papillary thyroid carcinoma with anterior microscopic extra-thyroidal extension into peri-thyroidal skeletal muscle. Surgical margins were clear of tumor and there was no lymphovascular invasion. The completion thyroidectomy was free of malignancy. She presents for discussion of further treatment options. Prior to the diagnosis of thyroid cancer, the patient and her husband were attempting pregnancy and wish to conceive as soon as possible.

Assessment and Literature Review

There are clear prognostic differences between microscopic extra-thyroidal extension, macroscopic invasion of strap muscles, and major extra-thyroidal extension. In the absence of prospective and experimental evidence, observational, mostly retrospective, studies help to clarify potential risks of microscopic extra-thyroidal extension and the possible utility of treatment approaches.

D. S. A. McLeod (✉)
Department of Endocrinology & Diabetes, Royal Brisbane & Women's Hospital, Herston, QLD, Australia

Department of Population Health, QIMR Berghofer Medical Research Institute, Herston, QLD, Australia
e-mail: Donald.mcleod@qimrberghofer.edu.au

G. Grani et al. (eds.), *Thyroid Cancer*,
https://doi.org/10.1007/978-3-030-61919-0_6

Definition and Prevalence

Microscopic extra-thyroidal extension occurs when thyroid cancer advances beyond the thyroid capsule into surrounding peri-thyroidal soft tissues of fat and/or skeletal muscle (sternothyroid), but without macroscopic skeletal muscle invasion. Until recently, a commonly synonymous term was minimal extra-thyroidal extension [1]; however, because risk stratification systems distinguish macroscopic from microscopic extension, continued use of minimal extra-thyroidal extension could be misleading. Microscopic extra-thyroidal extension should also be distinguished from major (or extensive) extra-thyroidal extension. Here, the tumor directly invades one or more of the surrounding organs, including the subcutaneous soft tissues, larynx, trachea, esophagus, recurrent laryngeal nerve, prevertebral fascia, and vascular structures including the mediastinal vessels or carotid arteries [1]. While there remains inadequate data to determine the exact level of risk for patients with macroscopic extension to skeletal muscle, a reasonable response to the uncertainty is to treat this small subgroup similarly to patients with tumors demonstrating major extra-thyroidal extension when considering postoperative treatment options.

These distinctions are codified in TNM staging systems. Before the sixth edition of the American Joint Committee on Cancer staging manual, any extra-thyroidal extension was classified as T4 [2], but for the sixth and seventh editions, minimal extra-thyroidal extension was T3, while major extra-thyroidal extension remained T4 (either T4a or T4b) [3, 4]. In the current eighth edition, microscopic extra-thyroidal extension does not impact on T stage; macroscopic extension to surrounding strap skeletal muscles remains T3; and major extra-thyroidal extension remains T4 (either T4a or T5b) [5].

Microscopic extra-thyroidal extension is common. Estimates vary in the order of 11–44% (Table 6.1) [6–12]. It is therefore important to have a clear concept of risks related to this pathologic feature, to ensure adequate but not overtreatment of patients.

Table 6.1 Ranges of microscopic extra-thyroidal extension prevalence

Institution (country) year [ref]	% with microscopic extra-thyroidal extension
Memorial Sloan-Kettering Cancer Center (USA) 2011 [6]	11.6
Walter Reed National Military Medical Center (USA) 2014 [7]	14.1
New York Presbyterian Hospital-Weill Cornell Medical College (USA) 2008 [8]	22.6
Cancer Institute Hospital (Japan) 2012 [9]	29.6
Kuma Hospital (Japan) 2006 [10]	30.5
Busan Paik Hospital (Korea) 2013 [11]	31.0
Samsung Medical Center (Korea) 2013 [12]	44.0

Comparison of Microscopic with Major Extra-thyroidal Extension

Older studies rarely distinguished microscopic and major extra-thyroidal extension and concluded that extra-thyroidal extension was associated with poor prognosis [13–17]. However, other large series gave clues that the most critical factor was major extra-thyroidal extension. The Mayo Clinic and Memorial Sloan-Kettering Cancer Center did this by defining extra-thyroidal extension based on visual operative findings (hence classifying patients with microscopic extension as having intra-thyroidal tumors) and showed that macroscopic extra-thyroidal extension had markedly impaired prognosis while patients with only microscopic extra-thyroidal extension had overall very good prognosis [18, 19].

More recent analyses have confirmed large differences in outcome between microscopic and major extra-thyroidal extension. Arora and colleagues assessed 212 patients with papillary thyroid cancer for disease-free survival, finding a 6.4 (95% confidence interval = 1.6–25.9) times increased recurrence risk for patients with major extra-thyroidal extension compared with those who had microscopic extension on multivariate analysis [8]. The European Multicentre Study of Differentiated Thyroid Cancer prospectively recruited 351 patients with either microscopic or major extra-thyroidal extension [20]. Major extra-thyroidal extension was independently associated with a 3.23 (1.10–9.51)-fold higher risk of progression. In 930 patients, Hotomi and colleagues from Japan found that recurrence was 6.76 (4.25–10.76) times more likely and death was 7.97 (4.20–15.14) times more likely, for patients with major extra-thyroidal extension than for patients with microscopic or no extra-thyroidal extension [9]. Consistent with the clinical outcome data, tumors with more extensive extra-thyroidal extension have been found to harbor higher rates of angioinvasion and are of higher proliferative grade [21].

Given that major extra-thyroidal extension appears to denote more aggressive disease and a significantly poorer prognosis than microscopic extra-thyroidal extension, it is therefore important to consider whether microscopic extra-thyroidal extension holds any prognostic influence for both survival and risk of recurrent disease.

Survival with Microscopic Extra-thyroidal Extension

In the absence of other negative prognostic factors, survival of patients with microscopic extra-thyroidal extension is excellent. The National Thyroid Cancer Treatment Cooperative Study is a large multicenter registry of thyroid cancer patients from 11 hospitals in North America. For papillary cancer patients with microscopic extra-thyroidal extension but no additional risk features (i.e., tumor size >4 cm, positive cervical lymph nodes, or distant metastases), the disease-specific survival approaches 100% [22–24], with the most recent published analysis assessing long-term disease-specific survival including 3572 patients totaling 16,683 person years (2728 patients stage low-risk patients including those with microscopic extra-thyroidal extension) [24]. Disease-specific survival of 100% has also been reported in 115 otherwise low-risk patients with microscopic extra-thyroidal extension treated at Memorial Sloan-Kettering Cancer Center (at 10 years) [6] and 127 patients with microscopic extra-thyroidal extension and no distant metastases treated at the Mayo Clinic (at 20 years) [25]. Hotomi and colleagues reported a 97.3% 10-year disease-specific survival in 275 patients prospectively followed with "minimal" extra-thyroidal extension (a group which also included large proportions of patients with major extra-thyroidal extension based on standard definitions) [9]. Because of this excellent survival, microscopic extra-thyroidal extension has been removed from the eighth edition of TNM staging [5].

Only one study has reported an impaired prognosis in patients with microscopic extra-thyroidal extension. This analysis included 21,907 patients with "minimal" extra-thyroidal extension (including both microscopic extra-thyroidal extension and macroscopic extension to skeletal muscle) from differentiated thyroid cancer recorded in the US National Cancer Database, finding a 13% (5–22%) lower overall survival compared with patients without extra-thyroidal extension [26]. Interpreting the significance of these data for tumors with isolated microscopic extra-thyroidal extension is difficult. Firstly, because the disease-specific survival of these patients is likely to be very high, a 13% higher disease-specific mortality rate would be negligible in absolute risk difference. Secondly, it was not possible to separate patients with microscopic extra-thyroidal extension from macroscopic extra-thyroidal extension to skeletal muscle, which may be important. Thirdly, while the analysis was carefully performed and adjustments made for available confounders, there is great potential for unmeasured confounding due to associated higher-risk features not being captured in the database.

Recurrence Risk with Microscopic Extra-thyroidal Extension

Table 6.2 describes studies assessing the risk of recurrence for papillary thyroid cancers with microscopic extra-thyroidal extension, compared to those with intra-thyroidal primary tumors [6–12, 27–31]. What could account for this variability in results? The most likely explanation is that microscopic extra-thyroidal extension is a marker of slightly more aggressive tumor biology, although, in the presence of careful (pre-)operative evaluation and adequate surgical clearance, it loses importance as an independent prognostic factor. Several lines of evidence support this hypothesis. Firstly, tumors with microscopic extra-thyroidal extension are more likely to have other high-risk features (Table 6.3) [6–9, 11, 12, 27, 29–33]. The one study to report significantly higher recurrence risk with microscopic extra-thyroidal extension did not perform a multivariate analysis to determine if it independently predicted recurrence [12]. Likewise, the apparent trend in other studies could well

Table 6.2 Studies assessing the risk of recurrence of papillary cancers with microscopic extrathyroidal extension, compared to tumors without microscopic extra-thyroidal extension

Institution/cohort (country) year [ref]	Study population/groups examined	Evidence
No increased risk		
Kuma Hospital (Japan) 2006 [10, 27]	1167 patients undergoing curative intent surgery followed for a minimum of 5 years, including 356 with microscopic extra-thyroidal extension	No difference in recurrence in patients with microscopic extra-thyroidal extension compared to those without; the recurrence-free survival at 15 years was >90%. In the 215 patients with microscopic extra-thyroidal extension aged >45 years, the results were the same
Memorial Sloan-Kettering Cancer Center (USA) 2011 [6]	984 patients with clinical T1/T2 N0 disease, including 115 with microscopic extra-thyroidal extension	Recurrence at 10 years was no different in those with or without extra-thyroidal extension (95% vs. 98%; $P = 0.188$)
Yonsei University College of Medicine (Korea) 2011 [29]	288 patients with papillary microcarcinoma, including 89 patients with microscopic extra-thyroidal extension	During mean follow-up of 6 years, 3.4% of patients with microscopic extra-extrathyroidal extension had recurrence, vs. 4.5% of patients without ($P = 0.67$)
Asan Medical Center (Korea) ePub 2019 [28]	571 patients treated with lobectomy, including 182 patients with microscopic extra-thyroidal extension but no other higher-risk clinical or histologic features	During median follow-up of 8.4 years, 2.7% of patients with microscopic extra-thyroidal extension had recurrence, vs. 5% of patients with low-risk intrathyroidal tumors
Numerically higher but not statistically significant increased risk		
New York Presbyterian Hospital-Weill Cornell Medical College (USA) 2008 [8]	48 patients with microscopic extra-thyroidal extension. A comparison group was 141 patients with no extra-thyroidal extension	On univariate analysis, 21% of patients with microscopic extra-thyroidal extension had recurrence, compared to 13% of the patients without ($P = 0.2$)
Cancer Institute Hospital (Japan) 2012 [9]	265 patients with >1 cm cancers and "minimal" extra-thyroidal extension. A comparison group was 412 patients without extra-thyroidal extension	10-year recurrence-free survival of patients with "minimal" extra-thyroidal extension was 91.5%, compared to 96% for those without (univariate analysis)
Busan Paik Hospital (Korea) 2013 [11]	332 patients without macroscopic extra-thyroidal extension, including 103 with microscopic extra-thyroidal extension	Recurrence at 5 years was 13.6% of patients with microscopic extra-thyroidal extension, vs. 7.9% of 229 patients without ($P = 0.153$; univariate analysis)
Walter Reed National Military Medical Center (USA) 2014 [7]	Various, but the groups of interest were 33 patients followed with microscopic extra-thyroidal extension vs. 164 patients with intrathyroidal tumors	9% of patients with microscopic extra-thyroidal extension had recurrent disease (median follow-up 4.5 years, compared to 4% of those without (median follow-up 6.8 years; not statistically compared)

(continued)

Table 6.2 (continued)

Institution/cohort (country) year [ref]	Study population/groups examined	Evidence
Pitié-Salpêtrière Hospital (France) 2014 [30]	124 patients with papillary microcarcinoma plus microscopic extra-thyroidal extension and no nodal metastases. Various other groups but most comparable 1220 patients with intrathyroidal papillary microcarcinoma	During median follow-up of 6.7 years, 4.8% of patients with microscopic extra-extrathyroidal extension had recurrent disease, vs. 1.3% of patients without (not statistically compared)
Asan Medical Center (Korea) 2015 [31]	546 patients with solitary primary tumors and no major extra-thyroidal extension, including 259 patients with extension to peri-thyroidal soft tissues and 91 to sternothyroid (it is unclear how many of these were macroscopic extension)	On a limited multivariate analysis, risk of recurrence in those with "minimal" extra-thyroidal extension (compared with no extension) was 1.88 (0.99–3.56). Some overlap in cohort with ref [28] above
Statistically significant increased risk		
Samsung Medical Center (Korea) 2013 [12]	Various papillary thyroid cancer patients, but the compared groups were 378 patients with microscopic extra-thyroidal extension vs. 445 patients without	378 patients with microscopic extra-thyroidal extension had recurrence at median follow-up of 4.5 years, compared with 1.2% of 445 patients without ($P = 0.012$; univariate analysis)

Table 6.3 Tumor features more commonly present in patients with microscopic extra-thyroidal extension

Older age [6, 9, 31]
Tumor size >1 cm [6, 12, 27, 31]
Angioinvasion [8]
Higher-risk histologic subtypes [32]
Lymph node metastasis [7–9, 11, 29–31]
Extra-nodal extension [33]
Positive surgical margins [8, 12]
$BRAF^{V600E}$ mutation [32]

be explained by these other prognostic factors. Secondly, the studies showing very low recurrence rates and no increased recurrence risk from microscopic extra-thyroidal extension apparently had careful pre- and intraoperative assessment, in addition to surgical clearance of all identified tumor (± radioiodine).

Management of the Case

The above literature review highlights that while major extra-thyroidal extension is an important risk factor for poor outcome, microscopic extra-thyroidal extension can have an excellent prognosis in the absence of other high-risk features.

Returning to our case, we should therefore ask the following questions:

- Was completion thyroidectomy required?
- Is a postoperative thyroglobulin useful in determining further treatment?
- Will radioiodine ablation be helpful?
- What should the thyrotropin (TSH) target be?
- Would molecular testing of our patient's thyroid cancer assist in decision-making?

Was Completion Thyroidectomy Required?

Until recently, most authorities recommended total thyroidectomy when microscopic extra-thyroidal extension was present [34–36]. However, excellent results have been reported with lobectomy where careful patient selection was performed [37–39]. Nixon and colleagues reported a 100% 10-year recurrence-free survival in 26 patients treated with lobectomy (who also had tumors <4 cm diameter, without evidence of lymph node metastases) [6], and Song and colleagues reported a 2.7% risk of recurrence over median follow-up of 8.4 years in 182 Korean patients with microscopic extra-thyroidal but no other higher-risk features.

So, while the most recent American Thyroid Association [40], British Thyroid Association [41], and Italian [42] guidelines continue to recommend completion thyroidectomy when extra-thyroidal extension is identified, others suggest that lobectomy may be appropriate for many patients with microscopic extra-thyroidal extension. Japanese guidelines recommend lobectomy where nodal disease is absent and primary tumor size is <2 cm and an individualized approach for others without defined high-risk features [43]. The National Comprehensive Cancer Network (United States) guidelines also do not recommend completion thyroidectomy in the absence of high-risk features [44].

Is a Postoperative Thyroglobulin Useful in Determining Further Treatment?

Dynamic risk stratification, a biochemical (serum thyroglobulin) and structural (imaging) assessment of response-to-therapy [45], was first described for monitoring patients following total thyroidectomy and radioiodine ablation, but multiple studies have validated the approach for patients following total thyroidectomy alone. An undetectable or very low serum thyroglobulin postsurgery (i.e., 6–8 weeks after) is associated with extremely low recurrence risk of recurrence [46–49], as is a decreasing or stable postoperative serum thyroglobulin when thyroglobulin is initially detectable [46]. For our patient, the postoperative serum thyroglobulin could be especially helpful. An undetectable serum thyroglobulin on levothyroxine therapy would suggest significant volume disease has not been left behind and build a case that recurrence risk will be low.

Will Radioiodine Remnant Ablation Be Helpful?

The main potential rationale for radioiodine remnant ablation in our patient is to improve recurrence risk. Unfortunately, few data are available to help guide this decision. The National Thyroid Cancer Treatment Cooperative Study's data on radioiodine confirm no difference in survival or recurrence risk on multivariate analyses for their stage I (our patient's stage) or II patients [23, 50]. Nixon and colleagues from Memorial Sloan-Kettering reported that in 23 thyroidectomized patients with microscopic extra-thyroidal extension of tumors <4 cm diameter and without evidence of lymph node metastases, recurrence-free survival to 10 years was 100% [6]. In the corresponding 63 patients who received radioiodine ablation, recurrence free survival was 90% ($P = 0.29$). This work highlights the possibility of safely selecting patients for less intensive therapy. One retrospective Korean study has assessed recurrence in 121 patients with microscopic extra-thyroidal extension receiving radioiodine ablation, compared with 108 patients who did not [51]. Here, Jeon and colleagues found that 13.2% of patients receiving radioiodine had recurrence, vs. 9.3% of those without radioiodine ($P = 0.44$). Radioiodine status remained nonsignificant for recurrence on multivariate analysis. Finally, radioiodine is rarely used in Japan, yet the Japanese studies of microscopic extra-thyroidal extension report excellent recurrence-free survival [9, 10, 27]. One of the two ongoing trials for radioiodine allows inclusion of patients with microscopic extra-thyroidal extension (IoN; NCT01398085). This may help illuminate the role of radioiodine remnant ablation in patients with microscopic extra-thyroidal extension, although the trial is unlikely to be powered for this specific subgroup.

Until further data are published, an individualized approach to decision-making, taking into account confidence in available surgical skill, other tumor prognostic features, the postoperative serum thyroglobulin level, patient preference, and availability of quality follow-up, is reasonable. If radioiodine is to be used for minimal extra-thyroidal extension, low administered activity therapy (i.e., 30 mCi) appears adequate [52].

What Should the Thyrotropin (TSH) Target Be?

TSH suppression has a role in the treatment of high-risk differentiated thyroid cancer [53]. Assuming a low postoperative serum thyroglobulin, the above discussion does not support this label for our patient's thyroid cancer. The National

Thyroid Cancer Treatment Cooperative Study did not find any significant differences in survival or recurrence for their stage I patients (our patient's stage) based on serum TSH variations during follow-up [23]. A Dutch study including mostly low-risk patients found that recurrence and death were significantly increased above a serum TSH threshold of 2 mU/L [54]. Therefore, a long-term goal of a low normal serum TSH that ensures euthyroidism, i.e., 0.5–2.0 mU/L, would be reasonable here. Some authorities recommend commencing treatment with a lower serum TSH target before subsequently re-stratifying risk, although an early undetectable postoperative serum thyroglobulin would suggest an "excellent response" using dynamic risk stratification [45], and may allow for earlier arrival at long-term TSH targets.

Would Molecular Testing of Our Patient's Thyroid Cancer Assist in Decision-Making?

An intriguing prospect would be to use genomic/molecular markers of higher risk to guide the extent of treatment. The American Thyroid Association thyroid cancer treatment guidelines mention *BRAF* mutational status in the newest initial risk stratification system [40]. $BRAF^{V600E}$ mutation is more common in tumors with extra-thyroidal extension, in addition to being associated with other higher-risk features [32]. However, *BRAF* mutation is a common event in papillary thyroid cancers, and papillary cancers with isolated microscopic extra-thyroidal extension rarely recur after surgical excision. Thus, a benefit from using *BRAF* mutational status here is uncertain; relying on *BRAF* status could potentially lead to overtreatment with additional surgery/radioiodine in those at very low risk of recurrence. Additional markers will likely be required to optimize clinical decision-making.

Case Progress

The postoperative thyroglobulin on levothyroxine was undetectable (<0.5 ng/mL). Based on this result, the other low-risk tumor features, and the confidence that an effective pre- and intraoperative assessment of disease burden had been performed, the patient and her clinicians were comfortable to recommend against postoperative radioiodine ablation. Avoiding radioiodine also had the advantage in potentially preventing delay in attempting pregnancy. On 6-month review, the patient was well without clinical, biochemical (serum thyroglobulin <0.5 ng/mL), or ultrasound signs of recurrence disease. Serum TSH was 0.8 mU/L on levothyroxine replacement. She was not yet pregnant.

Clinical Pearls/Pitfalls

- Not all extra-thyroidal extension is equal. Major extra-thyroidal extension has clear prognostic importance. Microscopic extra-thyroidal extension more often occurs in tumors with other adverse prognostic features, but its role as an independent prognostic marker is questionable.
- When other high-risk features are absent, survival and recurrence-free survival of patients with microscopic extra-thyroidal extension may approach those of patients with intrathyroidal tumors.
- Some authorities recommend completion thyroidectomy when microscopic extra-thyroidal extension is present, although other guidelines do not mandate this.
- Where other high-risk features are absent, a benefit from radioiodine remnant ablation is unclear. An individualized approach to decision-making is reasonable. When radioiodine ablation is performed, low activity therapy (i.e., 30 mCi) appears adequate.
- TSH suppression is not required for most patients with microscopic extra-thyroidal extension, unless other high-risk features are present.
- The role of molecular markers in determining optimal treatment remains unclear.

References

1. Ghossein R. Update to the College of American Pathologists reporting on thyroid carcinomas. Head Neck Pathol. 2009;3(1):86–93.
2. Fleming ID, Cooper JS, Henson DE, Hutter RVP, Kennedy BJ, Murphy GP, et al. AJCC cancer staging manual. 5th ed. Philadelphia: Lippincott-Raven; 1997.
3. Greene FL, Page DL, Fleming ID, Fritz AG, Balch CM, Haller DG, et al. AJCC cancer staging manual. 6th ed. New York: Springer; 2002.
4. Edge SB, Byrd DR, Compton CC, Fritz AG, Greene FL, Trotti A, editors. AJCC cancer staging manual. 7th ed. New York: Springer; 2010.
5. Amin MB, Edge S, Greene F, Byrd DR, Brookland RK, Washington MK, et al. AJCC cancer staging manual. 8th ed. Chicago: American Joint Committee on Cancer, Springer; 2017.
6. Nixon IJ, Ganly I, Patel S, Palmer FL, Whitcher MM, Tuttle RM, et al. The impact of microscopic extrathyroid extension on outcome in patients with clinical T1 and T2 well-differentiated thyroid cancer. Surgery. 2011;150(6):1242–9.
7. Radowsky JS, Howard RS, Burch HB, Stojadinovic A. Impact of degree of extrathyroidal extension of disease on papillary thyroid cancer outcome. Thyroid. 2014;24(2):241–4.
8. Arora N, Turbendian HK, Scognamiglio T, Wagner PL, Goldsmith SJ, Zarnegar R, et al. Extrathyroidal extension is not all equal: implications of macroscopic versus microscopic extent in papillary thyroid carcinoma. Surgery. 2008;144(6):942–7; discussion 7–8.
9. Hotomi M, Sugitani I, Toda K, Kawabata K, Fujimoto Y. A novel definition of extrathyroidal invasion for patients with papillary thyroid carcinoma for predicting prognosis. World J Surg. 2012;36(6):1231–40.
10. Ito Y, Tomoda C, Uruno T, Takamura Y, Miya A, Kobayashi K, et al. Prognostic significance of extrathyroid extension of papillary thyroid carcinoma: massive but not minimal extension affects the relapse-free survival. World J Surg. 2006;30(5):780–6.

11. Shin JH, Ha TK, Park HK, Ahn MS, Kim KH, Bae KB, et al. Implication of minimal extrathyroidal extension as a prognostic factor in papillary thyroid carcinoma. Int J Surg. 2013;11(9):944–7.
12. Jung SP, Kim M, Choe JH, Kim JS, Nam SJ, Kim JH. Clinical implication of cancer adhesion in papillary thyroid carcinoma: clinicopathologic characteristics and prognosis analyzed with degree of extrathyroidal extension. World J Surg. 2013;37(7):1606–13.
13. Carcangiu ML, Zampi G, Pupi A, Castagnoli A, Rosai J. Papillary carcinoma of the thyroid. A clinicopathologic study of 241 cases treated at the University of Florence, Italy. Cancer. 1985;55(4):805–28.
14. Simpson WJ, McKinney SE, Carruthers JS, Gospodarowicz MK, Sutcliffe SB, Panzarella T. Papillary and follicular thyroid cancer. Prognostic factors in 1,578 patients. Am J Med. 1987;83(3):479–88.
15. Cady B, Rossi R. An expanded view of risk-group definition in differentiated thyroid carcinoma. Surgery. 1988;104(6):947–53.
16. DeGroot LJ, Kaplan EL, McCormick M, Straus FH. Natural history, treatment, and course of papillary thyroid carcinoma. J Clin Endocrinol Metab. 1990;71(2):414–24.
17. Mazzaferri EL, Jhiang SM. Long-term impact of initial surgical and medical therapy on papillary and follicular thyroid cancer. Am J Med. 1994;97(5):418–28.
18. Hay ID, Bergstralh EJ, Goellner JR, Ebersold JR, Grant CS. Predicting outcome in papillary thyroid carcinoma: development of a reliable prognostic scoring system in a cohort of 1779 patients surgically treated at one institution during 1940 through 1989. Surgery. 1993;114(6):1050–7; discussion 7–8.
19. Andersen PE, Kinsella J, Loree TR, Shaha AR, Shah JP. Differentiated carcinoma of the thyroid with extrathyroidal extension. Am J Surg. 1995;170(5):467–70.
20. Kramer JA, Schmid KW, Dralle H, Dietlein M, Schicha H, Lerch H, et al. Primary tumour size is a prognostic parameter in patients suffering from differentiated thyroid carcinoma with extrathyroidal growth: results of the MSDS trial. Eur J Endocrinol/Eur Fed Endocrine Soc. 2010;163(4):637–44.
21. Rivera M, Ricarte-Filho J, Tuttle RM, Ganly I, Shaha A, Knauf J, et al. Molecular, morphologic, and outcome analysis of thyroid carcinomas according to degree of extrathyroid extension. Thyroid. 2010;20(10):1085–93.
22. Sherman SI, Brierley JD, Sperling M, Ain KB, Bigos ST, Cooper DS, et al. Prospective multicenter study of thyroid carcinoma treatment: initial analysis of staging and outcome. National Thyroid Cancer Treatment Cooperative Study Registry Group. Cancer. 1998;83(5):1012–21.
23. Jonklaas J, Sarlis NJ, Litofsky D, Ain KB, Bigos ST, Brierley JD, et al. Outcomes of patients with differentiated thyroid carcinoma following initial therapy. Thyroid. 2006;16(12):1229–42.
24. Jonklaas J, Nogueras-Gonzalez G, Munsell M, Litofsky D, Ain KB, Bigos ST, et al. The impact of age and gender on papillary thyroid cancer survival. J Clin Endocrinol Metab. 2012;97(6):E878–87.
25. Hay ID, Johnson TR, Thompson GB, Sebo TJ, Reinalda MS. Minimal extrathyroid extension in papillary thyroid carcinoma does not result in increased rates of either cause-specific mortality or postoperative tumor recurrence. Surgery. 2016;159(1):11–9.
26. Youngwirth LM, Adam MA, Scheri RP, Roman SA, Sosa JA. Extrathyroidal extension is associated with compromised survival in patients with thyroid cancer. Thyroid. 2017;27(5):626–31.
27. Ito Y, Tomoda C, Uruno T, Takamura Y, Miya A, Kobayashi K, et al. Minimal extrathyroid extension does not affect the relapse-free survival of patients with papillary thyroid carcinoma measuring 4 cm or less over the age of 45 years. Surg Today. 2006;36(1):12–8.
28. Song E, Ahn J, Song DE, Kim WW, Jeon MJ, Sung TY, et al. Modified risk stratification based on cervical lymph node metastases following lobectomy for papillary thyroid carcinoma. Clin Endocrinol (Oxf). 2019. https://doi.org/10.1111/cen.14115.
29. Moon HJ, Kim EK, Chung WY, Yoon JH, Kwak JY. Minimal extrathyroidal extension in patients with papillary thyroid microcarcinoma: is it a real prognostic factor? Ann Surg Oncol. 2011;18(7):1916–23.

30. Chereau N, Buffet C, Tresallet C, Tissier F, Golmard JL, Leenhardt L, et al. Does extracapsular extension impact the prognosis of papillary thyroid microcarcinoma? Ann Surg Oncol. 2014;21(5):1659–64.
31. Woo CG, Sung CO, Choi YM, Kim WG, Kim TY, Shong YK, et al. Clinicopathological significance of minimal extrathyroid extension in solitary papillary thyroid carcinomas. Ann Surg Oncol. 2015;22(Suppl 3):S728–33.
32. Krasner JR, Alyouha N, Pusztaszeri M, Forest VI, Hier MP, Avior G, et al. Molecular mutations as a possible factor for determining extent of thyroid surgery. J Otolaryngol Head Neck Surg. 2019;48(1):51.
33. Clain JB, Scherl S, Dos Reis L, Turk A, Wenig BM, Mehra S, et al. Extrathyroidal extension predicts extranodal extension in patients with positive lymph nodes: an important association that may affect clinical management. Thyroid. 2014;24(6):951–7.
34. Pacini F, Schlumberger M, Dralle H, Elisei R, Smit JW, Wiersinga W. European consensus for the management of patients with differentiated thyroid carcinoma of the follicular epithelium. European J Endocrinol/Eur Fed Endocrine Soc. 2006;154(6):787–803.
35. Cooper DS, Doherty GM, Haugen BR, Kloos RT, Lee SL, Mandel SJ, et al. Revised American Thyroid Association management guidelines for patients with thyroid nodules and differentiated thyroid cancer. Thyroid. 2009;19(11):1167–214.
36. Pitoia F, Ward L, Wohllk N, Friguglietti C, Tomimori E, Gauna A, et al. Recommendations of the Latin American Thyroid Society on diagnosis and management of differentiated thyroid cancer. Arq Bras Endocrinol Metabol. 2009;53(7):884–97.
37. Shaha AR, Shah JP, Loree TR. Low-risk differentiated thyroid cancer: the need for selective treatment. Ann Surg Oncol. 1997;4(4):328–33.
38. Cross S, Wei JP, Kim S, Brams DM. Selective surgery and adjuvant therapy based on risk classifications of well-differentiated thyroid cancer. J Surg Oncol. 2006;94(8):678–82.
39. Nixon IJ, Ganly I, Patel SG, Palmer FL, Whitcher MM, Tuttle RM, et al. Thyroid lobectomy for treatment of well differentiated intrathyroid malignancy. Surgery. 2012;151(4):571–9.
40. Haugen BR, Alexander EK, Bible KC, Doherty GM, Mandel SJ, Nikiforov YE, et al. 2015 American Thyroid Association management guidelines for adult patients with thyroid nodules and differentiated thyroid cancer: the American Thyroid Association guidelines task force on thyroid nodules and differentiated thyroid cancer. Thyroid. 2016;26(1):1–133.
41. Perros P, Boelaert K, Colley S, Evans C, Evans RM, Gerrard Ba G, et al. Guidelines for the management of thyroid cancer. Clin Endocrinol (Oxf). 2014;81(Suppl 1):1–122.
42. Pacini F, Basolo F, Bellantone R, Boni G, Cannizzaro MA, De Palma M, et al. Italian consensus on diagnosis and treatment of differentiated thyroid cancer: joint statements of six Italian societies. J Endocrinol Invest. 2018;41(7):849–76.
43. Ito Y, Miyauchi A, Oda H, Masuoka H, Higashiyama T, Kihara M, et al. Appropriateness of the revised Japanese guidelines' risk classification for the prognosis of papillary thyroid carcinoma: a retrospective analysis of 5,845 papillary thyroid carcinoma patients. Endocr J. 2019;66(2):127–34.
44. Haddad RI, Bischoff L, Busaidy NL, Dickson P, Duh QY, Ehya H, et al. National comprehensive cancer network. Thyroid carcinoma (version 2.2019) 2019. December 20, 2019. Available from: https://www.nccn.org/professionals/physician_gls/pdf/thyroid.pdf.
45. Momesso DP, Tuttle RM. Update on differentiated thyroid cancer staging. Endocrinol Metab Clin North Am. 2014;43(2):401–21.
46. Durante C, Montesano T, Attard M, Torlontano M, Monzani F, Costante G, et al. Long-term surveillance of papillary thyroid cancer patients who do not undergo postoperative radioiodine remnant ablation: is there a role for serum thyroglobulin measurement? J Clin Endocrinol Metab. 2012;97(8):2748–53.
47. Sung TY, Cho JW, Lee YM, Lee YH, Kwon H, Jeon MJ, et al. Dynamic risk stratification in stage I papillary thyroid cancer patients younger than 45 years of age. Thyroid. 2017;27(11):1400–7.

48. Park S, Kim WG, Song E, Oh HS, Kim M, Kwon H, et al. Dynamic risk stratification for predicting recurrence in patients with differentiated thyroid cancer treated without radioactive iodine remnant ablation therapy. Thyroid. 2017;27(4):524–30.
49. Momesso DP, Vaisman F, Yang SP, Bulzico DA, Corbo R, Vaisman M, et al. Dynamic risk stratification in patients with differentiated thyroid cancer treated without radioactive iodine. J Clin Endocrinol Metab. 2016;101(7):2692–700.
50. Jonklaas J, Cooper DS, Ain KB, Bigos T, Brierley JD, Haugen BR, et al. Radioiodine therapy in patients with stage I differentiated thyroid cancer. Thyroid. 2010;20(12):1423–4.
51. Jeon YW, Ahn YE, Chung WS, Choi HJ, Suh YJ. Radioactive iodine treatment for node negative papillary thyroid cancer with capsular invasion only: results of a large retrospective study. Asia Pac J Clin Oncol. 2016;12(1):e167–73.
52. Han JM, Kim WG, Kim TY, Jeon MJ, Ryu JS, Song DE, et al. Effects of low-dose and high-dose postoperative radioiodine therapy on the clinical outcome in patients with small differentiated thyroid cancer having microscopic extrathyroidal extension. Thyroid. 2014;24(5):820–5.
53. McLeod DS. Thyrotropin in the development and management of differentiated thyroid cancer. Endocrinol Metab Clin North Am. 2014;43(2):367–83.
54. Hovens GC, Stokkel MP, Kievit J, Corssmit EP, Pereira AM, Romijn JA, et al. Associations of serum thyrotropin concentrations with recurrence and death in differentiated thyroid cancer. J Clin Endocrinol Metab. 2007;92(7):2610–5.

Chapter 7
A Small Papillary Thyroid Cancer with Angioinvasion

Michael E. Hopkins and Iain J. Nixon

Introduction

Papillary thyroid cancer (PTC) is a relatively non-aggressive cancer in comparison to other malignancies. Patients that are at highest risk of recurrence and death are generally older and have aggressive, large volume local, regional, and distant disease [1]. These patients are typically treated aggressively with total thyroidectomy, selective neck dissection, and adjuvant radioactive iodine (RAI) therapy. Patients with small papillary thyroid cancers (PTC) without many of these features are more challenging to manage, since the majority of patients have excellent outcomes in terms of both survival and recurrence [2]. Further risk stratification is therefore useful to avoid over- or under-treatment of patients within this cohort. The overwhelming majority of patients with a small PTC will present without advanced disease features, and the only variables available for risk stratification relate to the primary disease itself. This includes the presence of vascular invasion histologically, which presents a management challenge.

Case Presentation (Diagnosis and Investigation)

A 35-year-old female music teacher underwent a right thyroid lobectomy for an enlarging thyroid nodule which was causing increasing dysphagia. A pre-operative thyroid ultrasound had demonstrated this to be 1.5 cm and suspicious for malignancy in ultrasound appearance and on fine needle aspiration cytology. There was

M. E. Hopkins (✉) · I. J. Nixon
Department of Otolaryngology, Head and Neck Surgery, NHS Lothian, Edinburgh, UK
e-mail: Michael.hopkins6@nhs.net; Iain.Nixon@nhs.net

G. Grani et al. (eds.), *Thyroid Cancer*,
https://doi.org/10.1007/978-3-030-61919-0_7

no evidence of pathological cervical lymph nodes on pre-operative imaging. The operation went without complication, the lobe was removed intact, and there were no adverse intraoperative features. A nerve monitor was used, and at the end of the procedure, both the vagus and recurrent laryngeal nerves (RLN) stimulated; furthermore, both parathyroid glands were reported to have remained in situ. Post-operative assessment of the vocal cords revealed good function bilaterally, and the patient's serum-adjusted calcium was 9.0 mg/dl (8.5–10 mg/dl). The post-operative thyroid-stimulating hormone was measured at 6-week follow-up and found to be 6.2 mU/L (0.5–5 mU/L); this was an increase compared to her pre-operative baseline of 3.8 mU/L, and not unexpected following excision of a thyroid lobe. The post-excision histopathological assessment of the lobe revealed evidence of a 1.5 cm, of encapsulated PTC with one focus of vascular invasion in a background of Hashimoto's thyroiditis. The patient was notified of the findings, and her case was discussed at the regional multidisciplinary team (MDT) meeting to decide on the need for further therapy.

Literature Review

For small PTC, in general, clinical outcomes are excellent. Indeed, in both Japan and the USA, there is a move towards active observation rather than surgery for such cases [1, 3]. Only one third of patients go on to require surgery because of growth or the development of regional metastases, and therefore, histological details in the contralateral lobe or central neck are not known for the majority of cases.

There are no prospective studies that have examined the treatment of patients with angioinvasion in PTC. Professional groups such as the American Thyroid Association (ATA) and the British Thyroid Association (BTA) recognize that vascular invasion is an adverse risk feature in PTC, which, if present, increases the risk of recurrence of up to 30% [1]. Consequently, international guidelines recommend consideration of RAI, which requires total thyroidectomy, in such cases. Gross macroscopic angioinvasion, as observed in the operating theatre or on histology, is a significant adverse prognostic indicator and is generally rare in PTC. However, when present, there is an association with more advanced disease and adverse outcome [4], due to the increased propensity for regional or distant disease to occur.

Although there is an association between vascular invasion and adverse outcome [4], most patients who have vascular invasion also have additional disease features which place them at higher risk of recurrence already [5, 6]. Wreesman et al. found that the presence of angioinvasion alone, in the absence of additional high-risk features (e.g. tumour size >4 cm, extra-thyroidal extension, distant metastases, or age over 45 years), was not predictive of an increased risk of recurrence [7]. The extent of angioinvasion is also a factor that has been shown to impact the prognosis. Multiple studies have outlined that the number of identified sites of vascular invasion is correlated with outcome. Therefore, some experts recommend a cut-off of ≤4 foci as being clinically significant, accepting that a binary scale is suboptimal [8].

Although this subject is contentious, the evidence does suggest if findings of angioinvasion are seen at a microscopic level; moreover if there are four or less foci of invasion, then excellent outcomes are likely to be achieved, even without contralateral lobectomy and RAI [4]. This notion accepts that the probability of occult disease being present in the contralateral lobe and central neck compartment is high [1]. However, such putative disease may never become clinically evident [9].

Case Summary

Two justifiable options exist for this patient who has already undergone surgery: close clinical surveillance including periodic neck ultrasound *or* proceeding to completion thyroidectomy + RAI. It must be recognized that, in the absence of suspicious nodules on pre-operative ultrasound, completion thyroidectomy is performed with the sole purpose of facilitating RAI, as the contralateral lobe rarely harbours disease which alters clinical decision-making in small well-differentiated thyroid carcinomas (WDTC) (<4 cm) [10].

Ultimately, numerous factors from the case need to be considered before deciding on further treatment, and these can be broken down into (1) patient factors and (2) tumour-related factors. Clearly, if the patient had sustained a RLN palsy or permanent hypoparathyroidism after the initial operation, one would avoid further surgery. However, this was not the case here; indeed the procedure went without complication. Considering patient factors, as a music teacher, her lifestyle places demands on her voice, giving her more to lose in the event of surgical injury to the nerve and from side effects of adjuvant therapy (xerostomia, sialadenitis) [11]. She is also young, with low-risk disease, and therefore likely to do well regardless of further treatment as mortality risk in stage I well-differentiated thyroid cancer approaches 0%. However, the fact that her TSH level has increased on a background of Hashimoto's thyroiditis and her pre-operative TSH level suggests that she is likely to require lifelong thyroxine replacement following lobectomy, mitigating one of the adverse effects of completion surgery [12]. With regard to the tumour, the lesion is a small classic PTC with a reassuring pre-operative ultrasound. This would certainly be in favour of no further active treatment. However, if suspicious contralateral nodules were observed subsequently, then lobectomy and RAI could be advocated. If there is significant vascular invasion, patients should be considered to be at low-intermediate risk of recurrence. At this patient's age, her risk of clinical recurrence and disease-related mortality is extraordinarily low, and the ATA does not routinely recommend RAI [1]. Therefore, although further treatment with completion thyroidectomy and RAI therapy could be considered, active monitoring may be recommended instead [1].

In summary, whichever option is chosen for the patient, she is likely to have an excellent outcome as she is young and has a small-volume PTC, and there are no macroscopic regional or distant metastases or extra-thyroidal extension. Therefore, her risk of disease-related mortality, even without adjuvant treatment, is <1%. It is imperative that risks of treatment are minimized and that the patient is comfortable with the treatment strategy that is proposed. We must also consider that if the patient opts for a conservative approach, initially this decision can be changed during follow-up. In addition, the patient is of childbearing age and may wish to avoid RAI until after any planned pregnancy.

In this case, the patient and clinical team opted for thyroid lobectomy and surveillance. With a single focus of vascular invasion and a low-risk patient, both the patient and clinical team were happy with an approach that included annual clinical assessment, thyroid function testing, and ultrasound surveillance.

This case highlights the importance of individualized decision-making in patients with low-risk DTC (in this case a small PTC with vascular invasion). In such cases a balanced approach to management should address both patient- and tumour-related factors to achieve an outcome which optimizes both oncological and functional outcomes.

References

1. Haugen BR, Alexander BR, Bible KC, et al. 2015 American Thyroid Association management guidelines for adult patients with thyroid nodules and differentiated thyroid cancer: the American Thyroid Association guidelines task force on thyroid nodules and differentiated thyroid cancer. Thyroid. 2016;26(1):1–133.
2. Sanabria A, Kowalski LP, Shah JP, et al. Growing incidence of thyroid carcinoma in recent years: factors underlying overdiagnosis. Head Neck. 2018;40:855–66.
3. Ito Y, Miyauchi A, Oda H. Low-risk papillary microcarcinoma of the thyroid: a review of active surveillance trials. Eur J Surg Oncol. 2018;44(3):307–15.
4. Nixon IJ, Simo RS, Kim D. Refining definitions within low-risk differentiated thyroid cancers. Clin Otolaryngol. 2018;43:1195–200.
5. Gardner RE, Tuttle RM, Burman KD, et al. Prognostic importance of vascular invasion in papillary thyroid carcinoma. Arch Otolaryngol Head Neck Surg. 2000;126:309–12.
6. Nishida T, Katayama S, Tsujimoto M. The clinicopathological significance of histologic vascular invasion in differentiated thyroid carcinoma. Am J Surg. 2002;183:80–6.
7. Wreesman VB, Nixon IJ, Rivera M, et al. Prognostic value of vascular invasion in well-differentiated papillary thyroid carcinoma. Thyroid. 2015;25:503–8.
8. Xu B, Wang L, Tuttle RM, et al. Prognostic impact of extent of vascular invasion in low-grade encapsulated follicular cell-derived thyroid carcinomas: a clinicopathological study of 276 cases. Hum Pathol. 2015;46:1789–98.
9. Vaisman F, Momesso D, Bulzico DA, et al. Thyroid lobectomy is associated with excellent clinical outcomes in properly selected differentiated thyroid cancer patients with tumors greater than 1cm. J Thyroid Res. 2013;2013:398194.
10. Williamson AG, Wilmot V, Ntala C, et al. Differentiated thyroid cancer: a retrospective evaluation of the impact of changes to disease management guidelines on patients in south East Scotland. Surgeon. 2019;17(2):73–9.
11. Bhayani MK, Acharya V, Kongkiatkamon S, et al. Sialendoscopy for patient with radioiodine-induced sialadenitis and xerostomia. Thyroid. 2015;25(7):834–8.
12. Lee DY, Seok J, Jeong WJ, et al. Prediction of thyroid hormone supplementation after thyroid lobectomy. J Surg Res. 2015;193(1):273–8.

Chapter 8
A Patient with a Pathological Diagnosis of Noninvasive Follicular Thyroid Neoplasm with Papillary-Like Nuclear Features (NIFTP)

David Carruthers and Steven P. Hodak

Case Presentation

The patient is a 34-year-old woman who presented with an asymptomatic left-sided thyroid nodule. The nodule was first noted 2 years prior to presentation, and ultrasonography at that time showed a mixed hypoechoic solid and cystic nodule, with solid components measuring 13 × 10 × 8 mm. Fine-needle aspiration (FNA) demonstrated benign cytology.

On follow-up ultrasonography 2 years later, the solid component of the nodule had increased in size to 17 × 16 × 20 mm, and the entire nodule now measured 20 × 15 × 20 mm. The nodule remained mixed solid and cystic, hypoechoic, homogeneous with well-defined borders without microcalcifications or other high-risk features (Fig. 8.1). The TSH was 1.9 mU/L (0.4–4.0 mU/L). Cytology from a repeat FNA was Bethesda IV/suspicious for a follicular neoplasm, and reflex molecular diagnostic testing with Thyroseq (UPMC and CBL Pathology Inc.), a next-generation genomic classifier (GC), was performed. The GC result showed an NRAS p.Q61R mutation which is associated with a 70–80% probability of follicular-pattern cancer or noninvasive follicular thyroid neoplasm with papillary-like nuclear features (NIFTP). The patient underwent an uncomplicated left lobectomy, and final pathology confirmed a 2.1 cm noninvasive follicular thyroid neoplasm with papillary-like nuclear features (NIFTP) (Fig. 8.2).

D. Carruthers · S. P. Hodak (✉)
Department of Endocrinology, Diabetes, and Metabolism, New York University, New York, NY, USA
e-mail: steven.hodak@nyulangone.org

G. Grani et al. (eds.), *Thyroid Cancer*,
https://doi.org/10.1007/978-3-030-61919-0_8

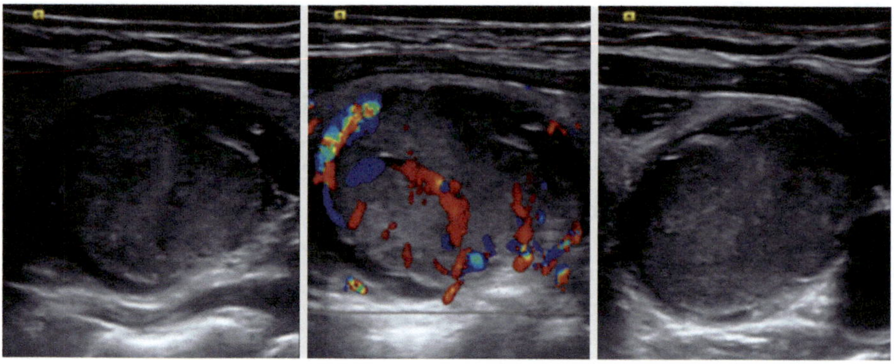

Fig. 8.1 Ultrasound of the left thyroid lobe nodule. Left to right: longitudinal, longitudinal with Doppler, transverse

Fig. 8.2 NIFTP gross specimen

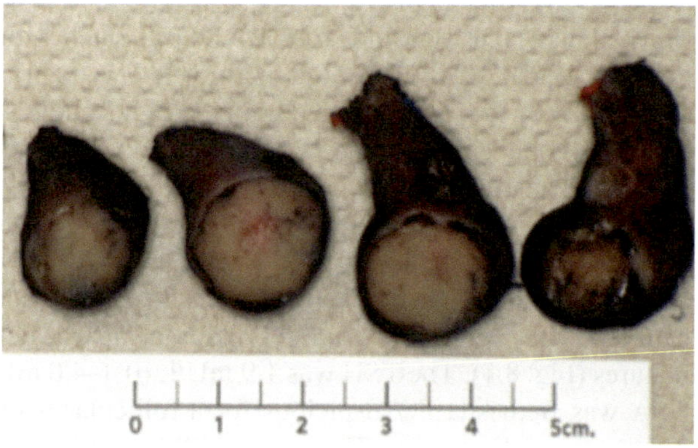

Literature Review

In 2012, the National Cancer Institute convened a conference to discuss a paradigm shift in how we view and categorize cancer. The conference leads to a publication calling for changes in terminology to better distinguish indolent and aggressive tumors, with the goal of reducing overdiagnosis and overtreatment of those lesions with low malignant potential [1]. Thyroid cancer was identified as a type of neoplasm that could be sufficiently indolent to justify revision of existing nomenclature to reflect exceedingly low malignant potential.

Epidemiologic data show that increased screening and more frequent imaging have led to a significant rise in thyroid cancer incidence with no change in mortality. This is primarily driven by detection of low-grade papillary thyroid cancers (PTC) [2–4]. This includes an increased prevalence of the follicular variant of papillary thyroid cancer (FVPTC) in the USA [5, 6].

FVPTC is defined as a tumor with neoplastic follicles, but with nuclear features of PTC. FVPTC is further subdivided based on the presence of capsular and vascular invasion as encapsulated noninvasive FVPTC (NIEFVPTC), encapsulated invasive FVPTC (EFVPTC), and infiltrative margins FVPTC (IFVPTC) [7, 8]. Altogether, FVPTC accounted for >20% of thyroid cancers in Europe and the USA, quadrupling in prevalence from 1974 to 2009 [6, 9], though prevalence varies by race [10]. Prior to 2016, many of these cancers were treated aggressively with total thyroidectomy and radioactive iodine (RAI) remnant ablation, but retrospective studies showed FVPTC's risk of metastasis and recurrence to be dependent on invasion. NIEFVPTC demonstrated very low malignant potential, with <1% local, regional, or distant metastases up to 10-year follow-up in >300 published cases, despite the majority of these patients being treated conservatively with lobectomy and without RAI, whereas capsular or vascular invasion was associated with an increased risk of recurrence and metastasis. On a molecular level, NIEFVPTC is found to have a high rate of RAS or RAS-like mutations, whereas IFVPTC is more likely to have BRAFV600E mutations [7, 11]. This distinction is important, as it shows the former to be more genetically similar to follicular thyroid cancer, while the latter BRAF-driven neoplasms are more similar to classical variant PTC.

Given the indolent behavior and favorable prognosis of the NIEFVPTC, in 2016 an international consensus group consisting of 24 experienced thyroid pathologists, 2 endocrinologists (including SPH), 1 surgeon, and 1 psychiatrist convened to discuss possible reclassification of NIEFVPTC and to consider removing the word "cancer" from its name. They reviewed 268 tumors diagnosed previously as encapsulated FVPTC and divided them into groups based on the presence or absence of invasion. Group 1 was composed of 138 cases of NIEFVPTC with 10-year follow-up. Group 2 contained 130 cases demonstrating vascular or capsular invasion with at least 1-year follow-up. At 10–16 years' follow-up, 100% of the patients in group 1 were alive with no evidence of recurrence. Group 2 had 1–18 years' follow-up, and 12% had a disease-specific adverse event including 2 % with locoregional recurrence or persistent disease, 5 % lung and/or bone metastases, and 5 % with indeterminate or biochemically incomplete response with detectable serum thyroglobulin.

Based on the favorable prognosis of NIEFVPTC, they renamed this clinical entity to emphasize its indolent clinical behavior, ultimately settling on noninvasive follicular thyroid neoplasm with papillary-like nuclear features (NIFTP). Additionally, they promulgated the inclusion and exclusion criteria for the diagnosis of NIFTP found in Table 8.1 [8]. These diagnostic criteria aim to exclude conventional PTC (true papillae <1% and psammoma bodies), invasive EFVPTC (invasion), poorly differentiated carcinoma (tumor necrosis and high mitotic activity), and other PTC variants (cellular/morphological characteristics of other PTC variants) [12]. In 2017, the American Thyroid Association (ATA) endorsed this nomenclature in an update statement to their 2015 guidelines [13]. The diagnostic category of NIFTP was subsequently codified by the World health Organization (WHO) in its 2017 update [14].

Table 8.1 Diagnostic Criteria for NIFTP

2016 NIFTP Diagnostic Criteria[a]	2018 NIFTP Diagnosis Revision[b]
1. The tumor is fully encapsulated with clear demarcation 2. Follicular growth pattern with *<1% papillae*[c] No psammoma bodies present <30% solid growth or other PTC variant morphological pattern 3. *Nuclear score 2–3 (papillary-like features present)*[c] 4. No vascular or capsular invasion with sufficient microscopic examination of the capsule 5. No tumor necrosis 6. No high mitotic activity (<3 mitoses per 10 high-power fields)	1. The tumor is fully encapsulated with clear demarcation 2. Follicular growth pattern with *No true papillae*[c] No psammoma bodies present <30% solid growth or other PTC variant morphological pattern 3. *Nuclear score 2–3 (papillary-like features present). Nuclear score of 3, rarely seen without true papillae. If nuclear score is 3, recommend full tumor analysis and molecular testing. BRAFV600E mutation would exclude NIFTP*[c] 4. No vascular or capsular invasion with sufficient microscopic examination of the capsule 5. No tumor necrosis 6. No high mitotic activity (<3 mitoses per 10 high-power fields)

[a]Criteria from 2016 Nikiforov et al. NIFTP *JAMA Oncology* publication [7]
[b]Refined NIFTP criteria from 2018 Kakudo et al. editorial [17]
[c]Refined NIFTP criteria proposed by the authors of the original 2016 diagnostic criteria. <1% papillae were accepted in the original diagnosis to account for poorly formed hyperplastic papillae, not true papillae which are seen in classical PTC [17]

Changing the nomenclature by removing the term "cancer" acknowledges the low risk of metastasis and was intended to remove associated cultural and psychological stigma and stress. It was also anticipated that this would decrease confusion among providers, patients, and families, who might otherwise opt for more aggressive and therapeutically unnecessary treatments such as completion thyroidectomy and use of radioactive iodine. It was anticipated that this would also reduce the risk of iatrogenic harm including recurrent laryngeal nerve injury, superior laryngeal nerve injury, hypoparathyroidism associated with completion thyroidectomy as well as the risks of secondary malignancy, and salivary gland and lacrimal duct injuries associated with RAI [15, 16]. Further, the change in nomenclature was also anticipated to decrease the known financial burden associated with completion thyroidectomy, RAI, and greater intensity of follow-up that the diagnosis of thyroid cancer typically conveys [17–19]. Whether or not the new NIFTP diagnosis will effectively reduce medical costs remains to be seen. It is most likely to impact populations where the prevalence of NIEFVPTC is significant and may be less significant in Asia where NIEFVPTC represents only 1.6% of all PTC vs. 13.3% in non-Asian series [20].

Since the introduction of the NIFTP diagnosis, most follow-up studies have confirmed the benignity of NIFTP even in tumors >4 cm [21–26]. However, there have also been reports of NIFTP with metastases [12, 22, 25, 27–31]. Valderrabano et al. reported two metastatic tumors classified as NIFTP. However, upon rereview, these tumors were found to have capsular or vascular invasion, which are definitive exclusion criteria for NIFTP diagnosis [12]. Rosario et al. reported a case of NIFTP with lymph node metastasis, but a conventional variant papillary microcarcinoma was also present in the surgical specimen [25]. Parente et al. found on retrospective review of 102 tumors reclassified as NIFTP that 5 (4.9%) had lymph node metastasis and 1 (1%) had distant metastasis [30].

Several publications from Korea report cases of NIFTP with BRAFV600E mutations on molecular analysis and lymph node metastases [22, 27–30]. Kim et al. reported lymph node metastasis in 9 of 74 (12%) cases of NIFTP, but 5 of these 9 cases were also noted to have concomitant conventional PTCs in the surgical specimen [28]. Lee et al reported five patients with NIFTP with BRAFV600E mutations, one of which had lymph node metastases [29]. Of these five cases, four were examined by a second pathologist who found one case had true papillae and another case showed capsular invasion, both of which are exclusion criteria for NIFTP diagnosis. The remaining two cases demonstrated no exclusion criteria, but the reviewer noted an insufficient number of tissue sections to adequately make an adequate assessment [12].

Lastly, Cho et al. reviewed 6269 PTCs, of which 152 cases without evidence of invasion met criteria for NIEFVPTC. They then divided the encapsulated follicular variant PTC by <1% papillae or 0% papillae as a cutoff. They found in the 1% papillae cutoff group that 3 of 105 (3%) had lymph node metastases, 1 of 105 (1%) had a distant metastasis, and 10 of 105 (10%) had BRAFV600E mutations. In the 0% papillae group, no BRAFV600E mutations were found, but central lymph node metastasis still occurred in 2 of 95 (3%) [27].

The original 2016 NIFTP criteria allowed for <1% papillary structures in order to allow for "few delicate, poorly formed, hyperplastic-type papillae" [12]. However, these guidelines had been interpreted to allow inclusion of true papillae, a feature typical of classical PTC. Due to this point of confusion, in 2018 the authors of the NIFTP working group proposed to addend the NIFTP definition, adding:

1. No true papillae are allowed for the diagnosis of NIFTP. The previous exclusion criteria "true papillae < 1%" should be replaced with "no true papillae."
2. Florid nuclear features of PTC [8] is not an exclusion criterion but is typically accompanied by true papillae. If such nuclear features are seen, examination of the entire tumor, not just the capsule, with optional, but recommended, analyses for BRAFV600E using either immunohistochemical methods or molecular techniques may be necessary (see Table 8.1) [12].

It is also essential when evaluating NIFTP tumors that they are adequately sectioned to fully evaluate the capsule and nuclei, as an incomplete evaluation of the tumor and capsule may allow invasive features to escape detection, leading to inappropriate diagnosis as NIFTP [12].

Lastly, it is important to reemphasize that NIFTP is a histologically follicular neoplasm typically driven by RAS or RAS-like mutations. Tumors harboring genetic alterations such as BRAFV600E, BRAFV600E-like mutations [32], RET/PTC rearrangements, or TERT mutations are very unlikely to be NIFTP, and in these cases, scrupulous examination of these tumors will likely demonstrate features that invalidate a NIFTP diagnosis.

Though the NIFTP diagnosis requires surgical excision and pathologic review, it has been demonstrated that the mRNA molecular profiling of NIFTP tumors may promise the possibility to further risk stratify these tumors. This is based on the observation that the mRNA profile of follicular adenomas and IFVPTC are distinct, whereas NIFTP mRNA profiles can either be follicular adenoma-like or IFVPTC-like, suggesting that it may be possible to identify a subset of NIFTP tumors at high risk for progression to IFVPTC. Whether such mRNA profiling could further inform the intensity of postsurgical follow-up or perhaps even identify tumors amenable to observational management without surgery will require further investigation [33].

There are no long-term prospective studies or consensus guidelines regarding outcomes and appropriate follow-up of patients with a NIFTP diagnosis. However, a NIFTP is by definition a noninvasive transitional lesion. Any evidence of invasion on final pathology excludes the NIFTP diagnosis. Therefore, surgical excision is curative, and these patients should be followed in very much the same manner as a patient who has undergone revision of a benign follicular adenoma. However, this recommendation must depend on confidence that the NIFTP diagnosis has been correctly made.

Our approach to management of patients with NIFTP tumors is as follows:

- Patients with small, typical NIFTP tumors (we arbitrarily define "small" as <2 cm) that have been correctly classified using the most stringent criteria by an experienced pathologist may be considered surgically cured. These patients may be discharged from further specific specialty care.
- For NIFTP tumors 2–4 cm in size, we recommend confirming with the reading pathologist that both the entire capsule and parenchyma of the tumor have been adequately sectioned to ensure the NIFTP diagnosis is correctly made. In these cases we also consider these patients to be surgically cured, and they may be discharged from further specific specialty care as well.
- Though not definitively proven, we believe that certain features increase the risk that a NIFTP diagnosis may be made incorrectly. We therefore recommend heightened surveillance if any of the following are present:
  - Large NIFTP tumors (arbitrarily defined as >4 cm)
  - Presence of florid nuclear features
  - Presence of a high-grade oncogenic driver gene alterations such as BRAF*V660E* or BRAF*V600E*-like genetic profiles [32]
  - Inability to confirm that the diagnosis of NIFTP was made based on stringent criteria

  In these cases, we recommend establishing a baseline thyroglobulin level and postoperative neck ultrasound examination 6–12 months after surgery. Subsequently, we recommend assessment with annual thyroglobulin screening indefinitely, as well as follow-up neck ultrasound examination every 2–3 years for the next 5 years and then every 3–5 years thereafter as long as there are no new clinical concerns.
- Postsurgical hypothyroidism should always be treated as needed to a clinically appropriate goal TSH, which we define as lower to mid-normal range.

Back to the Patient

Following uncomplicated left lobectomy, final pathology confirmed a 2.1 × 1.8 × 1.6 cm NIFTP (Figs. 8.2 and 8.3). Postoperatively she was discharged from the endocrine surgery clinic and returned to her community endocrine practice. Her TSH remained normal at 2 years' follow-up without the use of thyroid hormone replacement.

Clinical Pearls/Pitfalls

- NIFTP is a diagnosis made after complete resection of the tumor with lobectomy.
- Following definitive resection, NIFTP has a favorable prognosis even without completion thyroidectomy and RAI, with <1% tumor recurrence or metastasis, even in tumors >4 cm in size.
- NIFTP tumors often are low suspicion nodules on ultrasonography and indeterminate cytology on fine-needle aspiration.
- There are strict inclusion and exclusion criteria for diagnosing NIFTP. Adequate tumor sections must be taken to fully evaluate the tumor and capsule to ensure they meet NIFTP criteria.
- NIFTP may not contain any true papillae. Fewer than 1% few delicate, poorly formed, hyperplastic-type papillae are allowed.
- On molecular analysis, NIFTP commonly have RAS and RAS-like mutations. Tumors with BRAFV600E or BRAFV600E-like mutations, RET/PTC rearrangements, should be excluded for NIFTP diagnosis.

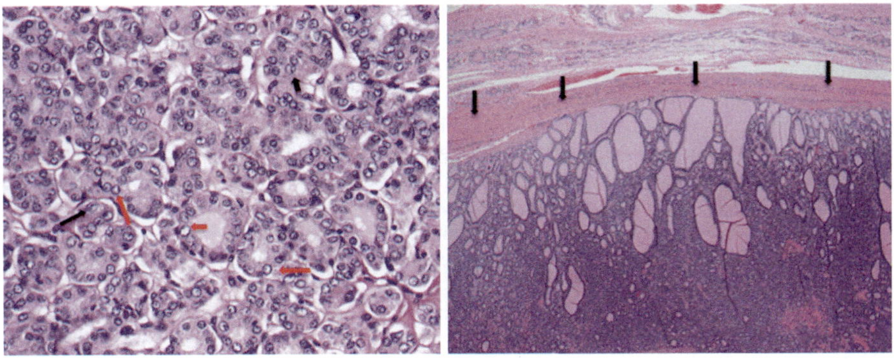

Fig. 8.3 Left: NIFTP at amplification x40 with characteristic nuclear enlargement, nuclear grooves (black arrows), and chromatin clearing (red arrows). Right: NIFTP at amplification ×4 showing a portion of the intact tumor capsule (black arrows)

References

1. Esserman LJ, Thompson IM, Reid B, Nelson P, Ransohoff DF, Welch HG, et al. Addressing overdiagnosis and overtreatment in cancer: a prescription for change. Lancet Oncol. 2014;15(6):e234–42.
2. Ahn HS, Kim HJ, Welch HG. Korea's thyroid-cancer "epidemic"--screening and overdiagnosis. N Engl J Med. 2014;371(19):1765–7.
3. Davies L, Welch HG. Increasing incidence of thyroid cancer in the United States, 1973–2002. JAMA. 2006;295(18):2164–7.
4. Morris LG, Sikora AG, Tosteson TD, Davies L. The increasing incidence of thyroid cancer: the influence of access to care. Thyroid. 2013;23(7):885–91.
5. Albores-Saavedra J, Henson DE, Glazer E, Schwartz AM. Changing patterns in the incidence and survival of thyroid cancer with follicular phenotype--papillary, follicular, and anaplastic: a morphological and epidemiological study. Endocr Pathol. 2007;18(1):1–7.
6. Jung CK, Little MP, Lubin JH, Brenner AV, Wells SA Jr, Sigurdson AJ, et al. The increase in thyroid cancer incidence during the last four decades is accompanied by a high frequency of BRAF mutations and a sharp increase in RAS mutations. J Clin Endocrinol Metab. 2014;99(2):E276–85.
7. Liu J, Singh B, Tallini G, Carlson DL, Katabi N, Shaha A, et al. Follicular variant of papillary thyroid carcinoma: a clinicopathologic study of a problematic entity. Cancer. 2006;107(6):1255–64.
8. Nikiforov YE, Seethala RR, Tallini G, Baloch ZW, Basolo F, Thompson LD, et al. Nomenclature revision for encapsulated follicular variant of papillary thyroid carcinoma: a paradigm shift to reduce overtreatment of indolent tumors. JAMA Oncol. 2016;2(8):1023–9.
9. Lupi C, Giannini R, Ugolini C, Proietti A, Berti P, Minuto M, et al. Association of BRAF V600E mutation with poor clinicopathological outcomes in 500 consecutive cases of papillary thyroid carcinoma. J Clin Endocrinol Metab. 2007;92(11):4085–90.
10. Mehta V, Ow TJ, Kim S, Tharakan T, Schiff B, Smith RV, et al. Significant racial differences in the incidence and behavior of the follicular variant of papillary thyroid carcinoma. Head Neck. 2019;41(5):1403–11.
11. Rivera M, Ricarte-Filho J, Knauf J, Shaha A, Tuttle M, Fagin JA, et al. Molecular genotyping of papillary thyroid carcinoma follicular variant according to its histological subtypes (encapsulated vs infiltrative) reveals distinct BRAF and RAS mutation patterns. Mod Pathol. 2010;23(9):1191–200.
12. Kakudo K, El-Naggar AK, Hodak SP, Khanafshar E, Nikiforov YE, Nose V, et al. Noninvasive follicular thyroid neoplasm with papillary-like nuclear features (NIFTP) in thyroid tumor classification. Pathol Int. 2018;68(6):327–33.
13. Haugen BR, Sawka AM, Alexander EK, Bible KC, Caturegli P, Doherty GM, et al. American Thyroid Association guidelines on the management of thyroid nodules and differentiated thyroid cancer task force review and recommendation on the proposed renaming of encapsulated follicular variant papillary thyroid carcinoma without invasion to noninvasive follicular thyroid neoplasm with papillary-like nuclear features. Thyroid. 2017;27(4):481–3.
14. Lloyd RV, Osamura R, Kloppel G, Rosai J (editors). WHO classification of tumours of endocrine organs. 4th ed: Lyon, IARC; 2017.
15. Hauch A, Al-Qurayshi Z, Randolph G, Kandil E. Total thyroidectomy is associated with increased risk of complications for low- and high-volume surgeons. Ann Surg Oncol. 2014;21(12):3844–52.
16. Iyer NG, Morris LG, Tuttle RM, Shaha AR, Ganly I. Rising incidence of second cancers in patients with low-risk (T1N0) thyroid cancer who receive radioactive iodine therapy. Cancer. 2011;117(19):4439–46.
17. Hodak S, Tuttle RM, Maytal G, Nikiforov YE, Randolph G. Changing the cancer diagnosis: the case of follicular variant of papillary thyroid cancer-Primum non nocere and NIFTP. Thyroid. 2016;26(7):869–71.

18. Ramsey S, Blough D, Kirchhoff A, Kreizenbeck K, Fedorenko C, Snell K, et al. Washington State cancer patients found to be at greater risk for bankruptcy than people without a cancer diagnosis. Health Aff. 2013;32(6):1143–52.
19. Agrawal N, Abbott CE, Liu C, Kang S, Tipton L, Patel K, et al. Noninvasive follicular tumor with papillary-like nuclear features: not a tempest in a teapot. Endocr Pract. 2017;23(4):451–7.
20. Bychkov A, Jung CK, Liu Z, Kakudo K. Noninvasive follicular thyroid neoplasm with papillary-like nuclear features in Asian practice: perspectives for surgical pathology and cytopathology. Endocr Pathol. 2018;29(3):276–88.
21. Faquin WC, Wong LQ, Afrogheh AH, Ali SZ, Bishop JA, Bongiovanni M, et al. Impact of reclassifying noninvasive follicular variant of papillary thyroid carcinoma on the risk of malignancy in The Bethesda System for Reporting Thyroid Cytopathology. Cancer Cytopathol. 2016;124(3):181–7.
22. Hahn SY, Shin JH, Lim HK, Jung SL, Oh YL, Choi IH, et al. Preoperative differentiation between noninvasive follicular thyroid neoplasm with papillary-like nuclear features (NIFTP) and non-NIFTP. Clin Endocrinol (Oxf). 2017;86(3):444–50.
23. Ibrahim AA, Wu HH. Fine-needle aspiration cytology of noninvasive follicular variant of papillary thyroid carcinoma is cytomorphologically distinct from the invasive counterpart. Am J Clin Pathol. 2016;146(3):373–7.
24. Maletta F, Massa F, Torregrossa L, Duregon E, Casadei GP, Basolo F, et al. Cytological features of "noninvasive follicular thyroid neoplasm with papillary-like nuclear features" and their correlation with tumor histology. Hum Pathol. 2016;54:134–42.
25. Rosario PW, Mourao GF, Nunes MB, Nunes MS, Calsolari MR. Noninvasive follicular thyroid neoplasm with papillary-like nuclear features. Endocr Relat Cancer. 2016;23(12):893–7.
26. Yang GCH, Fried KO, Scognamiglio T. Sonographic and cytologic differences of NIFTP from infiltrative or invasive encapsulated follicular variant of papillary thyroid carcinoma: a review of 179 cases. Diagn Cytopathol. 2017;45(6):533–41.
27. Cho U, Mete O, Kim MH, Bae JS, Jung CK. Molecular correlates and rate of lymph node metastasis of non-invasive follicular thyroid neoplasm with papillary-like nuclear features and invasive follicular variant papillary thyroid carcinoma: the impact of rigid criteria to distinguish non-invasive follicular thyroid neoplasm with papillary-like nuclear features. Mod Pathol. 2017;30(6):810–25.
28. Kim TH, Lee M, Kwon AY, Choe JH, Kim JH, Kim JS, et al. Molecular genotyping of the non-invasive encapsulated follicular variant of papillary thyroid carcinoma. Histopathology. 2018;72(4):648–61.
29. Lee SE, Hwang TS, Choi YL, Kim WY, Han HS, Lim SD, et al. Molecular profiling of papillary thyroid carcinoma in Korea with a high prevalence of BRAF(V600E) mutation. Thyroid. 2017;27(6):802–10.
30. Parente DN, Kluijfhout WP, Bongers PJ, Verzijl R, Devon KM, Rotstein LE, et al. Clinical safety of renaming encapsulated follicular variant of papillary thyroid carcinoma: is NIFTP truly benign? World J Surg. 2018;42(2):321–6.
31. Xu B, Tallini G, Scognamiglio T, Roman BR, Tuttle RM, Ghossein RA. Outcome of large noninvasive follicular thyroid neoplasm with papillary-like nuclear features. Thyroid. 2017;27(4):512–7.
32. Cancer Genome Atlas Research Network. Integrated genomic characterization of papillary thyroid carcinoma. Cell. 2014;159(3):676–90.
33. Giannini R, Ugolini C, Poma AM, Urpi M, Niccoli C, Elisei R, et al. Identification of two distinct molecular subtypes of non-invasive follicular neoplasm with papillary-like nuclear features by digital RNA counting. Thyroid. 2017;27(10):1267–76.

Chapter 9
Papillary Thyroid Cancer with Central Neck Lymph Node Metastases

Alyse S. Goldberg, Lorne E. Rotstein, and Anna M. Sawka

Abbreviations

PMC Papillary microcarcinoma
RAI Radioactive iodine
TSH Thyroid-stimulating hormone concentration

Case Presentation

A previously healthy 30-year-old female was seen by her family physician for a general medical exam. As part of this evaluation, she underwent measurement of thyroid-stimulating hormone (TSH) concentration and a neck ultrasound. It was not clear why the ultrasound was ordered, as the patient was not aware of any abnormality in her thyroid exam. The patient had no compressive symptoms (i.e., no hoarseness, dysphagia, nor dyspnea). There was no family history of thyroid cancer nor thyroid disorders. The patient had no significant history of head and neck radiation exposure.

A. S. Goldberg
Division of Endocrinology, Department of Medicine, Sunnybrook Health Sciences Centre, Toronto, Ontario, Canada
e-mail: agoldberg@utoronto.ca

L. E. Rotstein
Department of Surgery, University Health Network and University of Toronto, Toronto, Ontario, Canada
e-mail: Lorne.Rotstein@uhn.ca

A. M. Sawka (✉)
Division of Endocrinology, University Health Network and University of Toronto, Toronto, Ontario, Canada
e-mail: Annie.Sawka@uhn.ca

G. Grani et al. (eds.), *Thyroid Cancer*,
https://doi.org/10.1007/978-3-030-61919-0_9

Diagnosis/Assessment

For the case presented, the baseline TSH level was normal (2.49 mU/L), and a neck ultrasound showed a left-sided solid, 1.0 cm hypoechoic thyroid nodule with smooth margins and no microcalcifications; there were no other thyroid nodules and no enlarged/suspicious lymph nodes. Ultrasound-guided fine-needle aspiration biopsy of the thyroid nodule was positive for papillary thyroid cancer. She underwent total thyroidectomy, and the intraoperative detection of an enlarged paratracheal lymph node prompted therapeutic left pretracheal and left paratracheal nodal dissection as part of the same procedure. The final surgical pathology showed multifocal micropapillary thyroid cancer (PMC, follicular variant), with two foci, measuring in maximal diameter 0.9 cm (in the left lobe) and 0.2 cm (in the right lobe), respectively. There was no extrathyroidal extension of the primary tumor, with no lymphatic, vascular, nor capsular invasion. The resection margins were clear. There was evidence of chronic lymphocytic thyroiditis. Upon examination of the eight resected central neck lymph nodes, two of them were positive for PTC, the foci measuring 8 mm and 3 mm, respectively, in maximal diameter, without extranodal extension.

The clinicopathologic stage of disease in this case was interpreted as follows:

- T1aN1aMx (Stage I) per the AJCC/TNM VIII system [1, 2]
- Low risk (for thyroid cancer-related mortality) by the MACIS system (score 3.37) [3]
- American Thyroid Association (ATA) intermediate risk of recurrence using the 2009 classification system [4]

Postoperatively, the patient started taking levothyroxine and recovered uneventfully, with normal calcium and parathyroid hormone levels, and had no problems with her voice. Approximately 11 weeks following surgery, while on levothyroxine therapy (TSH 7.24 mU/L with a normal free thyroxine concentration), the thyroglobulin was <0.9 ng/ml, but thyroglobulin antibodies were present at a level of 97 IU/L (thyroglobulin antibody reference range <39 IU/L and the assay detection limit 20 IU/L). Given the presence of thyroglobulin antibodies, the thyroglobulin measurement was considered unreliable, due to potential assay interference [5]. A postoperative ultrasound of the neck 12 weeks after surgery was negative. Her levothyroxine dose was increased, with the intention of suppressing the TSH concentration (<0.1 mU/L). The patient's endocrinologist recommended radioactive iodine (RAI) adjuvant treatment, suggesting that this may reduce disease recurrence and facilitate disease follow-up (with thyroglobulin measurements and radioactive iodine scans). However, the patient did not want to take RAI, unless there was proof that it could reduce her risk of dying from thyroid cancer or distant metastatic recurrence. She strongly disliked the idea of taking any form of "radiation," unless it was clear that it could prevent death or distant metastases (which were her primary concerns). She was then referred an endocrinologist at a tertiary care center for further counseling.

Literature Review

Classification of Lymph Node Disease

Randolph et al. of the American Thyroid Association's Surgical Affairs Committee have reviewed the literature on prognostic significance of nodal metastases of papillary thyroid carcinoma and have proposed a categorization system for nodal disease [6]. Pathologic N1 (pN1) is any metastatic papillary thyroid cancer detected on the pathologic specimen of any resected lymph nodes [6]. Clinically apparent nodal disease, referred to as clinical N1 (cN1), is defined as metastatic lymph nodes identified on either physical examination, diagnostic imaging studies, or intraoperative inspection by the surgeon, and the absence of such features is clinical N0 (cN0) [6]. The presence of one or more metastatic lymph nodes that are visible on preoperative physical examination, ultrasound, or during surgery (the latter according to surgical and pathologic reports) has been independently associated with increased risk of recurrence of disease in a multivariable analysis, including data from 545 patients [7]. However, in the central neck, the accuracy of intraoperative surgical inspection is only about 60% [8], with larger affected nodes being more readily clinically detected [9]. Moreover, the significance of subclinical, low-volume nodal disease in the central neck is not clear.

Regardless of how cN1 disease is detected, resection of such affected nodes and relevant nodal compartments is termed "therapeutic neck dissection" [6]. In contrast, "prophylactic neck dissection" is defined as nodal dissection in the absence of any evidence of cN1 disease prior to the procedure [6]. Randolph et al. divided nodal disease into two categories: lower-risk N1 disease and higher-risk N1 disease [6]. Lower-risk N1 disease has been defined by the presence of the following criteria: (a) clinical N0; (b) low-volume nodal disease, specifically micrometastatic nodes (i.e., largest focus of thyroid cancer in the node <0.2 cm in diameter) or small nodal metastases (0.2 to <1.0 cm in diameter); and (c) ≤5 small lymph node metastases (i.e., each measuring <1.0 cm in diameter) [6]. Higher-risk N1 disease has been defined by the presence of the following criteria: (a) clinically detectable lymph node metastases (cN1), (b) metastatic lymph node(s) >3 cm, and (c) >5 metastatic lymph nodes [6]. Randolph et al. have also reported that gross extranodal extension, increasing number of metastatic lymph nodes with microscopic extranodal extension, or the combination of microscopic extranodal extension and metastatic lymph nodes >1 cm is also predictive of a higher risk of disease recurrence [6]. The location of nodal disease has been reported to be associated with the size of involved nodes in papillary thyroid cancer, particularly for bulky enlarged nodes. For example, Chow et al. reported that 13% of N1a and 56% of N1b papillary thyroid cancer patients had involved nodes >2 cm in diameter ($p < 0.001$) [10]. Ito et al. suggested that for papillary thyroid cancer patients whose nodal disease is detected on preoperative imaging, the cause-specific survival of patients with N1b level nodal involvement is not significantly different from that of those with N1a nodal involvement [11]. However, in this study [11], the disease-free survival was adversely affected in papillary thyroid cancer patients with N1b level nodal involvement who had pathologic evidence of aggressive nodal disease, including the lymph nodes measuring >3 cm in diameter, extranodal extension, or ≥5 or more involved nodes [11]. Furthermore, the presence of two or more such adverse features in N1b disease was associated with reduced cause-specific survival [11]. Age also appears to be an important prognostic variable in N1 disease. For example, Verburg et al. reported that in differentiated thyroid cancer, patients aged ≥45 years who have lateral neck lymph node metastases have a reduced long-term life expectancy, but life expectancy is not significantly impacted in younger patients with similar disease features [12]. Furthermore, Hughes et al. have reported that in differentiated thyroid cancer patients with N1 disease, the recurrence rate was 8% in those <45 years of age, as compared with 31% in those ≥45 years of age [13]. In this study, all disease recurrences were successfully treated in the N1 patients aged <45 years, but only about a third of those aged ≥45 years of age [13]. In conclusion, the size and number, location of metastatic lymph nodes, the presence of extranodal extension, and patient age are relevant considerations in risk stratification of N1 disease.

Epidemiology of N1 Disease in Patients with PMC

Lymph node metastases are evident at the time of diagnosis in approximately 12–64% of cases of PMC [14–26]. If nodal metastases are present in this situation, the ipsilateral paratracheal compartments, followed by the pretracheal compartments, are the levels most frequently affected [20]. Lateral neck nodal metastases may be present in about 3–7% of individuals with PMC [15, 20, 24, 27, 28]. The presence of primary tumor extrathyroidal extension [14, 19, 29] and tumor multifocality [19, 29, 30] are risk factors for the presence of lymph node metastases with PMC. In summary, N1 disease is not uncommon in patients with PMC, and if it is present, it is most frequent in the central neck.

Prognosis of N1 Disease in Patients with PMC

The overall risk of disease recurrence or persistence in patients with papillary thyroid microcarcinoma and positive lymph nodes (without distant metastases at presentation) has been reported to range between 3.0% and 22% [15–17, 19]. The risk of dying of thyroid cancer and developing distant metastatic recurrence in this context are important considerations. In a recent retrospective review of PMCs, Mercante et al. reported that in a subgroup of 27 patients with T1aN1a disease, none of the patients died of disease nor developed distant metastases (follow-up about 8 years) [19]. Similarly, Kim et al. found that in a subgroup of 168 individuals with

PMC with no evidence of macroscopic extrathyroidal extension nor distant metastases at initial presentation, no patient died of thyroid cancer nor developed distant metastatic disease (mean follow-up about 5 years) [15]. In a retrospective review of PMC cases from a hospital in Hong Kong, Chow et al. [22] reported that in a subgroup of 48 patients with PMC and various degrees of severity of lymph node disease without distant metastases, 2% died due to thyroid cancer (1/50) and 4.0% (two patients) developed distant metastatic recurrence (mean follow-up about 8 years) [22]. In a retrospective chart review of patients with differentiated thyroid carcinoma ≤1 cm in diameter treated in the years 1962–1995 in France, Baudin et al. reported that in node-positive PMC patients without distant metastases at primary presentation, none of the patients died from thyroid cancer (0/113) and only 1% developed distant metastatic recurrence (1/113) (mean follow-up of about 7 years) [21]. Also, in a retrospective review of PMC cases at the Mayo Clinic, Hay et al. studied that the outcomes of a subgroup of 273 patients had positive lymph nodes at diagnosis [17]. Hay et al. indicated that no female with initial disease confined to the neck ultimately died of disease or developed distant metastases, but one male with extensive bulky lateral neck disease at presentation developed bone metastases and died of the disease, approximately 30 years after presentation (mean study follow-up 17 years) [17]. In summary, in papillary thyroid microcarcinoma patients with limited nodal involvement, no evidence of other adverse disease features, and no distant metastatic disease at the time of presentation, the risk of dying of thyroid cancer is likely about 0–2%, and the risk of developing distant metastatic recurrence is likely about 0–4%.

In patients with papillary thyroid microcarcinoma and lymph node metastases (T1aN1), the risk of local-regional recurrence of disease in the neck or lymph nodes is another relevant consideration. The risk of local-regional recurrence in T1aN1 PMC has been reported to range from 3% to 16% [15, 17, 21]. Furthermore, the incidence rate of local-regional recurrence has been subdivided according to the level of nodal involvement at the time of initial diagnosis as follows, in two of the more recent studies: N1a (central neck) 0–3% and N1b (lateral neck or mediastinum) 2–11% (excluding individuals with extrathyroidal extension of the primary tumor at initial diagnosis) [15, 19]. Based on these limited data, it appears that nodal recurrence of disease is relatively uncommon in patients with PMC whose initial nodal disease is confined to the central neck, in the absence of other adverse disease characteristics.

Does RAI Adjuvant Treatment Reduce the Risk of Disease Recurrence in T1aN1 Disease?

There are limited data from observational studies examining whether radioactive adjuvant treatment reduces the risk of recurrence after total thyroidectomy in patients with node-positive PMC. Hay et al. reported that of 253 node-positive patients with PMC, RAI adjuvant treatment did not significantly reduce local recurrence in the neck ($p = 0.81$) nor distant metastatic recurrence ($p = 0.68$) [17]. Ross et al. of the National Thyroid Cancer Treatment Cooperative Study Group also reported that in a subgroup analysis of 135 node-positive patients with PMC who were followed prospectively, RAI treatment did not significantly improve recurrence-free survival in node-positive patients (17% without RAI, 11% with RAI, $p > 0.05$) [16]. Kim et al. reported that in a subgroup of 168 PMC patients who either had nodal disease, microscopic extrathyroidal extension of the primary tumor, or multifocality, RAI treatment did not significantly improve recurrence-free survival ($p = 0.52$) [15]. Chow et al. reported that in 50 PMC patients with N1 disease, the administration of RAI did not significantly impact the risk of lymph node recurrence (nodal relapse rate 12.2% (5/41) in the RAI-treated patients and 22.2% (2/9) in those who did not receive RAI, $p = 0.6$) [22]. Creach et al. published a retrospective study of PMC patients, which included a subgroup analysis of 153 individuals with N1 disease [26]. In this study, the 5-year recurrence-free survival rate was significantly higher in node-positive PMC patients treated with RAI (93.2%) compared to those not treated with RAI (42.9%) ($p < 0.0001$) [26]. An important limitation of the latter study is that not all of the patients had total thyroidectomy, so it is not clear if the surgical extent was the same in both groups [26]. Hu et al. performed a systematic review of the published observational literature, comparing patients with papillary microcarcinoma post-total or near-total thyroidectomy who were treated with radioactive iodine to those who were not, after statistical adjustment for other prognostic factors (including presence of nodal metastases) [31]. Hu et al. reported no significant RAI treatment benefit in papillary microcarcinoma patients in meta-analyses of the following 10-year outcomes: any tumor recurrence, locoregional disease recurrence, distant metastatic recurrence, or thyroid cancer-specific mortality [31]. Important limitations of these data include the retrospective nature of included studies and a lack of risk stratification for degree of nodal involvement [31]. Randomized controlled trials are clearly needed to better define the role of RAI adjuvant treatment in node-positive PMC patients, with attention to risk stratification of nodal disease.

Management Considerations and Outcomes

Our patient presented with PMC, with no preoperative evidence of nodal metastases, but with intraoperative palpation of a suspicious paratracheal lymph node. This prompted ipsilateral para- and pretracheal lymph node dissection, yielding two small metastatic lymph nodes (maximal diameter 8 mm) out of eight nodes that were removed. The finding of the largest node being palpable intraoperatively in this case would technically upstage the disease to the "higher-risk" nodal disease category as defined by Randolph et al. [6], but the relatively small size and number of involved nodes and negative pre- and postoperative imaging would be more suggestive of a lower-risk nodal disease. The inherent limitations of accuracy of intraoperative detection of nodal disease in the central neck [7, 8], and the lack of data on independent prognostic significance of this finding, are important considerations. The risk stratification of this case was largely based on the number, size, and levels of involved lymph nodes, in the context of the patient's young age, the absence of an adverse histologic subtype, the lack of extrathyroidal extension or vascular invasion of the primary tumor, and negative postoperative ultrasound imaging of the neck. Diagnostic I-123 scanning was not available at the treating institution, and I-131 pretherapy scans were generally not employed in the treating institution. However, there are some data suggesting that such imaging may be helpful in evaluating disease status and other relevant variables, in patients being considered for RAI remnant ablation or treatment [32, 33]. The addition of single-photon emission computed tomography–computed tomography (SPECT-CT) to iodine radioisotope planar imaging may provide additional information, clarifying the structural correlates of areas of increased uptake [34]. If an interfering thyroglobulin antibody were not present, measurement of serum thyroglobulin, either stimulated (by recombinant human thyrotropin or thyroid hormone withdrawal) thyroglobulin could be helpful [35]. Ibrahimpasic et al. have also suggested that an unstimulated thyroglobulin <1 ng/ml in select low- and intermediate-risk papillary thyroid cancer after total thyroidectomy is a positive prognostic factor and have questioned the benefit of radioactive iodine treatment in this context based on retrospectively collected data from the Memorial Sloan Kettering Cancer Center [36]. The potential strengths and limitations of various postsurgical diagnostic test options for patients being considered for RAI remnant ablation or therapy are weighed in the most recent ATA guidelines on the management of thyroid nodules and differentiated thyroid cancer in adults [37].

The patient was counseled on disease prognosis, risks, benefits, and evidence uncertainties relating to RAI treatment in the context of her disease stage. Follow-up implications, including the limitation of biochemical follow-up in the presence of thyroglobulin antibodies, were also explained. The patient ultimately declined RAI treatment, reiterating her general opposition to "radiation" and indicating that the available evidence was not sufficiently convincing, in terms of reducing the risk of dying of thyroid cancer or developing distant metastatic disease in her situation. She was less concerned about the potential for local-regional recurrence and understood the possibility of needing additional surgery in the event of a recurrence. The patient agreed to close surveillance by ultrasound imaging of the neck and measurement of thyroglobulin and thyroglobulin antibody levels, with the intention of accepting additional treatment in the event of disease recurrence. She also accepted initial thyroid hormone suppressive treatment, with the intention of suppressing TSH to levels <0.1 mIU/L. In subsequent years, given the absence of structural recurrence of disease, despite of a borderline detectable thyroglobulin antibody, the goal TSH was modified to 0.1–0.5 mIU/L, in keeping with concurrent clinical practice guideline recommendations [37]. Serial neck ultrasounds have been completely negative for disease.

The thyroglobulin antibody positivity at the time of diagnosis was consistent with the pathologic evidence of Hashimoto's thyroiditis. The baseline thyroglobulin antibody titer (97 IU/L) decreased by 67% within 10 months following surgery and continued to slowly decrease to undetectable or borderline detectable levels over the next 10 years (i.e. 21 IU/L with a detection limit of 20 IU/L approximately 10 years after thyroidectomy). The serum thyroglobulin measurements remained undetectable over the next 10 years, using a high-sensitivity thyroglobulin assay in most recent years (i.e., level < 0.1 ng/dl). The patient was maintained on mild thyroid hormone suppressive therapy, keeping the TSH 0.1–0.5 mIU/L with normal free thyroxine levels in most recent years (TSH 0.42 mIU/L at last measurement). The continuing presence of thyroglobulin antibody has been reported to be associated with the presence of residual disease [38, 39]. However, a decrease in thyroglobulin antibody titers of ≥50% in the first postoperative year after total thyroidectomy is associated with a risk of disease recurrence or persistence of 0–2% [38, 39]. Furthermore, Tsushima et al. reported that in a multivariable model adjusted for other relevant prognostic factors, a thyroglobulin antibody reduction of <50% from baseline or rise in this measurement over 1–2 years following thyroidectomy was independently associated with significantly increased risk of recurrence in lymph nodes [40].

Spencer and Fatemi have proposed a classification system for thyroglobulin antibody trends during long-term follow-up of papillary thyroid cancer, including the following categories: (a) falling thyroglobulin antibody trend (>50% reduction from initial value, associated with <3% risk of recurrence), (b) stable but significantly elevated thyroglobulin antibody (<50% change from initial value, approximately 20% risk of disease recurrence), and (c) rising thyroglobulin antibody trend (progressive, sustained rise in thyroglobulin antibody of >50% from initial value, approximately 40% risk of disease recurrence) [41]. It is important to note that the time to disappearance of thyroglobulin antibodies after total thyroidectomy may be increased in the presence of higher baseline levels of thyroglobulin antibodies and a higher degree of lymphocytic infiltration noted at thyroidectomy specimen [42]. Our patient continues to be followed, but as of 10 years after her thyroidectomy (with no radioactive iodine treatment), she has had no evidence of structural disease on ultrasound imaging, and her thyroglobulin antibodies are consistently either undetectable or within the coefficient of variability of the border of the detection limit of our assay (detection limit 20 mIU/L); there has been no change in her undetectable thyroglobulin levels, even with the availability of a more sensitive assay in recent years. In follow-up visits, she asserts that she is satisfied and she made the right choice for her, relating to not taking RAI, and she is highly compliant with close surveillance and TSH suppressive therapy (with a current goal TSH of 0.1–0.5 mIU/L).

Clinical Pearls/Pitfalls

- The risk of recurrence of patients with papillary thyroid carcinoma who have nodal metastases is dependent on factors such as the size, number, and presence or absence of extranodal extension of involved nodes and patient age, in addition to consideration of other disease features.
- Lymph node metastases are not uncommon in patients with PMC.
- The risk of disease recurrence or persistence in node-positive patients with papillary thyroid microcarcinoma is variable; however, some of the lowest recurrence rates in this group appear to be in patients with relatively low-volume nodal disease confined to the central neck, in the absence of other adverse prognostic features or clinically detectable disease preoperatively.
- There is important uncertainty as to whether adjuvant RAI treatment significantly impacts the risk of disease recurrence in node-positive PMC patients, particularly for lower-risk (low-volume central neck) nodal disease. The existing evidence base on this topic is largely based on reports from retrospective studies where the extent of nodal involvement or other important confounders were not accounted for in the analysis. Results of ongoing randomized controlled trials of radioactive iodine treatment in low- and intermediate-risk papillary thyroid cancer will inform future disease management (43, 44).
- Thyroglobulin antibodies interfere with thyroglobulin interpretation, but monitoring changes in antithyroglobulin antibody titers, in conjunction with structural imaging, may be helpful in disease surveillance.
- Patient preferences are important to consider in RAI decision-making, especially when there is conflicting or unclear evidence of long-term outcome benefit in the body of existing observational evidence. Long-term randomized controlled trials are needed to clarify the role of RAI treatment in low-volume central neck nodal disease.

References

1. Brierley JD, Gospodarowicz MK, Wittekind C. The TNM classification of malignant tumours. 8th ed. Oxford: Wiley Blackwell; 2017.
2. Amin MB. AJCC cancer staging manual. 8th ed. Switerland: Springer Nature; 2017.
3. Hay ID, Bergstralh EJ, Goellner JR, Ebersold JR, Grant CS. Predicting outcome in papillary thyroid carcinoma: development of a reliable prognostic scoring system in a cohort of 1779 patients surgically treated at one institution during 1940 through 1989. Surgery. 1993;114:1050–7.

4. Cooper DS, Doherty GM, Haugen BR, Kloos RT, Lee SL, American Thyroid Association (ATA) Guidelines Taskforce on Thyroid Nodules and Differentiated Thyroid Cancer, et al. Revised American thyroid association management guidelines for patients with thyroid nodules and differentiated thyroid cancer. Thyroid. 2009;19:1167–214.
5. Spencer CA, Takeuchi M, Kazarosyan M, Wang CC, Guttler RB, Singer PA, et al. Serum thyroglobulin autoantibodies: prevalence, influence on serum thyroglobulin measurement, and prognostic significance in patients with differentiated thyroid carcinoma. J Clin Endocrinol Metab. 1998;83:1121–7.
6. Randolph GW, Duh QY, Heller KS, LiVolsi VA, Mandel SJ, Steward DL, American Thyroid Association Surgical Affairs Committee's Taskforce on Thyroid Cancer Nodal Surgery, et al. The prognostic significance of nodal metastases from papillary thyroid carcinoma can be stratified based on the size and number of metastatic lymph nodes, as well as the presence of extranodal extension. Thyroid. 2012;22:1144–52.
7. Bardet S, Malville E, Rame JP, Babin E, Samama G, De Raucourt D, et al. Macroscopic lymph-node involvement and neck dissection predict lymph-node recurrence in papillary thyroid carcinoma. Eur J Endocrinol. 2008;158(4):551–60.
8. Ji YB, Lee DW, Song CM, Kim KR, Park CW, Tae K. Accuracy of intraoperative determination of central node metastasis by the surgeon in papillary thyroid carcinoma. Otolaryngol Head Neck Surg. 2014;150(4):542–7.
9. Scherl S, Mehra S, Clain J, Dos Reis LL, Persky M, Turk A, et al. The effect of surgeon experience on the detection of metastatic lymph nodes in the central compartment and the pathologic features of clinically unapparent metastatic lymph nodes: what are we missing when we don't perform a prophylactic dissection of central compartment lymph nodes in papillary thyroid cancer? Thyroid. 2014;24(8):1282–8.
10. Chow SM, Yau S, Kwan CK, Poon PC, Law SC. Local and regional control in patients with papillary thyroid carcinoma: specific indications of external radiotherapy and radioactive iodine according to T and N categories in AJCC 6th edition. Endocr Relat Cancer. 2006;13:1159–72.
11. Ito Y, Fukushima M, Tomoda C, Inoue H, Kihara M, Higashiyama T, et al. Prognosis of patients with papillary thyroid carcinoma having clinically apparent metastasis to the lateral compartment. Endocr J. 2009;56(6):759–66.
12. Verburg FA, Mäder U, Tanase K, Thies ED, Diessl S, Buck AK, et al. Life expectancy is reduced in differentiated thyroid cancer patients ≥45 years old with extensive local tumor invasion, lateral lymph node, or distant metastases at diagnosis and normal in all other DTC patients. J Clin Endocrinol Metab. 2013;98:172–80.
13. Hughes CJ, Shaha AR, Shah JP, Loree TR. Impact of lymph node metastasis in differentiated carcinoma of the thyroid: a matched-pair analysis. Head Neck. 1996;18:127–32.
14. Varshney R, Pakdaman MN, Sands N, Hier MP, Rochon L, Black MJ, et al. Lymph node metastasis in thyroid papillary microcarcinoma: a study of 170 patients. J Laryngol Otol. 2014;128(10):922–5.
15. Kim HJ, Kim NK, Choi JH, Kim SW, Jin SM, Suh S, et al. Radioactive iodine ablation does not prevent recurrences in patients with papillary thyroid microcarcinoma. Clin Endocrinol. 2013;78:614–20.
16. Ross DS, Litofsky D, Ain KB, Bigos T, Brierley JD, Cooper DS, et al. Recurrence after treatment of micropapillary thyroid cancer. Thyroid. 2009;19:1043–8.
17. Hay ID, Hutchinson ME, Gonzalez-Losada T, McIver B, Reinalda ME, Grant CS, et al. Papillary thyroid microcarcinoma: a study of 900 cases observed in a 60-year period. Surgery. 2008;144:980–8.
18. Wada N, Duh QY, Sugino K, Iwasaki H, Kameyama K, Mimura T, et al. Lymph node metastasis from 259 papillary thyroid microcarcinomas: frequency, pattern of occurrence and recurrence, and optimal strategy for neck dissection. Ann Surg. 2003;237:399–407.
19. Mercante G, Frasoldati A, Pedroni C, Formisano D, Renna L, Piana S, et al. Prognostic factors affecting neck lymph node recurrence and distant metastasis in papillary microcarcinoma of the thyroid: results of a study in 445 patients. Thyroid. 2009;19:707–16.

20. Roh JL, Kim JM, Park CI. Central cervical nodal metastasis from papillary thyroid microcarcinoma: pattern and factors predictive of nodal metastasis. Ann Surg Oncol. 2008;15(9):2482–6.
21. Baudin E, Travagli JP, Ropers J, Mancusi F, Bruno-Bossio G, Caillou B, et al. Microcarcinoma of the thyroid gland: the Gustave-Roussy Institute experience. Cancer. 1998;83(3):553–9.
22. Chow SM, Law SC, Chan JK, Au SK, Yau S, Lau WH. Papillary microcarcinoma of the thyroid-prognostic significance of lymph node metastasis and multifocality. Cancer. 2003;98(1):31–40.
23. Roti E, degli Uberti EC, Bondanelli M, Braverman LE. Thyroid papillary microcarcinoma: a descriptive and meta-analysis study. Eur J Endocrinol. 2008;159(6):659–73.
24. Pelizzo MR, Boschin IM, Toniato A, Piotto A, Bernante P, Pagetta C, et al. Papillary thyroid microcarcinoma (PTMC): prognostic factors, management and outcome in 403 patients. Eur J Surg Oncol. 2006;32(10):1144–8.
25. Yu XM, Wan Y, Sippel RS, Chen H. Should all papillary thyroid microcarcinomas be aggressively treated? An analysis of 18,445 cases. Ann Surg. 2011;254(4):653–60.
26. Creach KM, Siegel BA, Nussenbaum B, Grigsby PW. Radioactive iodine therapy decreases recurrence in thyroid papillary microcarcinoma. ISRN Endocrinol. 2012;2012:816386.
27. Kwak JY, Kim EK, Kim MJ, Son EJ, Chung WY, Park CS, et al. Papillary microcarcinoma of the thyroid: predicting factors of lateral neck node metastasis. Ann Surg Oncol. 2009;16:1348–55.
28. Kim YS. Patterns and predictive factors of lateral lymph node metastasis in papillary thyroid microcarcinoma. Otolaryngol Head Neck Surg. 2012;147:15–9.
29. Zhang L, Wei WJ, Ji QH, Zhu YX, Wang ZY, Wang Y, et al. Risk factors for neck nodal metastasis in papillary thyroid microcarcinoma: a study of 1066 patients. J Clin Endocrinol Metab. 2012;97:1250–7.
30. Vasileiadis I, Karakostas E, Charitoudis G, Stavrianaki A, Kapetanakis S, Kouraklis G, et al. Papillary thyroid microcarcinoma: clinicopathological characteristics and implications for treatment in 276 patients. Eur J Clin Investig. 2012;42:657–64.
31. Hu G, Zhu W, Yang W, Wang H, Shen L, Zhang H. The effectiveness of radioactive iodine remnant ablation for papillary thyroid microcarcinoma: a systematic review and meta-analysis. World J Surg. 2016;40(1):100–9.
32. Van Nostrand D, Aiken M, Atkins F, Moreau S, Garcia C, Acio E, et al. The utility of radioiodine scans prior to iodine 131 ablation in patients with well-differentiated thyroid cancer. Thyroid. 2009;19:849–55.
33. Chen MK, Yasrebi M, Samii J, Staib LH, Doddamane I, Cheng DW. The utility of I-123 pretherapy scan in 1-131 radioiodine therapy for thyroid cancer. Thyroid. 2012;22:304–9.
34. Wong K, Sisson JC, Koral KF, Frey KA, Avram AM. Staging of differentiated thyroid carcinoma using diagnostic 131I SPECT/CT. Am J Roentgenol. 2010;195:730–6.
35. Vaisman A, Orlov S, Yip J, Hu C, Lim T, Dowar M, et al. Application of post-surgical stimulated thyroglobulin for radioiodine remnant ablation selection in low-risk papillary thyroid carcinoma. Head Neck. 2010;32(6):689–98.
36. Ibrahimpasic T, Nixon IJ, Palmer FL, Whitcher MM, Tuttle RM, Shaha A, Patel SG, Shah JP, Ganly I. Undetectable thyroglobulin after total thyroidectomy in patients with low- and intermediate-risk papillary thyroid cancer – is there a need for radioactive iodine therapy? Surgery. 2012;152(6):1096–105.
37. Haugen BR, Alexander EK, Bible KC, Doherty GM, Mandel SJ, Nikiforov YE, Pacini F, Randolph GW, Sawka AM, Schlumberger M, Schuff KG, Sherman SI, Sosa JA, Steward DL, Tuttle RM, Wartofsky L. 2015 American Thyroid Association management guidelines for adult patients with thyroid nodules and differentiated thyroid cancer: the American Thyroid Association Guidelines Task Force on Thyroid Nodules and Differentiated Thyroid Cancer. Thyroid. 2016;26(1):1–133.
38. Yamada O, Miyauchi A, Ito Y, Nakayama A, Yabuta T, Masuoka H, et al. Changes in serum thyroglobulin antibody levels as a dynamic prognostic factor for early-phase recurrence of thyroglobulin antibody-positive papillary thyroid carcinoma after total thyroidectomy. Endocr J. 2014;61:961–5.

39. Kim WG, Yoon JH, Kim WB, Kim TY, Kim EY, Kim JM, et al. Change of serum antithyroglobulin antibody levels is useful for prediction of clinical recurrence in thyroglobulin-negative patients with differentiated thyroid carcinoma. J Clin Endocrinol Metab. 2008;93:4683–9.
40. Tsushima Y, Miyauchi A, Ito Y, Kudo T, Masuoka H, Yabuta T, et al. Prognostic significance of changes in serum thyroglobulin antibody levels of pre- and post-total thyroidectomy in thyroglobulin antibody-positive papillary thyroid carcinoma patients. Endocr J. 2013;60:871–6.
41. Spencer C, Fatemi S. Thyroglobulin antibody (TgAb) methods – strengths, pitfalls and clinical utility for monitoring TgAb-positive patients with differentiated thyroid cancer. Best Pract Res Clin Endocrinol Metab. 2013;27:701–12.
42. Matrone A, Latrofa F, Torregrossa L, Piaggi P, Gambale C, Faranda A, Ricci D, Agate L, Molinaro E, Basolo F, Vitti P, Elisei R. Changing trend of thyroglobulin antibodies in patients with differentiated thyroid cancer treated with total thyroidectomy without (131)I ablation. Thyroid. 2018;28(7):871–9.
43. Mallick U, Harmer C, Hackshaw A, Moss L, IoN Trial Management Group. Iodine or Not (IoN) for low-risk differentiated thyroid cancer: the next UK National Cancer Research Network randomised trial following HiLo. Clin Oncol (R Coll Radiol). 2012;24(3):159–61.
44. Leboulleux S. Differentiated thyroid cancer: is there a need for radioiodine ablation in low risk patients? (ESTIMABL2). Available at: https://clinicaltrials.gov/ct2/show/NCT01837745. Accessed 3 Feb 2020.

Chapter 10
A Patient with a Large Minimally Invasive Follicular Thyroid Cancer

Jina Kim, Wen T. Shen, and Julie Ann Sosa

Case Presentation

A 42-year-old woman with a history of multinodular goiter was noted to have a progressively enlarging right thyroid nodule. She was asymptomatic and biochemically and clinically euthyroid. Thyroid ultrasound demonstrated a right solid, isoechoic thyroid nodule with smooth margins and no echogenic foci (intermediate suspicion according to the American Thyroid Association guidelines, TR3 according to the Thyroid Imaging Reporting and Data System), measuring 3.5 × 3.0 × 2.0 cm. Fine-needle aspiration demonstrated a follicular neoplasm (Bethesda category IV). Molecular testing was not performed. There was no evidence of cervical lymphadenopathy on ultrasound. A right thyroid lobectomy was performed.

Epidemiology

Follicular thyroid cancer (FTC) is a differentiated thyroid cancer that represents approximately 10% of all thyroid malignancies in the United States [1]. Since the 1970s, the overall incidence rate of FTC has increased by 0.6% per year. Between 2000 and 2006, the FTC incidence rate saw the greatest increase by 6.0% per year. More recently, between 2006 and 2013, the FTC incidence rate has *decreased* by 3.0% per year [1].

J. Kim · W. T. Shen · J. A. Sosa (✉)
Department of Surgery, University of California San Francisco, San Francisco, CA, USA
e-mail: julie.sosa@ucsf.edu

G. Grani et al. (eds.), *Thyroid Cancer*,
https://doi.org/10.1007/978-3-030-61919-0_10

Iodine deficiency and obesity have been identified as risk factors for the development of FTC. Compared to the United States, which is considered an iodine-replete area, iodine-deficient regions have observed a higher incidence of FTC [2]. In a meta-analysis of adiposity and thyroid cancer, obesity (BMI $\geq$ 30 kg/m^2) was found to confer a 61% increased risk of FTC compared to matched patients of normal weight [3].

Staging

As a differentiated thyroid cancer, FTC is staged based on the same staging systems as papillary thyroid cancer (PTC). In 2018, the 8th edition of the American Joint Committee on Cancer (AJCC)/tumor-node-metastasis (TNM) cancer staging system was introduced into clinical practice. Three important differences between the 7th and 8th editions of the AJCC/TNM system for differentiated thyroid cancer were:

- The threshold age for prognostic staging increased from 45 years to 55 years. While the 7th edition used 45 years of age as the cutoff to designate patients who were at higher risk of dying from thyroid cancer, the 8th edition increases the threshold to 55 years.
- Minor extrathyroidal extension on histological examination no longer affects T stage or overall stage.
- N1 disease is now stage II (rather than stage III) for patients ≥55 years of age. Previously, in the 7th edition, N1 disease was at least stage III for patients ≥45 years of age.

With these changes, a significant number of patients with FTC were downstaged to better reflect their low risk of dying from thyroid cancer. By providing a more accurate assessment of the risk of mortality related to thyroid cancer, the authors expect these changes to reshape treatment patterns, such as extent of thyroid surgery and/or need for radioactive iodine therapy [4]. The 8th edition of the AJCC/TNM staging system has been validated specifically for FTC in small retrospective studies [5, 6]. For example, in a 2018 retrospective European study of 164 patients with FTC, the 8th AJCC/TNM staging system was a better predictor of overall survival and disease-specific survival for FTC compared to the 7th edition [5].

In addition to the AJCC/TNM system, histologic characteristics also provide important prognostic information for FTC. In 2017, the World Health Organization changed the histological subclassification of FTC to more accurately reflect the risk of mortality and recurrence associated with FTC [7]. The new histological subclassification is discussed in the next section.

Histology

FTC is characterized by the absence of nuclear features of PTC and the presence of capsular and/or vascular invasion. Therefore, histologic rather than cytologic evaluation of tumors is mandatory to discern between malignant lesions and benign adenomas [8, 9]. Traditionally, FTC was classified as either minimally invasive or widely invasive based on the presence of vascular or capsular infiltration [9]. In 2017, the WHO modified classification of FTC into three groups based on the degree of invasion: minimally invasive FTC (miFTC), encapsulated angioinvasive FTC (eaFTC), and widely invasive FTC (wiFTC) [7].

- miFTC includes tumors with invasion of the tumor capsule only, without vascular invasion (Fig. 10.1). However, there is no consensus around the definition of capsular invasion. Some consider even a focal extension into the capsule to be diagnostic for malignancy [10, 11]. This diagnosis is made more difficult by the potential for disruption of the nodule at the time of FNA, by an intraoperative disruption of the capsule during thyroidectomy, or pathologic artifacts; all of these factors may be difficult to distinguish from neoplastic capsular invasion. Hence, the integrity of the tumor capsule is fundamental to allow proper diagnosis [12].

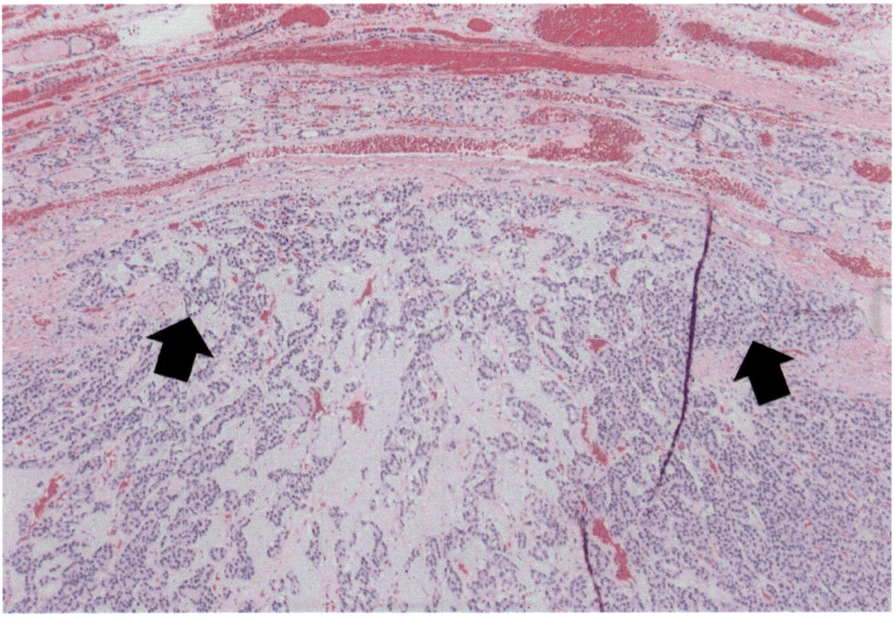

Fig. 10.1 Follicular thyroid cancer with capsular invasion only is considered minimally invasive. Arrows show the area of invasion through the capsule, forming a characteristic "mushroom" (H&E, × 400)

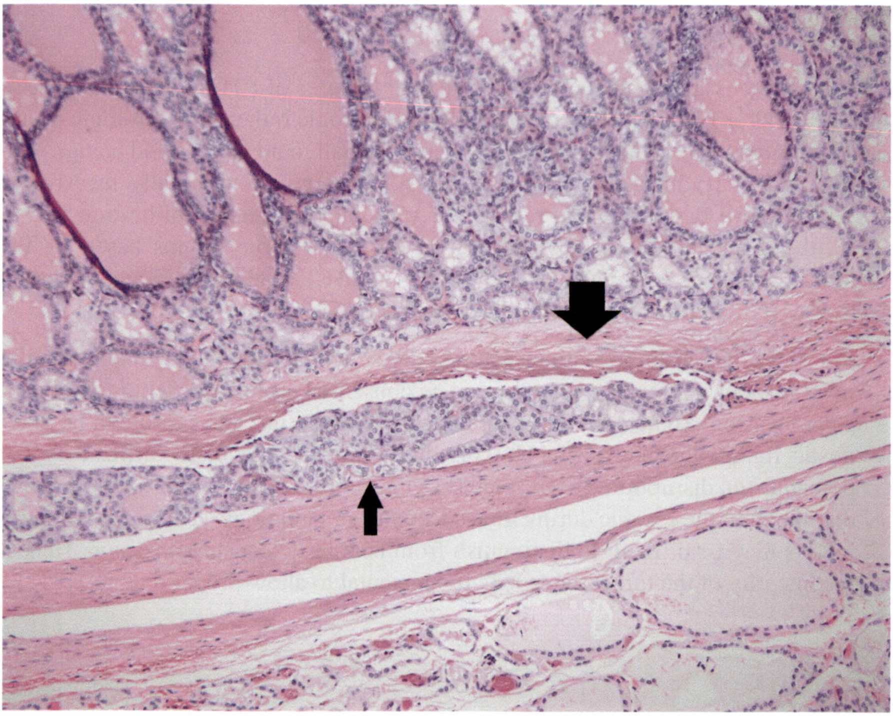

Fig. 10.2 Follicular thyroid cancer that demonstrates any vascular invasion is considered an encapsulated angioinvasive follicular thyroid cancer based on the 2017 World Health Organization classification. Thin arrow shows tumor attachment to the vessel wall, and thick arrow shows the vascular space (H&E, × 100)

- eaFTC includes tumors with any evidence of vascular invasion (Fig. 10.2). Even a single focus of angioinvasion assigns the tumor as eaFTC [13, 14].
- wiFTC includes tumors with gross invasion of the thyroid gland and extrathyroidal tissues, often with extensive vascular invasion.

The recent modifications to both the WHO classification and the AJCC/TNM staging system reflect the dynamic conversation among experts to better define prognosis in FTC. In the future, molecular testing may be another mechanism to provide prognostic information in FTC. Our current understanding of the molecular characteristics of FTC is discussed next.

Molecular Characteristics of FTC

RAS mutations are markers for follicular-type thyroid lesions (follicular adenomas, follicular thyroid cancer, non-invasive follicular thyroid neoplasm with papillary-like nuclear features [15–17]). Two prior meta-analyses have found *RAS* mutations to be more common in FTC (frequency of 25–27%) and relatively rare in PTC (frequency of 5–6%) [18, 19]. The *RAS* gene encodes three isoforms (*NRAS*, *HRAS*, and *KRAS*), which are ultimately involved in mediating cell differentiation and proliferation [20, 21]. *HRAS* mutations are associated with the greatest risk of cancer [22]. It has been proposed that RAS mutation predisposes differentiated cancers to dedifferentiation, and therefore, RAS-positive follicular adenomas are precursors to RAS-positive FTC and possibly follicular variant of PTC [23].

The *PAX8/PPARγ* rearrangement is a fusion of the *PAX8* gene and the peroxisome proliferator-activated receptor (*PPARγ*) gene. It is present in 30–35% of conventional FTC and in 2–13% of follicular adenomas [24, 25]. Follicular tumors with *PAX8/PPARγ* rearrangements often have invasion, and therefore, detection of this rearrangement should compel a thorough investigation for vascular and/or capsular invasion in the tumor [24, 26]. Tumors with *PAX8/PPARγ* rearrangement do not have *RAS* mutations, which suggests that two separate biological pathways may contribute to the development of FTC [16].

In light of the new 2017 WHO classification of FTC, Nicolson et al. performed whole-exome sequencing of 12 miFTC, 17 eaFTC, and 10 wiFTC to compare genetic makeup of these histopathologically different forms of FTC. Of this cohort, 20.5% had a *RAS* mutation, and there was a trend toward more mutations observed in eaFTC and wiFTC, although these were not statistically significant findings. Higher mutation burden was associated with worse survival, independent of histopathological classification. The authors propose that the longer a tumor is present, the more likely it is to accumulate mutations and become more aggressive, rather than acquiring a single specific genetic alteration conferring compromised prognosis [27].

miFTC

Compared to more invasive subtypes of FTC, miFTC has been shown to have favorable outcomes with low risk of disease-related mortality. This understanding of the behavior of miFTC has guided management recommendations. However, studies from the United States and Japan have been conflicting [14, 28–31].

One of the earliest studies on the outcomes of patients with FTC was a review of 72 patients at the Mayo Clinic in 1992: 20 patients had capsular invasion only, and 45 patients had vascular invasion, with or without capsular invasion. After a median follow-up of 11 years, 10-year cause-specific mortality was 0% for patients with capsular invasion and 28% for patients with vascular invasion ($p = 0.019$); the 10-year rates of development of distant metastases were 0% and 19%, respectively ($p = 0.052$). This suggests that patients with FTC and only capsular invasion (the equivalent of the current definition of miFTC) represent a subgroup of patients that have excellent outcomes and therefore can be managed less aggressively [14].

In a 2011 study by O'Neill et al., 124 patients with FTC were compared in three groups: miFTC, miFTC with vascular invasion, and wiFTC. Overall, the disease-free survival rate was 85% at a median follow-up of 40 months, but disease-free survival differed significantly among the groups. Disease-free survival was 97% for the miFTC group, 81% for the miFTC with vascular invasion group, and 46% for the wiFTC group. Only patients aged <45 years with miFTC (no vascular invasion) had 100% disease-free survival, suggesting that thyroid lobectomy alone may be sufficient in these patients and that total thyroidectomy (with or without radioactive iodine ablation [RAI]) should be performed in all other patients with FTC [28].

In a 2000–2009 retrospective study from the Surveillance, Epidemiology, and End Results (SEER) database, a total of 1200 patients with miFTC and 4208 with wiFTC were identified. miFTC tumors were less likely than wiFTC tumors to involve lymph nodes (0.9 vs. 3.6%; $p < 0.001$) and metastasize (0.5 vs. 8.9%; $p < 0001$). At last follow-up, a significantly greater proportion of patients with miFTC were alive (96.8 vs. 86.5% with wiFTC; $p < 0.001$). Of particular interest was that only two miFTC patients died of disease-specific causes (disease-specific survival rate, 99.8%), compared to a disease-specific survival rate of 94.8% in patients with wiFTC ($p < 0.001$). The overall survival rate of patients with miFTC was found to be comparable to that of the general US population [29].

In contrast, other studies – albeit from single centers – have suggested that miFTC has a higher rate of metastasis and is associated with compromised patient survival [30–33]. In a 2012 retrospective, single-center study of 251 Japanese patients diagnosed with miFTC from 1989 to 2006, Sugino et al. found a compromised cause-specific survival of 95.2, 89.5, and 84.5% at 10, 15, and 20 years, respectively [31]. Distant metastases were identified in 54 patients (22%), including 22 patients (8.8%) with metastases identified at the time of initial surgery. In a subsequent 2014 study, Sugino et al. focused on the outcomes of miFTC patients who had a completion thyroidectomy at their institution. Of 324 patients who underwent thyroid lobectomy for miFTC, 101 patients underwent completion thyroidectomy within 6 months of initial surgery, and 81 patients had radioiodine ablation. The remaining patients did not undergo further treatment. Distant metastasis-free survival rates were 85.5, 75.2, and 73.5% at 10, 15, and 20 years, respectively. On multivariable analysis, lack of completion thyroidectomy was independently associated with compromised distant metastasis-free survival (odds ratio 2.93, 95% confidence interval [CI] 1.16–8.95, $p = 0.0222$) [30]. These data – albeit from a single institution – would support performing completion thyroidectomy for patients with miFTC.

Unfortunately, these data on the prognosis of miFTC do not reflect the 2017 WHO classification schema, which means that the study cohort may include those who have eaFTC based on current definitions. Moving forward, as clinicians and researchers differentiate between miFTC and eaFTC, we may be able to provide more accurate prognostic information for miFTC.

Treatment of miFTC

Although the optimal management of low-risk tumors like miFTC remains controversial, many support thyroid lobectomy (with or without isthmusectomy) as adequate treatment for miFTC based on the low rate of metastatic disease and mortality [14, 34–36]. A 2014 consensus report on miFTC by the European Society of Endocrine Surgeons (ESES) recommended that thyroid lobectomy be performed for miFTC with capsular invasion at diagnosis, without vascular invasion, without any lymph node or distant metastases, tumors <4.0 cm, and in patients <45 years [37]. Candidates for total thyroidectomy are patients ≥45 years, tumor size ≥4.0 cm, vascular invasion, and presence of lymph node or distant metastases. Lymphadenectomy was considered only when clinical evidence of lymph node metastasis was present. ESES also recommended RAI when criteria for total thyroidectomy were met and if recurrence was observed on follow-up. However, as with the prognostic information related to miFTC, these recommendations may serve a limited role since they predate the 2017 WHO histologic reclassification and introduction of the 2018 AJCC/TNM staging system.

Despite recommendations for a more conservative approach toward miFTC, a recent US study shows that miFTC remains aggressively treated. In a 2010–2011 National Cancer Data Base study of 617 patients, the rate of total thyroidectomy was similar for miFTC with vascular invasion compared to miFTC with capsular invasion only (72.9 vs. 75.1%, $p = 0.537$). RAI was administered to 52.6% of patients with miFTC with capsular invasion only and to 62.1% of patients with miFTC with vascular invasion ($p = 0.017$) [38].

Lymph Node and Distant Metastases in miFTC

Compared to PTC, lymph node metastases are less common in FTC and occur in fewer than 5% of miFTC cases [14, 31, 37, 39, 40]. While the authors of the 2014 ESES consensus report found no difference in miFTC outcomes based on lymph node metastases, some studies have demonstrated that the presence of lymph node metastases portends compromised survival for FTC in general [40–43]. For example, in a study of the 1988–2003 Surveillance, Epidemiology, and End Results dataset, lymph node metastases occurred in 2% of FTC patients (compared to 22% of PTC patients). Lymph node metastasis in FTC was associated with increased risk of death, regardless of age (hazard ratio [HR] 11.23, 95% CI 2.44–61.69, $p = 0.002$ for age <45 years; HR 2.86, 95% CI 1.71–4.78, $p < 0.001$ for age ≥ 45 years) [40]. On the other hand, lymph node involvement in PTC was associated with increased risk of death only for patients ≥45 years, suggesting nodal involvement may carry different prognostic value for FTC and PTC. This difference remains to be fully elucidated.

Currently, lymph node management for miFTC should follow guidelines for DTC. According to the 2015 ATA guidelines for DTC, prophylactic lymphadenectomy is not indicated for small, clinically node-negative PTC and for most FTC. Therapeutic central and/or lateral compartmental neck dissection is indicated for patients with clinical evidence of nodal disease by physical exam or preoperative imaging and cytology [44]. RAI should be administered postoperatively for patients with regional nodal metastases [44].

On the other hand, FTC is more likely to present with distant metastases than PTC, and even miFTC cases may present with or develop distant metastases [32, 45, 46]. Based on retrospective data, approximately 10% of patients with miFTC will have distant metastases at the time of presentation [31, 47].

For miFTC with distant metastases, treatment should begin with total thyroidectomy to allow for total body I-131 scanning [48]. RAI is then used after total thyroidectomy if distant metastases are detected [37]. For single resectable metastases, surgical resection may be considered. Chemotherapy or external beam radiation can also be used. In a retrospective, single-center study of 251 Japanese patients with miFTC, 8.8% had distant metastases at the time of initial surgery, and 21.5% of patients were diagnosed with distant metastases within a median follow-up time of 90 months. The lung and bone were the most common sites of metastases. While 57% of patients demonstrated radioiodine uptake in their metastases on scintigraphy, complete response to RAI was seen in only one patient and partial response in two patients. The other patients had stable or progressive disease [31].

Molecular Characteristics of miFTC

Beyond histopathological observations and clinical outcomes, more recent studies have evaluated various molecular analyses that may help to predict aggressiveness in miFTC. Investigators have examined frequency of allelic loss as well as alterations in gene, RNA, and protein expression in miFTC in efforts to better characterize malignant potential of miFTC.

Hunt et al. assessed a panel of ten tumor suppressor genes (*L-MYC*, *CMM*, *hOGG1*, *VHL*, *APC*, *MCC*, *MTS1/p16*, *pTEN*, *p53*, and *NF2*) to study loss of heterozygosity mutations, with the hypothesis that genotyping follicular-derived thyroid neoplasms may predict histologic FTC aggressiveness [49]. Despite a limited sample size (8 follicular adenomas, 5 miFTC, and 5 wiFTC), the authors found that the frequency of allelic loss (FAL) did correlate with histologic aggressiveness: follicular adenomas had a FAL of only 9%, compared with a FAL of 30% for miFTC and 53% for wiFTC. In another study, Lubitz et al. found that while many miFTCs were genetically similar, miFTC had 223 differently expressed genes compared to follicular adenomas and 365 differently expressed genes compared to wiFTC [50].

In a 2016 study, Ito et al. investigated the utility of Ki-67 labeling index (LI) ≥5% in predicting miFTC recurrence. Ki-67 immunostaining was used on formalin-fixed, paraffin-embedded tissues from 192 patients with miFTC. Patients with higher Ki-67 LI had worse disease-free survival, compared to patients with low Ki-67 LI. On multivariable analysis, Ki-67 LI ≥5% was associated with a higher risk of disease recurrence (HR 6.061, 95% CI 1.263–29.412, $p = 0.0243$) [51]. This analysis suggests that Ki-67 LI may be used as a prognostic indicator in miFTC.

The utility of long non-coding RNA H19 expression as a prognostic indicator has also been studied in miFTC. Aberrant expression of RNA H19 has been associated with tumor progression in prior studies [52, 53]. In a study of 186 patients with miFTC, total microRNA was isolated from frozen tissues, and quantitative reverse transcription PCR was performed to determine expression levels of H19. Patients with lower H19 expression had a mean overall survival of 89 months, while those with higher H19 expression had a mean overall survival of 166 months [54].

Molecular analysis is a relatively new, dynamic area of research that may ultimately help us to better understand FTC [55]. Already, recent changes in the staging system and histologic classification reflect efforts to provide more accurate prognostic information related to FTC. In the future, the combination of clinical, histopathological, and molecular characteristics of miFTC may provide better information regarding the malignant potential of miFTC and allow clinicians to personalize treatment for patients.

Back to the Case

Surgical pathology demonstrated a unifocal, well-differentiated 3.4 cm follicular cancer with a single area of capsular invasion, consistent with a minimally invasive follicular thyroid cancer. The patient received no further surgery or adjuvant therapy. Planned surveillance includes neck ultrasound and serum TSH and thyroglobulin levels after 6 months and then periodically, depending on the patient's risk for recurrent disease and thyroglobulin status.

Clinical Pearls

- In 2017, the World Health Organization modified classification of FTC into three groups: minimally invasive follicular cancer, encapsulated angioinvasive FTC, and widely invasive follicular thyroid cancer.
- Compared to wiFTC, miFTC portends a more favorable prognosis, with a disease-specific survival rate of 99.8% in the United States.
- Extent of surgery remains controversial for miFTC, but thyroid lobectomy is recommended for tumors with only capsular invasion at diagnosis, without vascular invasion, without lymph node or distant metastases, tumors <4.0 cm, and in patients <45 years, according to the 2014 consensus report from the European Society of Endocrine Surgeons.

References

1. Lim H, Devesa SS, Sosa JA, Check D, Kitahara CM. Trends in thyroid cancer incidence and mortality in the United States, 1974-2013. JAMA. 2017;317:1338–48.
2. Kim J, Gosnell JE, Roman SA. Geographic influences in the global rise of thyroid cancer. Nat Rev Endocrinol. 2019. https://doi.org/10.1038/s41574-019-0263-x.
3. Schmid D, Ricci C, Behrens G, Leitzmann MF. Adiposity and risk of thyroid cancer: a systematic review and meta-analysis. Obes Rev. 2015;16:1042–54.
4. Tuttle RM, Michael Tuttle R, Haugen B, Perrier ND. Updated American Joint Committee on Cancer/tumor-node-metastasis staging system for differentiated and anaplastic thyroid cancer (Eighth Edition): what changed and why? Thyroid. 2017:751–6. https://doi.org/10.1089/thy.2017.0102.
5. van Velsen EFS, Stegenga MT, van Kemenade FJ, Kam BLR, van Ginhoven TM, Edward Visser W, et al. Comparing the prognostic value of the eighth edition of the American Joint Committee on Cancer/tumor node metastasis staging system between papillary and follicular thyroid cancer. Thyroid. 2018:976–81. https://doi.org/10.1089/thy.2018.0066.
6. Ito Y, Miyauchi A, Hirokawa M, Yamamoto M, Oda H, Masuoka H, et al. Prognostic value of the 8th tumor-node-metastasis classification for follicular carcinoma and poorly differentiated carcinoma of the thyroid in Japan. Endocr J. 2018;65:621–7.
7. International Agency for Research on Cancer. WHO classification of tumours of endocrine organs. Lyon: International Agency for Research on Cancer; 2017.
8. Franssila KO, Ackerman LV, Brown CL, Hedinger CE. Follicular carcinoma. Semin Diagn Pathol. 1985;2:101–22.
9. International Agency for Research on Cancer, World Health Organization, International Academy of Pathology. Pathology and genetics of tumours of endocrine organs. Lyon: IARC; 2004.
10. Heffess CS, Thompson LD. Minimally invasive follicular thyroid carcinoma. Endocr Pathol. 2001;12:417–22.
11. Thompson LD, Wieneke JA, Paal E, Frommelt RA, Adair CF, Heffess CS. A clinicopathologic study of minimally invasive follicular carcinoma of the thyroid gland with a review of the English literature. Cancer. 2001;91:505–24.
12. Hermann M, Tonninger K, Kober F, Furtlehner E-M, Schultheis A, Neuhold N. [Minimally invasive follicular thyroid carcinoma : not always total thyroidectomy]. Chirurg. 2010;81:627–30, 632–5.
13. Nikiforov YE, Biddinger PW, Thompson LDR. Diagnostic pathology and molecular genetics of the thyroid: a comprehensive guide for practicing thyroid pathology. Philadelphia: Lippincott Williams & Wilkins; 2012.
14. van Heerden JA, Hay ID, Goellner JR, Salomao D, Ebersold JR, Bergstralh EJ, et al. Follicular thyroid carcinoma with capsular invasion alone: a nonthreatening malignancy. Surgery. 1992;112:1130–6; discussion 1136–8.
15. Nikiforov YE, Nikiforova MN. Molecular genetics and diagnosis of thyroid cancer. Nat Rev Endocrinol. 2011;7:569–80.
16. Nikiforova MN, Lynch RA, Biddinger PW, Alexander EK, Dorn GW 2nd, Tallini G, et al. RAS point mutations and PAX8-PPAR gamma rearrangement in thyroid tumors: evidence for distinct molecular pathways in thyroid follicular carcinoma. J Clin Endocrinol Metab. 2003;88:2318–26.
17. McFadden DG, Dias-Santagata D, Sadow PM, Lynch KD, Lubitz C, Donovan SE, et al. Identification of oncogenic mutations and gene fusions in the follicular variant of papillary thyroid carcinoma. J Clin Endocrinol Metab. 2014;99:E2457–62.
18. Vasko V, Ferrand M, Di Cristofaro J, Carayon P, Henry JF, de Micco C. Specific pattern of RAS oncogene mutations in follicular thyroid tumors. J Clin Endocrinol Metab. 2003;88:2745–52.

19. Liu R-T, Hou C-Y, You H-L, Huang C-C, Hock-Liew, Chou F-F, et al. Selective occurrence of ras mutations in benign and malignant thyroid follicular neoplasms in Taiwan. Thyroid. 2004;14:616–21.
20. Xing M. Genetic alterations in the phosphatidylinositol-3 kinase/Akt pathway in thyroid cancer. Thyroid. 2010;20:697–706.
21. Davis RJ. The mitogen-activated protein kinase signal transduction pathway. J Biol Chem. 1993;268:14553–6.
22. Patel SG, Carty SE, McCoy KL, Ohori NP, LeBeau SO, Seethala RR, et al. Preoperative detection of RAS mutation may guide extent of thyroidectomy. Surgery. 2017;161:168–75.
23. Ferrari SM, Fallahi P, Ruffilli I, Elia G, Ragusa F, Paparo SR, et al. Molecular testing in the diagnosis of differentiated thyroid carcinomas. Gland Surg. 2018;7:S19–29.
24. French CA, Alexander EK, Cibas ES, Nose V, Laguette J, Faquin W, et al. Genetic and biological subgroups of low-stage follicular thyroid cancer. Am J Pathol. 2003;162:1053–60.
25. Dwight T, Thoppe SR, Foukakis T, Lui WO, Wallin G, Höög A, et al. Involvement of the PAX8/Peroxisome proliferator-activated receptor γ rearrangement in follicular thyroid tumors. J Clin Endocrinol Metabol. 2003;88:4440–5. https://doi.org/10.1210/jc.2002-021690.
26. Nikiforova MN, Biddinger PW, Caudill CM, Kroll TG, Nikiforov YE. PAX8-PPARγ rearrangement in thyroid tumors: RT-PCR and immunohistochemical analyses. Am J Surg Pathol. 2002;26:1016.
27. Nicolson NG, Murtha TD, Dong W, Paulsson JO, Choi J, Barbieri AL, et al. Comprehensive genetic analysis of follicular thyroid carcinoma predicts prognosis independent of histology. J Clin Endocrinol Metab. 2018;103:2640–50.
28. O'Neill CJ, Vaughan L, Learoyd DL, Sidhu SB, Delbridge LW, Sywak MS. Management of follicular thyroid carcinoma should be individualised based on degree of capsular and vascular invasion. Eur J Surg Oncol. 2011;37:181–5.
29. Goffredo P, Cheung K, Roman SA, Sosa JA. Can minimally invasive follicular thyroid cancer be approached as a benign lesion? Ann Surg Oncol. 2013;20:767–72.
30. Sugino K, Kameyama K, Nagahama M, Kitagawa W, Shibuya H, Ohkuwa K, et al. Does completion thyroidectomy improve the outcome of patients with minimally invasive follicular carcinoma of the thyroid? Ann Surg Oncol. 2014;21:2981–6.
31. Sugino K, Kameyama K, Ito K, Nagahama M, Kitagawa W, Shibuya H, et al. Outcomes and prognostic factors of 251 patients with minimally invasive follicular thyroid carcinoma. Thyroid. 2012;22:798–804.
32. Ban EJ, Andrabi A, Grodski S, Yeung M, McLean C, Serpell J. Follicular thyroid cancer: minimally invasive tumours can give rise to metastases. ANZ J Surg. 2012;82:136–9.
33. Delbridge L, Parkyn R, Philips J, Barraclough B, Robinson B. Minimally invasive follicular thyroid carcinoma: completion thyroidectomy or not? ANZ J Surg. 2002;72:844–5.
34. Huang C-C, Hsueh C, Liu F-H, Chao T-C, Lin J-D. Diagnostic and therapeutic strategies for minimally and widely invasive follicular thyroid carcinomas. Surg Oncol. 2011;20:1–6.
35. Gemsenjäger E, Heitz PU, Martina B. Selective treatment of differentiated thyroid carcinoma. World J Surg. 1997;21:546–51; discussion 551–2.
36. Collini P, Sampietro G, Pilotti S. Extensive vascular invasion is a marker of risk of relapse in encapsulated non-Hürthle cell follicular carcinoma of the thyroid gland: a clinicopathological study of 18 consecutive cases from a single institution with a 11-year median follow-up. Histopathology. 2004;44:35–9.
37. Dionigi G, Kraimps J-L, Schmid KW, Hermann M, Sheu-Grabellus S-Y, De Wailly P, et al. Minimally invasive follicular thyroid cancer (MIFTC) – a consensus report of the European Society of Endocrine Surgeons (ESES). Langenbeck's Arch Surg. 2014;399:165–84.
38. Goffredo P, Jillard C, Thomas S, Scheri RP, Sosa JA, Roman S. Minimally invasive follicular carcinoma: predictors of vascular invasion and impact on patterns of care. Endocrine. 2016;51:123–30.

39. Brennan MD, Bergstralh EJ, van Heerden JA, McConahey WM. Follicular thyroid cancer treated at the Mayo Clinic, 1946 through 1970: initial manifestations, pathologic findings, therapy, and outcome. Mayo Clin Proc. 1991;66:11–22.
40. Zaydfudim V, Feurer ID, Griffin MR, Phay JE. The impact of lymph node involvement on survival in patients with papillary and follicular thyroid carcinoma. Surgery. 2008;144:1070–7; discussion 1077–8.
41. Ito Y, Hirokawa M, Masuoka H, Yabuta T, Kihara M, Higashiyama T, et al. Prognostic factors of minimally invasive follicular thyroid carcinoma: extensive vascular invasion significantly affects patient prognosis. Endocr J. 2013;60:637–42.
42. Podnos YD, Smith D, Wagman LD, Ellenhorn JDI. Radioactive iodine offers survival improvement in patients with follicular carcinoma of the thyroid. Surgery. 2005;138:1072–6; discussion 1076–7.
43. Grani G, Lamartina L, Durante C, Filetti S, Cooper DS. Follicular thyroid cancer and Hürthle cell carcinoma: challenges in diagnosis, treatment, and clinical management. Lancet Diabetes Endocrinol. 2018;6:500–14.
44. Haugen BR, Alexander EK, Bible KC, Doherty GM, Mandel SJ, Nikiforov YE, et al. 2015 American Thyroid Association management guidelines for adult patients with thyroid nodules and differentiated thyroid cancer: the American Thyroid Association guidelines task force on thyroid nodules and differentiated thyroid cancer. Thyroid. 2016;26:1–133.
45. Goffredo P, Sosa JA, Roman SA. Differentiated thyroid cancer presenting with distant metastases: a population analysis over two decades. World J Surg. 2013;37:1599–605.
46. Kuo EJ, Roman SA, Sosa JA. Patients with follicular and Hurthle cell microcarcinomas have compromised survival: a population level study of 22,738 patients. Surgery. 2013;154:1246–53; discussion 1253–4.
47. Asari R, Koperek O, Scheuba C, Riss P, Kaserer K, Hoffmann M, et al. Follicular thyroid carcinoma in an iodine-replete endemic goiter region: a prospectively collected, retrospectively analyzed clinical trial. Ann Surg. 2009;249:1023–31.
48. Doherty G. Follicular neoplasms of the thyroid. In: Textbook of endocrine surgery; 2005. p. 115–22. https://doi.org/10.1016/b978-0-7216-0139-7.50017-x.
49. Hunt JL, Livolsi VA, Baloch ZW, Swalsky PA, Bakker A, Sasatomi E, et al. A novel microdissection and genotyping of follicular-derived thyroid tumors to predict aggressiveness. Hum Pathol. 2003;34:375–80.
50. Lubitz CC, Gallagher LA, Finley DJ, Zhu B, Fahey TJ 3rd. Molecular analysis of minimally invasive follicular carcinomas by gene profiling. Surgery. 2005;138:1042–8; discussion 1048–9.
51. Ito Y, Hirokawa M, Miyauchi A, Masuoka H, Yabuta T, Fukushima M, et al. Prognostic impact of Ki-67 labeling index in minimally invasive follicular thyroid carcinoma. Endocr J. 2016;63:913–7.
52. Yoshimura H, Matsuda Y, Yamamoto M, Kamiya S, Ishiwata T. Expression and role of long non-coding RNA H19 in carcinogenesis. Front Biosci. 2018;23:614–25.
53. Weidle UH, Birzele F, Kollmorgen G, Rüger R. Long non-coding RNAs and their role in metastasis. Cancer Genomics Proteomics. 2017;14:143–60. https://doi.org/10.21873/cgp.20027.
54. Dai Y, Miao Y, Zhu Q, Gao M, Hao F. Expression of long non-coding RNA H19 predicts distant metastasis in minimally invasive follicular thyroid carcinoma. Bioengineered. 2019;10:383–9.
55. Yip L, Sosa JA. Molecular-directed treatment of differentiated thyroid cancer: advances in diagnosis and treatment. JAMA Surg. 2016;151:663–70.

Chapter 11
An Adolescent with Papillary Thyroid Carcinoma and Locally Metastatic Disease but No Distant Metastases

Sarah J. Bottomley and Steven G. Waguespack

Introduction

Papillary thyroid carcinoma (PTC) is the most common type of thyroid cancer in the pediatric population, representing 90% or more of cases in patients ≤18 years of age. Children with PTC are more likely than adults to present with regional lymph node involvement and extra-thyroidal extension. Despite often having advanced cervical disease at presentation, young patients have very favorable outcomes with long-term survival decades after diagnosis being the norm. The management of lymph node metastases is primarily surgical, and the role of radioactive iodine (RAI) in the treatment of cervical disease in children is diminishing.

Case Presentation

A 17-year-old female was found by her primary care provider to have a palpable right thyroid mass. She had no known personal risk factors for thyroid cancer, such as prior radiation exposure or family history, and was clinically and biochemically euthyroid. Neck ultrasound revealed a dominant solid nodule in the right lobe measuring 3.5 × 2.1 × 2.4 cm; cervical lymph nodes were not interrogated. The patient was seen by a local general surgeon, who performed a right thyroid lobectomy without a preoperative fine-needle aspiration biopsy (FNAB). Pathology revealed a T2N0Mx (AJCC 8th edition) PTC, classical subtype, with focal angioinvasion and positive surgical margins. There was one small lymph node adjacent to the gland

S. J. Bottomley · S. G. Waguespack (✉)
Department of Endocrine Neoplasia & Hormonal Disorders, University of Texas MD Anderson Cancer Center, Houston, TX, USA
e-mail: sjbottom@mdanderson.org; swagues@mdanderson.org

G. Grani et al. (eds.), *Thyroid Cancer*,
https://doi.org/10.1007/978-3-030-61919-0_11

that was negative for malignancy. Three days later the patient underwent a completion thyroidectomy and a central neck dissection by the same surgeon. The left lobe of the thyroid was without evidence of disease, and, in the central compartment, 16/26 lymph nodes (overall sizes ranging from 0.2 to 1.5 cm; no extranodal extension) were positive for PTC.

The patient presented to a tertiary cancer center for further evaluation. Neck US revealed a suspicious, 1.3 cm right level IV lymph node (Fig. 11.1a) that was positive for PTC on FNAB. Because the patient was already hypothyroid, a ^{123}I thyroid scan and a stimulated (TSH 86 mU/L) thyroglobulin (Tg) level were obtained after the patient followed a strict low-iodine diet for a week. There was uptake identified in the thyroid bed, but no lateral cervical uptake was seen (Fig. 11.1b). The stimulated Tg was 2.0 ng/ml with a concomitant Tg antibody that was mildly positive (46 IU/ml; normal $\leq$40). Despite the negative ^{123}I thyroid scan, the results of the US, FNA, and Tg and a pre-surgical CT neck were consistent with persistent neck disease. Therefore, a bilateral paratracheal, superior mediastinal, and right lateral

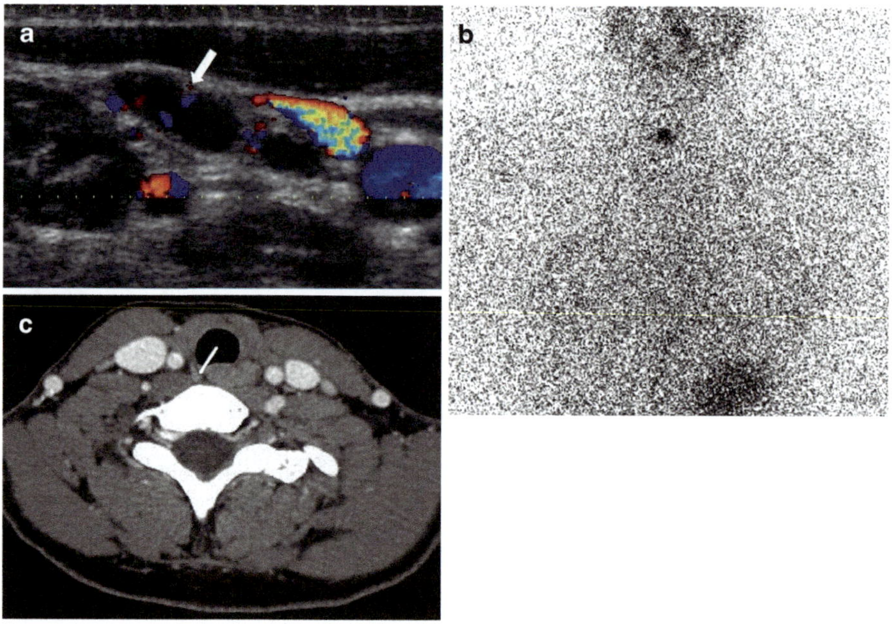

Fig. 11.1 A 17-year-old female with a locally metastatic PTC presented for further evaluation at a tertiary cancer center after having already had two surgeries by a general surgeon. Cervical ultrasonography revealed a suspicious, 1.3 cm right level IV lymph node (**a**, arrow), which was proven to be PTC after fine-needle aspiration biopsy. Despite the presence of residual lymph node disease, there was no indication of iodine-avid lateral neck metastases on a diagnostic ^{123}I thyroid scan (**b**). Preoperative contrast-enhanced CT also identified a suspicious lymph node in the right tracheoesophageal groove (**c**, arrow), which was resected and proven to be PTC. Subsequent to her third surgery, the patient had no evidence of residual PTC, and she remains disease-free 7 years after her last surgery

comprehensive neck dissection of levels 3, 4, and anterior 5 was undertaken, and pathology revealed 8/26 lymph nodes positive for PTC (overall sizes ranging from 0.1 to 1.6 cm; no extranodal extension); the tumor was negative for the *BRAF* V600E mutation. The right central compartment was re-explored because a preoperative contrast-enhanced CT neck suggested an abnormal lymph node in the right tracheoesophageal groove (Fig. 11.1c); on pathology, a single right paratracheal lymph node (0.5 cm; no extranodal extension) was positive for PTC.

Assessment and Literature Review

Thyroid cancer is rare in the pediatric population, but the incidence appears to be increasing, especially in adolescents, who represent the most commonly affected pediatric age group. In fact, thyroid cancer is the most prevalent cancer in older children and young adults, constituting 14% of all malignancies diagnosed at the ages of 15–19 years [1]. PTC is the most common type, accounting for 90% or more of childhood thyroid cancers, followed by follicular and, more rarely, medullary thyroid carcinomas. Primary risk factors for the development of thyroid cancer in children include thyroidal exposure to radiation and a family history of thyroid malignancy [2], but in reality, few children with differentiated thyroid cancer have a clearly identified risk factor.

PTC is frequently multifocal and bilateral, and, in children, regional lymph node metastases occur in up to 80% of cases [3–10]. Patients with a significant volume of cervical disease are at the highest risk of hematogenous lung metastases [5, 6], which occur in up to 25% of pediatric cases in some series [3, 5, 7, 11–16]. Despite more extensive disease at presentation, pediatric PTC is biologically distinct from PTC diagnosed in older adults. Children and young adults up to age 21 diagnosed with PTC have an extremely low disease-specific mortality (2% or less decades after diagnosis) [11, 14, 16–23]. This excellent prognosis, coupled with unique concerns regarding the possible long-term sequelae related to overzealous treatment during childhood, makes the management of pediatric PTC challenging. In 2015, formal guidelines for the management of pediatric PTC were published by the American Thyroid Association (ATA) [24]. Other available guidelines include those developed by the Polish National Societies [25].

Over the last few decades, the molecular pathogenesis of PTC has become better understood [26]. In pediatric PTC, chromosomal rearrangements involving the *RE*arranged during *T*ransfection (*RET*) proto-oncogene and the neurotrophic tyrosine receptor kinase (*NTRK*) genes (*NTRK1/3*) are the most common molecular events [27–34]. Although not as common as in adults, mutations in the v-raf murine sarcoma viral oncogene homolog B (*BRAF*) gene (namely, the $BRAF^{V600E}$ point mutation) are also prevalent in childhood PTC [10, 27–30, 32–38]. Knowledge regarding tumor genotype may inform the expected clinical course and response to RAI. For example, the $BRAF^{V600E}$ mutation results in constitutive activation of the mitogen-activated protein kinase pathway and downregulates the expression of genes involved in iodine metabolism, which has implications for disease responsiveness to therapeutic RAI [26, 39].

Children with PTC typically present with a palpable thyroid nodule and/or overt cervical lymphadenopathy [3, 4], which is not uncommonly treated with an antibiotic before the diagnosis of PTC is recognized. The initial workup of newly diagnosed or suspected PTC should include a comprehensive neck US (to include the lateral cervical lymph nodes) by an experienced ultrasonographer. US-guided FNAB in children is a highly sensitive and specific tool for the diagnosis and management of PTC; therefore, it is recommended in all children to confirm the diagnosis. FNAB of suspicious lymph nodes is essential for planning the appropriate surgical approach, which is the mainstay of therapy in pediatric PTC [24].

Contemporary guidelines recommend that children with PTC be cared for at centers where there is multidisciplinary expertise in the management of pediatric thyroid cancer. It is always preferred that surgery be performed by a high-volume thyroid surgeon [24, 40], defined in previous studies as a surgeon who performs 30 or more cervical endocrine procedures annually in adults and children [41], because the rate of permanent complications in children treated for thyroid cancer can be as high as 32% [42]. As anticipated, postoperative hypoparathyroidism is more likely to occur after a central neck dissection [42–44]. Most pediatric patients with PTC will require a total thyroidectomy (TT) with or without a compartment-oriented neck dissection. The type of surgery planned is based on the results of preoperative neck ultrasonography and FNAB. Additionally, cross-sectional imaging, using either a contrast-enhanced CT or MRI of the neck, is recommended for those with fixed thyroid masses, vocal cord paralysis, or bulky lymphadenopathy [2, 24, 25]. Although the use of iodinated CT contrast will delay the immediate postoperative evaluation and treatment with RAI, it is considered the optimal diagnostic study to inform the surgeon about the extent of cervical disease and its anatomic relationship with critical aerodigestive structures.

Numerous studies have shown that the extent of the initial surgery is the single most important factor for improving long-term disease-free survival, with more comprehensive surgery decreasing or eliminating the need for additional surgery and decreasing the risk of recurrence [6, 9, 14, 15, 17, 45, 46]. However, most previous studies are confounded by the routine use of RAI, so additional research is required in the contemporary era of PTC treatment in children, currently characterized by improved preoperative staging (leading to more appropriate initial oncologic surgery) and less utilization of adjuvant RAI therapy. Current guidelines recommend a central neck dissection (CND) in children who have gross extrathyroidal invasion and/or locoregional metastasis identified either pre- or intraoperatively [24, 25]. Comprehensive lateral neck dissection is recommended in those with FNAB-proven lateral neck disease. Patient age, tumor size and focality, vascular invasion, and the number and location of lymph node disease are some of the factors that can help to predict the presence of lymph node disease and the risk of persistent/recurrent cancer [10, 47–50]. Greater understanding of these prognostic factors may inform future guidelines as related to the optimal upfront surgical strategy.

The role of prophylactic CND in pediatric PTC without imaging evidence of lymph node metastases remains controversial. Due to the very high prevalence of cervical metastasis in children, prophylactic CND by a high-volume thyroid surgeon may be selectively considered based upon tumor size and focality. For patients with unifocal PTC, especially tumors >1 cm [10, 51], an ipsilateral CND, with pursuit of contralateral CND only if intraoperative findings suggest central compartment disease, may help to balance the risks and benefits [24, 48, 52]. In all cases, the plan for CND should be driven by the experience of the surgeon, recognizing that lymph node dissection is associated with higher rates of hypoparathyroidism and recurrent laryngeal nerve damage [42, 43]. Preservation of parathyroid and recurrent laryngeal nerve function is paramount, even if all central neck disease is not removed.

The inaugural ATA guidelines introduced a new risk categorization (ATA pediatric low-, intermediate-, and high risk) that helps to identify patients at risk of persistent cervical disease and to determine which patients should undergo more intensive postoperative staging [24]. Children with no or incidental, microscopic central lymph node disease are considered ATA low risk, with recommendations to monitor thyroglobulin (Tg) levels and neck US after the initial surgery. Children with more significant central or lateral neck disease are considered ATA pediatric intermediate risk (clinical N1a or microscopic N1b disease) or high risk (clinical N1b disease), and postoperative staging with a diagnostic RAI scan and a TSH-stimulated Tg is recommended to identify persistent locoregional and distantly metastatic disease [2, 24]. The Polish guidelines suggested a different risk stratification primarily based on tumor size and lymph node stage and, in contrast to the ATA guidelines, recommended that RAI be considered in all cases [25].

Children who are found or suspected to have iodine-avid nodal disease may benefit from ^{131}I therapy if the disease is not amenable to further surgery, as determined after consultation with a thyroid cancer surgeon. Despite RAI, complete remission for cervical disease is seen only in a minority of patients [53]. Children who have no scintigraphic or Tg evidence of residual cervical disease or distant metastases are unlikely to benefit from routine ^{131}I treatment [2, 24], but further research is needed regarding the optimal employment of adjuvant RAI. Nevertheless, clinicians making decisions regarding ^{131}I therapy in locally metastatic pediatric PTC should weigh the long-term risks of RAI (primarily second malignancies) [17, 19, 53–55] against the potential benefits of therapy while recognizing the excellent long-term survival in children with PTC regardless of initial therapy [16].

All children with PTC who have had a total thyroidectomy are replaced with thyroid hormone, and the goal TSH depends on the initial clinical and pathologic staging [2, 24, 25]. In most children with lymph node metastases, the TSH is initially maintained around 0.1 mU/L, and TSH suppression can eventually be reduced in children who have no evidence of disease after a 1–3 year period of follow-up. Similar to adults and even when ^{131}I therapy is not used, Tg levels can be used as a marker of residual or recurrent disease [56, 57], assuming there are no interfering Tg autoantibodies. However, the degree of Tg elevation that correlates to disease is not well studied in children, and current Tg cutoffs employed in the care of adults with PTC may not be applicable to young children. In any event, the trend of the Tg level over time is more informative than an isolated measurement. Finally, cervical US is a highly sensitive clinical tool to identify residual/recurrent PTC, and it is recommended at 6–12 month intervals early in the follow-up period and then with a frequency based upon the patient's perceived recurrence risk and clinical concern for disease [24, 25]. Dynamic risk stratification, similar to what is employed in adults, appears to better prognosticate final disease outcome and allows for a more personalized approach to follow-up in pediatric patients [58].

Back to the Case

Postoperatively, the patient was categorized as ATA pediatric intermediate risk due to extensive N1a and minimal N1b lymph node disease. Therefore, postoperative restaging was undertaken with a hypothyroid ^{123}I thyroid scan (2.2 mCi/81 MBq) and a stimulated Tg, which revealed 0.1% uptake in the right thyroid bed and a value of <0.9 ng/ml with an undetectable Tg antibody, respectively. ^{131}I therapy was not recommended due to the reassuring data, the unclear benefit of RAI in this young patient with an excellent long-term prognosis, as well as the knowledge that the previous lateral right neck disease did not concentrate iodine on a ^{123}I diagnostic scan, suggesting that RAI would not adequately treat any residual microscopic disease. Expectant monitoring and mild TSH suppression were recommended, and 7 years after her third surgery, she remained without evidence of disease based upon neck US and non-stimulated Tg and Tg antibody levels, both of which remained undetectable.

Clinical Pearls

- In the child presenting with a thyroid nodule, FNAB is safe and effective in making a diagnosis of PTC, which in turn allows for the most appropriate surgery (usually total thyroidectomy ± lymph node dissection) to be performed at the outset.
- Lymph node metastases are very common in children with PTC and are best treated by surgical resection.
- Preoperative staging with a comprehensive cervical US and FNAB of suspicious lymph nodes are essential; in addition, contrast-enhanced CT (preferred) or MRI may help to identify additional sites of disease and clarify anatomic relationships, both of which can enhance surgical planning and oncologic outcome.
- Comprehensive surgery, including a compartment-oriented lymph node resection dictated by imaging results, clinical presentation, and intraoperative findings, should be performed by a high-volume thyroid surgeon.

- ^{131}I therapy may not be necessary in all children with lymph node metastases, especially if there is no clinical evidence for residual cervical disease at the time of postoperative staging.
- Not all lymph node disease is iodine-avid, and the role of RAI in eradicating cervical disease in children remains poorly studied; for persistent macroscopic LN disease, repeat surgery by a high-volume thyroid surgeon is preferred over RAI in most cases.
- The follow-up of children with PTC incorporates routine cervical ultrasonography and the measurement of Tg levels; the goal of TSH suppression depends on the extent of initial disease and current disease status.

References

1. Howlader N, Noone AM, Krapcho M, Miller D, Brest A, Yu M, et al. SEER Cancer Statistics Review, 1975–2016, based on November 2018 SEER data submission, posted to the SEER web site, April 2019. Bethesda: National Cancer Institute; [cited 2020 March 31]. Available from: https://seer.cancer.gov/csr/1975_2016/.
2. Waguespack SG, Wasserman JD. Pediatric differentiated thyroid carcinoma. In: Mallick U, Harmer C, Mazzaferri EL, Kendall-Taylor P, editors. Practical management of thyroid cancer: a multidisciplinary approach. 2nd ed: Springer International Publishing; 2018. p. 273–94.
3. Zimmerman D, Hay ID, Gough IR, Goellner JR, Ryan JJ, Grant CS, et al. Papillary thyroid carcinoma in children and adults: long-term follow-up of 1039 patients conservatively treated at one institution during three decades. Surgery. 1988;104(6):1157–66.
4. Frankenthaler RA, Sellin RV, Cangir A, Goepfert H. Lymph node metastasis from papillary-follicular thyroid carcinoma in young patients. Am J Surg. 1990;160(4):341–3.
5. Wada N, Sugino K, Mimura T, Nagahama M, Kitagawa W, Shibuya H, et al. Treatment strategy of papillary thyroid carcinoma in children and adolescents: clinical significance of the initial nodal manifestation. Ann Surg Oncol. 2009;16(12):3442–9.
6. Machens A, Lorenz K, Nguyen Thanh P, Brauckhoff M, Dralle H. Papillary thyroid cancer in children and adolescents does not differ in growth pattern and metastatic behavior. J Pediatr. 2010;157(4):648–52.
7. Newman KD, Black T, Heller G, Azizkhan RG, Holcomb GW 3rd, Sklar C, et al. Differentiated thyroid cancer: determinants of disease progression in patients <21 years of age at diagnosis: a report from the Surgical Discipline Committee of the Children's Cancer Group. Ann Surg. 1998;227(4):533–41.
8. Popovtzer A, Shpitzer T, Bahar G, Feinmesser R, Segal K. Thyroid cancer in children: management and outcome experience of a referral center. Otolaryngol Head Neck Surg. 2006;135(4):581–4.
9. Savio R, Gosnell J, Palazzo FF, Sywak M, Agarwal G, Cowell C, et al. The role of a more extensive surgical approach in the initial multimodality management of papillary thyroid cancer in children. J Pediatr Surg. 2005;40(11):1696–700.
10. Byeon HK, Kim SB, Oh HS, Kim HK, Choi IH, Kim H, et al. Clinical analysis of pediatric thyroid cancer: a single medical institution experience of 18 years. Ann Otol Rhinol Laryngol. 2019;128(12):1152–7. https://doi.org/10.1177/0003489419868251.
11. Pawelczak M, David R, Franklin B, Kessler M, Lam L, Shah B. Outcomes of children and adolescents with well-differentiated thyroid carcinoma and pulmonary metastases following (1)(3)(1)I treatment: a systematic review. Thyroid. 2010;20(10):1095–101.

12. Vassilopoulou-Sellin R, Klein MJ, Smith TH, Samaan NA, Frankenthaler RA, Goepfert H, et al. Pulmonary metastases in children and young adults with differentiated thyroid cancer. Cancer. 1993;71(4):1348–52.
13. Bal CS, Kumar A, Chandra P, Dwivedi SN, Mukhopadhyaya S. Is chest x-ray or high-resolution computed tomography scan of the chest sufficient investigation to detect pulmonary metastasis in pediatric differentiated thyroid cancer? Thyroid. 2004;14(3):217–25.
14. Demidchik YE, Demidchik EP, Reiners C, Biko J, Mine M, Saenko VA, et al. Comprehensive clinical assessment of 740 cases of surgically treated thyroid cancer in children of Belarus. Ann Surg. 2006;243(4):525–32.
15. Handkiewicz-Junak D, Wloch J, Roskosz J, Krajewska J, Kropinska A, Pomorski L, et al. Total thyroidectomy and adjuvant radioiodine treatment independently decrease locoregional recurrence risk in childhood and adolescent differentiated thyroid cancer. J Nucl Med. 2007;48(6):879–88.
16. Golpanian S, Perez EA, Tashiro J, Lew JI, Sola JE, Hogan AR. Pediatric papillary thyroid carcinoma: outcomes and survival predictors in 2504 surgical patients. Pediatr Surg Int. 2016;32(3):201–8.
17. Hay ID, Gonzalez-Losada T, Reinalda MS, Honetschlager JA, Richards ML, Thompson GB. Long-term outcome in 215 children and adolescents with papillary thyroid cancer treated during 1940 through 2008. World J Surg. 2010;34(6):1192–202.
18. Hay ID, Johnson TR, Kaggal S, Reinalda MS, Iniguez-Ariza NM, Grant CS, et al. Papillary thyroid carcinoma (PTC) in children and adults: comparison of initial presentation and long-term postoperative outcome in 4432 patients consecutively treated at the Mayo Clinic during eight decades (1936-2015). World J Surg. 2018;42(2):329–42.
19. Vassilopoulou-Sellin R, Goepfert H, Raney B, Schultz PN. Differentiated thyroid cancer in children and adolescents: clinical outcome and mortality after long-term follow-up. Head Neck. 1998;20(6):549–55.
20. Hogan AR, Zhuge Y, Perez EA, Koniaris LG, Lew JI, Sola JE. Pediatric thyroid carcinoma: incidence and outcomes in 1753 patients. J Surg Res. 2009;156(1):167–72.
21. Bal CS, Garg A, Chopra S, Ballal S, Soundararajan R. Prognostic factors in pediatric differentiated thyroid cancer patients with pulmonary metastases. J Pediatr Endocrinol Metab. 2015;28(7-8):745–51.
22. Alzahrani AS, Alswailem M, Moria Y, Almutairi R, Alotaibi M, Murugan AK, et al. Lung metastasis in pediatric thyroid cancer: radiological pattern, molecular genetics, response to therapy, and outcome. J Clin Endocrinol Metab. 2019;104(1):103–10.
23. Samuel AM, Rajashekharrao B, Shah DH. Pulmonary metastases in children and adolescents with well-differentiated thyroid cancer. J Nucl Med. 1998;39(9):1531–6.
24. Francis GL, Waguespack SG, Bauer AJ, Angelos P, Benvenga S, Cerutti JM, et al. Management guidelines for children with thyroid nodules and differentiated thyroid cancer. Thyroid. 2015;25(7):716–59.
25. Niedziela M, Handkiewicz-Junak D, Malecka-Tendera E, Czarniecka A, Dedecjus M, Lange D, et al. Diagnostics and treatment of differentiated thyroid carcinoma in children - Guidelines of Polish National Societies. Endokrynol Pol. 2016;67(6):628–42.
26. Cancer Genome Atlas Research N. Integrated genomic characterization of papillary thyroid carcinoma. Cell. 2014;159(3):676–90.
27. Bauer AJ. Molecular genetics of thyroid cancer in children and adolescents. Endocrinol Metab Clin N Am. 2017;46(2):389–403.
28. Prasad ML, Vyas M, Horne MJ, Virk RK, Morotti R, Liu Z, et al. NTRK fusion oncogenes in pediatric papillary thyroid carcinoma in Northeast United States. Cancer. 2016;122(7):1097–107.
29. Picarsic JL, Buryk MA, Ozolek J, Ranganathan S, Monaco SE, Simons JP, et al. Molecular characterization of sporadic pediatric thyroid carcinoma with the DNA/RNA ThyroSeq v2 next-generation sequencing assay. Pediatr Dev Pathol. 2016;19(2):115–22.

30. Nikita ME, Jiang W, Cheng SM, Hantash FM, McPhaul MJ, Newbury RO, et al. Mutational analysis in pediatric thyroid cancer and correlations with age, ethnicity, and clinical presentation. Thyroid. 2016;26(2):227–34.
31. Cordioli MI, Moraes L, Bastos AU, Besson P, Alves MT, Delcelo R, et al. Fusion oncogenes are the main genetic events found in sporadic papillary thyroid carcinomas from children. Thyroid. 2017;27(2):182–8.
32. Vanden Borre P, Schrock AB, Anderson PM, Morris JC 3rd, Heilmann AM, Holmes O, et al. Pediatric, adolescent, and young adult thyroid carcinoma harbors frequent and diverse targetable genomic alterations, including kinase fusions. Oncologist. 2017;22(3):255–63.
33. Pekova B, Dvorakova S, Sykorova V, Vacinova G, Vaclavikova E, Moravcova J, et al. Somatic genetic alterations in a large cohort of pediatric thyroid nodules. Endocr Connect. 2019;8:796.
34. Mostoufi-Moab S, Labourier E, Sullivan L, LiVolsi V, Li Y, Xiao R, et al. Molecular testing for oncogenic gene alterations in pediatric thyroid lesions. Thyroid. 2018;28(1):60–7.
35. Cordioli MI, Moraes L, Cury AN, Cerutti JM. Are we really at the dawn of understanding sporadic pediatric thyroid carcinoma? Endocr Relat Cancer. 2015;22(6):R311–24.
36. Ballester LY, Sarabia SF, Sayeed H, Patel N, Baalwa J, Athanassaki I, et al. Integrating molecular testing in the diagnosis and management of children with thyroid lesions. Pediatr Dev Pathol. 2016;19(2):94–100.
37. Alzahrani AS, Murugan AK, Qasem E, Alswailem M, Al-Hindi H, Shi Y. Single point mutations in pediatric differentiated thyroid cancer. Thyroid. 2017;27(2):189–96.
38. Sisdelli L, Cordioli M, Vaisman F, Moraes L, Colozza-Gama GA, Alves PAG Jr, et al. AGK-BRAF is associated with distant metastasis and younger age in pediatric papillary thyroid carcinoma. Pediatr Blood Cancer. 2019;66(7):e27707.
39. Chakravarty D, Santos E, Ryder M, Knauf JA, Liao XH, West BL, et al. Small-molecule MAPK inhibitors restore radioiodine incorporation in mouse thyroid cancers with conditional BRAF activation. J Clin Invest. 2011;121(12):4700–11.
40. Baumgarten HD, Bauer AJ, Isaza A, Mostoufi-Moab S, Kazahaya K, Adzick NS. Surgical management of pediatric thyroid disease: complication rates after thyroidectomy at the Children's Hospital of Philadelphia high-volume Pediatric Thyroid Center. J Pediatr Surg. 2019;54:1969.
41. Tuggle CT, Roman SA, Wang TS, Boudourakis L, Thomas DC, Udelsman R, et al. Pediatric endocrine surgery: who is operating on our children? Surgery. 2008;144(6):869–77; discussion 77
42. Klein Hesselink MS, Nies M, Bocca G, Brouwers AH, Burgerhof JG, van Dam EW, et al. Pediatric differentiated thyroid carcinoma in the Netherlands: a nationwide follow-up study. J Clin Endocrinol Metab. 2016;101(5):2031–9.
43. Wu SY, Chiang YJ, Fisher SB, Sturgis EM, Zafereo ME, Nguyen S, et al. Risks of hypoparathyroidism after total thyroidectomy in children: a 21-year experience in a high-volume cancer center. World J Surg. 2020;44(2):442–51.
44. Zobel MJ, Long R, Gosnell J, Sosa JA, Padilla BE. Postoperative hypoparathyroidism after total thyroidectomy in children. J Surg Res. 2020;252:63–8.
45. Jarzab B, Handkiewicz Junak D, Wloch J, Kalemba B, Roskosz J, Kukulska A, et al. Multivariate analysis of prognostic factors for differentiated thyroid carcinoma in children. Eur J Nucl Med. 2000;27(7):833–41.
46. Sywak M, Cornford L, Roach P, Stalberg P, Sidhu S, Delbridge L. Routine ipsilateral level VI lymphadenectomy reduces postoperative thyroglobulin levels in papillary thyroid cancer. Surgery. 2006;140(6):1000–5; discussion 5–7.
47. Jain NK, Mostoufi-Moab S, Hawkes CP, Nelson ND, Surrey LF, Jones ZS, et al. Extrathyroidal extension is an important predictor of regional lymph node metastasis in pediatric differentiated thyroid cancer. Thyroid. 2020;30(7):1037–43.
48. Spinelli C, Tognetti F, Strambi S, Morganti R, Massimino M, Collini P. Cervical lymph node metastases of papillary thyroid carcinoma, in the central and lateral compartments, in children and adolescents: predictive factors. World J Surg. 2018;42(8):2444–53.

49. Jeon MJ, Kim YN, Sung TY, Hong SJ, Cho YY, Kim TY, et al. Practical initial risk stratification based on lymph node metastases in pediatric and adolescent differentiated thyroid cancer. Thyroid. 2018;28(2):193–200.
50. Lazar L, Lebenthal Y, Segal K, Steinmetz A, Strenov Y, Cohen M, et al. Pediatric thyroid cancer: postoperative classifications and response to initial therapy as prognostic factors. J Clin Endocrinol Metab. 2016;101(5):1970–9.
51. Lee KE, Chung IY, Kang E, Koo do H, Kim KH, Kim SW, et al. Ipsilateral and contralateral central lymph node metastasis in papillary thyroid cancer: patterns and predictive factors of nodal metastasis. Head Neck. 2013;35(5):672–6.
52. Verburg FA, Van Santen HM, Luster M. Pediatric papillary thyroid cancer: current management challenges. Onco Targets Ther. 2017;10:165–75.
53. Wu X, Gu H, Gao Y, Li B, Fan R. Clinical outcomes and prognostic factors of radioiodine ablation therapy for lymph node metastases from papillary thyroid carcinoma. Nucl Med Commun. 2018;39(1):22–7.
54. Albano D, Bertagna F, Panarotto MB, Giubbini R. Early and late adverse effects of radioiodine for pediatric differentiated thyroid cancer. Pediatr Blood Cancer. 2017;64.
55. Iyer NG, Morris LG, Tuttle RM, Shaha AR, Ganly I. Rising incidence of second cancers in patients with low-risk (T1N0) thyroid cancer who receive radioactive iodine therapy. Cancer. 2011;117(19):4439–46.
56. Durante C, Montesano T, Attard M, Torlontano M, Monzani F, Costante G, et al. Long-term surveillance of papillary thyroid cancer patients who do not undergo postoperative radioiodine remnant ablation: is there a role for serum thyroglobulin measurement? J Clin Endocrinol Metab. 2012;97(8):2748–53.
57. Evans C, Tennant S, Perros P. Thyroglobulin in differentiated thyroid cancer. Clin Chim Acta. 2015;444:310–7.
58. Ajdari SE, Shafiei B, Motazedian M, Qutbi M, Esmaeilzadeh P, Asli IN, et al. Shifting paradigms in the management of pediatric differentiated thyroid cancer from static to dynamic risk stratification: a step forward toward precision medicine. Nuklearmedizin. 2019;58(3):249–57.

Part II
Differentiated Thyroid Cancer: Postoperative Follow-Up

Chapter 12
A Patient with Papillary Thyroid Cancer and Biochemical Evidence of Possible Residual Disease at the One-Year Follow-Up Visit

Valeria Ramundo, Sebastiano Filetti, and Cosimo Durante

Case Presentation

A 54-year-old man with type 2 diabetes and hypertension underwent carotid arterial Doppler US assessment as part of a primary cardiovascular prevention program. He was referred to our center because of the incidental finding of an asymptomatic nodule in the right lobe of the thyroid. Thyroid and neck US revealed a 2.4 cm hypoechoic right thyroid nodule, with irregular margins and suspicion of extrathyroidal extension. No suspicious lymph nodes were observed. The patient was euthyroid (serum TSH level of 1.6 mU/L). Fine-needle aspiration biopsy (FNAB) revealed cytological findings suggestive of papillary thyroid cancer (PTC) (Bethesda class V) [1].

A total thyroidectomy was performed, and the surgical pathology showed a follicular-variant PTC measuring 2.2 cm without evidence of extrathyroidal extension or vascular invasion (pT2, N0b – stage 1, according to the AJCC/TNM VIII Edition) [2]. According to the 2015 ATA Initial Risk Stratification System, the patient's disease was considered to be at low risk for recurrence [3]. After discussing these findings with the patient, and the pros and cons of radioactive iodine remnant ablation (RRA), he decided to forego the RAI treatment and to be followed with surveillance. The neck US examination performed at the 1-year follow-up visit did not reveal evidence of residual tumor nor suspicious lymph nodes. However, biochemical evaluation showed serum thyroglobulin (Tg) level of 3.5 ng/mL (normal after total thyroidectomy <0.2 ng/mL) with a TSH level of 1.1 mU/L and negative antithyroglobulin antibodies.

V. Ramundo · S. Filetti · C. Durante (✉)
Department of Translational and Precision Medicine, Sapienza University of Rome, Rome, Italy
e-mail: cosimo.durante@uniroma1.it

G. Grani et al. (eds.), *Thyroid Cancer*,
https://doi.org/10.1007/978-3-030-61919-0_12

Literature Review

What Is the Role of Serum Tg Measurement in Patients Who Have Not Undergone Radioiodine Remnant Ablation?

The role played by serum Tg analysis in the postoperative management of patients with PTC continues to evolve. Because Tg is produced solely by cells of thyroid follicular origin, its presence in the serum of a patient with PTC who has undergone thyroidectomy followed by RRA is a highly specific marker of residual or recurrent tumor tissue [3, 4]. But, in the growing number of cases in which RRA is omitted (i.e., those characterized by a low-to-intermediate ATA risk for recurrence), the specificity of assay positivity is lost, since there is no reliable cutoff for distinguishing Tg production by recurrent tumor tissue from that synthesized by nests of normal thyrocytes left behind after surgery. The specificity has been further diminished by the introduction of increasingly sensitive immunometric Tg assays [5]. In the past, Tg levels <1 ng/mL were considered "undetectable," but most assays being used today have functional sensitivity limits of 0.2 ng/mL, and second-generation assays can detect serum concentrations as low as 0.1 ng/mL. The clinical significance of this low-level production is uncertain, and large prospective studies are needed to define the cutoff between benign and malignant Tg production.

While the clinical significance of a single positive serum Tg assay is obviously uncertain in a non-radioiodine-ablated patient, *serial* measurements can still provide valuable information on the likelihood of persistent/recurrent disease [6, 7]. Benign production by the normal thyroid remnant is characterized by progressive, spontaneous decline over time, and studies of ATA low-risk nonablated populations indicate that in well over half (60%) of all cases, unstimulated Tg levels will drop below 0.2 ng/mL during the first year after surgery. By 5 years, this subgroup will comprise close to 80% of the population [6]. Once these levels have been achieved, nonablated patients are on equal footing with their ablated counterparts in terms of the diagnostic value of serum Tg assays for detecting persistent/recurrent disease. In 20% of the low-risk patients studied, however, Tg production declined steadily and subsequently plateaued at low but still detectable levels, but this pattern was also associated with the absence of structural disease at the end of follow-up (median 5 years). The single case of recurrence observed in the entire study population (n = 290) was heralded by a progressive rise in previously stable Tg levels [6]. Indeed, increasing Tg production (in particular, a Tg doubling time of <1 year) has repeatedly emerged as a strong predictor of the presence of locoregional and/or distant recurrence, even if RRA has been omitted [8].

Technically speaking, serum thyroglobulin assays should always be calibrated against the international CRM457 standard, and serial measurements for a given patient should ideally be performed by the same laboratory with the same assay. Anti-Tg antibodies should also be quantitatively assessed with each measurement of serum Tg [3]. These autoantibodies are present in approximately 25% of all patients with differentiated thyroid cancer, and they can cause falsely low or undetectable levels in immunometric assays for Tg [3]. There is no method that can reliably eliminate this interference. Radioimmunoassays are advocated by some as a less susceptible alternative, but they have limitations of their own (low availability and sensitivity and potential for falsely elevated Tg values), and their role in patient management is uncertain [3]. Temporal trends in serum anti-Tg antibody titers (again, measured with the same assay) have been used to distinguish residual normal thyroid tissue from recurrent tumor, although they are less precise than serum Tg trends [9–12].

What Is the Role of Neck US or Other Imaging Techniques?

While the results of serum Tg assays in nonablated PTC patients become more informative as follow-up progresses, neck US provides valuable information right from the start, and it plays an indispensable role in the initial assessment of patients during the follow-up, when Tg assay results may be difficult to interpret. Disease spread or recurrence almost always begins in the cervical lymph nodes, where it can be readily detected by ultrasound imaging, especially after thyroidectomy. Sonographic criteria for identifying nodal metastases in the neck are well established [13–15], and in experienced hands, neck ultrasound consistently proves to be much more sensitive for detecting this type of involvement than diagnostic I^{131}WBS [16, 17]. Its negative predictive power is excellent, even with the first preoperative scan (3–12 months after surgery), approaching 100% in patients with an ATA low risk of recurrence [18]. Its specificity can be improved if suspicious nodes are subjected to fine-needle aspiration biopsy (FNAB) for cytologic confirmation (or assessment of Tg levels in the needle washout) [19]. Neck ultrasound examination also furnishes important information for surgeons on the location of involved nodes. It is important to note that neck ultrasound should ideally be performed only by experienced sonography technicians or physicians.

Patients with PTC belonging to low- and intermediate-risk categories, with negative US findings and unstimulated Tg levels <1 ng/mL at the 1-year follow-up visit, can be safely followed with clinical assessments and unstimulated serum Tg determinations. Neck US might be repeated if anti-Tg antibody levels rise or unstimulated Tg levels exceed 1 ng/mL [20].

In the absence of positive neck findings on the ultrasound, distant metastases are rare. However, if Tg levels are increasing or the patient has suspicious signs/symptoms, the presence of extracervical lesions should be excluded with second-line imaging studies. These include both cross-sectional modalities (computed tomography or magnetic resonance imaging) and nuclear medicine procedures (WBS and 2-[18F]fluoro-2-deoxyglucose–positron emission tomography, 18FDG–PET) [3, 4]. 18FDG–PET findings are also potentially helpful for treatment planning since FDG-avid lesions are almost invariably refractory to high-dose radioiodine therapy, and they are associated with very high rates of disease-specific mortality [21, 22].

What Are the Criteria for the Absence of Persistent Tumor?

According to the 2015 ATA guidelines [3], patients who have undergone RRA can be considered disease-free when the following three conditions have been met: (1) the absence of clinical evidence of disease, (2) negative imaging studies (i.e., no extra-thyroidal uptake on the initial postoperative WBS and/or outside the thyroid bed on the initial posttreatment WBS, if performed, or, if uptake outside the thyroid bed had been present, no imaging evidence of tumor on a recent diagnostic or post-therapy WBS) and/or neck US, and (3) serum Tg levels that are <0.2 ng/mL during TSH suppression and <1 ng/mL after stimulation in the absence of interfering antibodies. The final criterion cannot be applied to patients in whom RRA has been omitted: the persistence of low-level Tg production that exceeds these limits but remains stable over time may be indicative of "minimal residual disease," but it may also stem from the normal thyroid remnant. Various subsequent studies proposed different criteria and serum Tg thresholds for patients not undergoing RRA: a proposal was included in the 2019 Guidelines of the European Society for Medical Oncology [23] (Table 12.1). It is important to recall that PTCs are slow-growing tumors and the likelihood of distant metastases in the absence of cervical lymph node involvement is extremely low. Therefore, if there is no sonographic evidence of neck disease, most patients can be safely managed with watchful waiting based on yearly US and periodic Tg assays [24]. The risk declines after the first 5 years of follow-up: in an Italian cohort, 77% of all recurrences are observed during this interval [25]. According to a recent Japanese study, 36.9% of the recurrences were detected in this timeframe; however, late recurrences even 10 or more years after initial treatment are still possible, particularly in case of risk factors (age ≥ 55 years, male gender, tumor size >4 cm, lymph node metastases, and extranodal extension) [26]. The duration of long-term follow-up is not yet defined and should be refined by future studies evaluating the event rate in real-world cohorts, followed using contemporary tools (such as ultrasensitive Tg, neck US, cross-sectional and functional imaging).

Back to the Patient

The possibility of a detectable Tg result at the 1-year follow-up visit had already been discussed with the patient when he decided to avoid RRA after total thyroidectomy. When the results were back, the implications of the findings were reviewed and management options were discussed. Given the low risk of recurrence and the negative sonographic findings, the proposal was made to proceed with follow-up as originally planned, with yearly neck US and serum Tg assays, and the patient agreed. The imaging findings continued to be unequivocally negative, and the serum Tg levels were already lower by the second-year visit. They declined steadily thereafter and dropped below 0.2 ng/mL at the 4-year visit (Fig. 12.1). Five years have passed since the thyroidectomy, and the patient remains symptom-free with no evidence of disease.

Table 12.1 Responses to treatment categories

Responses to treatment	Treatments: TT+RRA	TT alone	Lobectomy
Excellent	Negative imaging AND	Negative imaging AND	Negative imaging AND
	Undetectable TgAb AND	Undetectable TgAb AND	Undetectable TgAb AND
	Tg < 0.2 ng/mL OR S-Tg < 1 ng/mL	Tg < 0.2 ng/mL	Stable Tg levels
Biochemical incomplete	Negative imaging AND	Negative imaging AND	Negative imaging AND
	Tg ≥ 1 ng/mL OR S-Tg ≥ 10 ng/mL OR Rising TgAb levels	Tg > 5 ng/mL OR Rising Tg values with similar TSH levels OR Rising TgAb levels	Rising Tg values with similar TSH levels OR Rising TgAb levels
Structural incomplete	Imaging evidence of disease (regardless of Tg or TgAb)		
Indeterminate	Nonspecific imaging findings OR	Nonspecific imaging findings OR	Nonspecific imaging findings
	Faint uptake in thyroid bed on RAI scanning OR		
	Tg 0.2–1 ng/mL OR S-Tg 1–10 ng/mL OR TgAb stable OR declining in patient with no imaging evidence of disease	Tg 0.2–5 ng/mL OR TgAb levels stable or declining in the absence of structural or functional disease	

Reprinted with permission from Filetti et al. [23]
Abbreviations: *ATA* American Thyroid Association, *RAI* radioactive iodine, *RRA* radioactive iodine remnant ablation, *S-Tg* TSH-stimulated serum thyroglobulin, *Tg* serum thyroglobulin, *TgAb* anti-Tg antibodies, *TT* total thyroidectomy

Clinical Pearls

- Neck ultrasound is the mainstay of follow-up for PTC patients who have not undergone post-thyroidectomy RRA, especially during the first 5 years when serum Tg levels may be relatively uninformative.
- In over half of all PTC patients who have not undergone RRA, benign Tg production is already undetectable (i.e., <0.2 ng/mL) at the 1-year follow-up visit, and the percentage approaches 80% by year 5. For this subset of patients, the specificity of a positive serum Tg assay for predicting persistent/recurrent disease is the same as it is in ablated patients.
- Roughly one out of five nonablated patients will have persistent, stable low-level production (≥0.2 ng/mL). In the absence of clinical or imaging evidence of disease, watchful waiting may be the most appropriate course in these cases.

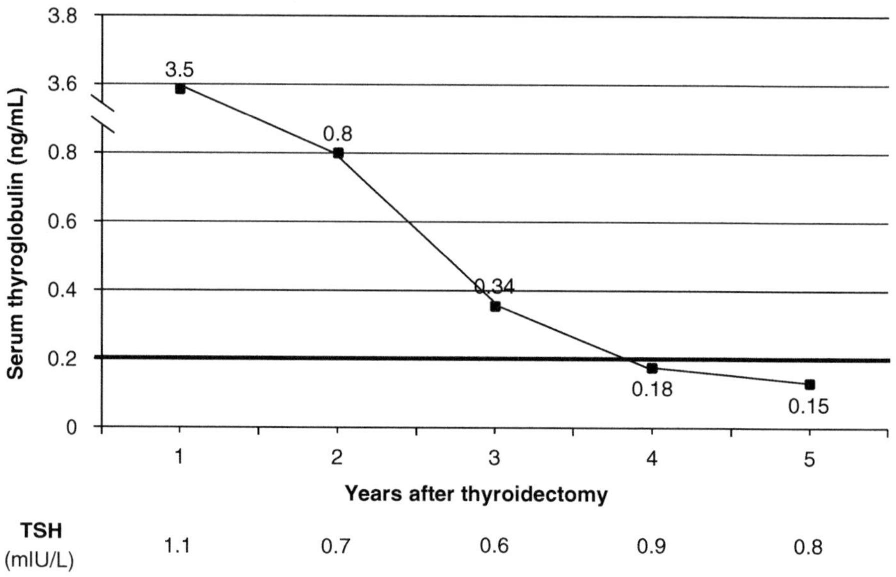

Fig. 12.1 Trend of serial basal Tg determination during the first 5 years after thyroidectomy. The graph line displays the Tg levels obtained with a highly sensitive immunometric assay (functional sensitivity, 0.2 ng/mL) at each annual visit. The corresponding TSH values are reported in the graph

References

1. Cibas ES, Ali SZ. The 2017 Bethesda system for reporting thyroid cytopathology. Thyroid. 2017;27(11):1341–6.
2. Amin MB, Greene FL, Edge SB, Compton CC, Gershenwald JE, Brookland RK, et al. The Eighth Edition AJCC Cancer Staging Manual: continuing to build a bridge from a population-based to a more "personalized" approach to cancer staging. CA Cancer J Clin. 2017;67(2):93–9.
3. Haugen BR, Alexander EK, Bible KC, Doherty GM, Mandel SJ, Nikiforov YE, et al. 2015 American Thyroid Association management guidelines for adult patients with thyroid nodules and differentiated thyroid cancer: the American Thyroid Association guidelines task force on thyroid nodules and differentiated thyroid cancer. Thyroid. 2016;26(1):1–133.
4. Pacini F, Schlumberger M, Dralle H, Elisei R, Smit JW, Wiersinga W. European consensus for the management of patients with differentiated thyroid carcinoma of the follicular epithelium. Eur J Endocrinol. 2006;154(6):787–803.
5. Schlumberger M, Hitzel A, Toubert ME, Corone C, Troalen F, Schlageter MH, et al. Comparison of seven serum thyroglobulin assays in the follow-up of papillary and follicular thyroid cancer patients. J Clin Endocrinol Metab. 2007;92(7):2487–95.
6. Durante C, Montesano T, Attard M, Torlontano M, Monzani F, Costante G, et al. Long-term surveillance of papillary thyroid cancer patients who do not undergo postoperative radioiodine remnant ablation: is there a role for serum thyroglobulin measurement? J Clin Endocrinol Metab. 2012;97(8):2748–53.
7. Angell TE, Spencer CA, Rubino BD, Nicoloff JT, LoPresti JS. In search of an unstimulated thyroglobulin baseline value in low-risk papillary thyroid carcinoma patients not receiving radioactive iodine ablation. Thyroid. 2014;24(7):1127–33.

8. Miyauchi A, Kudo T, Miya A, Kobayashi K, Ito Y, Takamura Y, et al. Prognostic impact of serum thyroglobulin doubling-time under thyrotropin suppression in patients with papillary thyroid carcinoma who underwent total thyroidectomy. Thyroid. 2011;21(7):707–16.
9. Spencer CA, Takeuchi M, Kazarosyan M, Wang CC, Guttler RB, Singer PA, et al. Serum thyroglobulin autoantibodies: prevalence, influence on serum thyroglobulin measurement, and prognostic significance in patients with differentiated thyroid carcinoma. J Clin Endocrinol Metab. 1998;83(4):1121–7.
10. Chiovato L, Latrofa F, Braverman LE, Pacini F, Capezzone M, Masserini L, et al. Disappearance of humoral thyroid autoimmunity after complete removal of thyroid antigens. Ann Intern Med. 2003;139(5 Pt 1):346–51.
11. Kim WG, Yoon JH, Kim WB, Kim TY, Kim EY, Kim JM, et al. Change of serum antithyroglobulin antibody levels is useful for prediction of clinical recurrence in thyroglobulin-negative patients with differentiated thyroid carcinoma. J Clin Endocrinol Metab. 2008;93(12):4683–9.
12. Durante C, Tognini S, Montesano T, Orlandi F, Torlontano M, Puxeddu E, et al. Clinical aggressiveness and long-term outcome in patients with papillary thyroid cancer and circulating anti-thyroglobulin autoantibodies. Thyroid. 2014;24(7):1139–45.
13. Leboulleux S, Girard E, Rose M, Travagli JP, Sabbah N, Caillou B, et al. Ultrasound criteria of malignancy for cervical lymph nodes in patients followed up for differentiated thyroid cancer. J Clin Endocrinol Metab. 2007;92(9):3590–4.
14. Leenhardt L, Erdogan MF, Hegedus L, Mandel SJ, Paschke R, Rago T, et al. 2013 European thyroid association guidelines for cervical ultrasound scan and ultrasound-guided techniques in the postoperative management of patients with thyroid cancer. Eur Thyroid J. 2013;2(3):147–59.
15. Lamartina L, Grani G, Biffoni M, Giacomelli L, Costante G, Lupo S, et al. Risk stratification of neck lesions detected sonographically during the follow-up of differentiated thyroid cancer. J Clin Endocrinol Metabol. 2016;101(8):3036–44.
16. Pacini F, Molinaro E, Castagna MG, Agate L, Elisei R, Ceccarelli C, et al. Recombinant human thyrotropin-stimulated serum thyroglobulin combined with neck ultrasonography has the highest sensitivity in monitoring differentiated thyroid carcinoma. J Clin Endocrinol Metab. 2003;88(8):3668–73.
17. Torlontano M, Attard M, Crocetti U, Tumino S, Bruno R, Costante G, et al. Follow-up of low risk patients with papillary thyroid cancer: role of neck ultrasonography in detecting lymph node metastases. J Clin Endocrinol Metab. 2004;89(7):3402–7.
18. Durante C, Attard M, Torlontano M, Ronga G, Monzani F, Costante G, et al. Identification and optimal postsurgical follow-up of patients with very low-risk papillary thyroid microcarcinomas. J Clin Endocrinol Metab. 2010;95(11):4882–8.
19. Grani G, Fumarola A. Thyroglobulin in lymph node fine-needle aspiration washout: a systematic review and meta-analysis of diagnostic accuracy. J Clin Endocrinol Metabol. 2014;99(6):1970–82.
20. Grani G, Ramundo V, Falcone R, Lamartina L, Montesano T, Biffoni M, et al. Thyroid cancer patients with no evidence of disease: the need for repeat neck ultrasound. J Clin Endocrinol Metab. 2019;104(11):4981–9.
21. Robbins RJ, Wan Q, Grewal RK, Reibke R, Gonen M, Strauss HW, et al. Real-time prognosis for metastatic thyroid carcinoma based on 2-[18F]fluoro-2-deoxy-D-glucose-positron emission tomography scanning. J Clin Endocrinol Metab. 2006;91(2):498–505.
22. Kang JH, Jung DW, Pak KJ, Kim IJ, Kim HJ, Cho JK, et al. Prognostic implication of fluorine-18 fluorodeoxyglucose positron emission tomography/computed tomography in patients with recurrent papillary thyroid cancer. Head Neck. 2018;40(1):94–102.
23. Filetti S, Durante C, Hartl D, Leboulleux S, Locati LD, Newbold K, et al. Thyroid cancer: ESMO Clinical Practice Guidelines for diagnosis, treatment and follow-up. Ann Oncol. 2019;30(12):1856–83.

24. Lamartina L, Grani G, Durante C, Borget I, Filetti S, Schlumberger M. Follow-up of differentiated thyroid cancer - what should (and what should not) be done. Nat Rev Endocrinol. 2018;14(9):538–51.
25. Durante C, Montesano T, Torlontano M, Attard M, Monzani F, Tumino S, et al. Papillary thyroid cancer: time course of recurrences during postsurgery surveillance. J Clin Endocrinol Metab. 2013;98(2):636–42.
26. Dong W, Horiuchi K, Tokumitsu H, Sakamoto A, Noguchi E, Ueda Y, et al. Time-varying pattern of mortality and recurrence from papillary thyroid cancer: lessons from a long-term follow-up. Thyroid. 2019;29(6):802–8.

Chapter 13
A Patient with Low-Risk Papillary Thyroid Cancer Who Has Undergone a Lobectomy: Monitoring for Recurrent Disease and Assessment of Thyroid Function

Fernanda Vaisman and Marcela Vaisberg Cohen

Clinical Case Presentation

A 22-year-old female was diagnosed with a 1.4 cm thyroid nodule in the right lobe, highly suspicious at ultrasound. FNA biopsy showed Bethesda VI, suggestive of papillary thyroid carcinoma. Neck ultrasound preoperatively showed no abnormal lymph nodes, and thyroid function tests showed serum TSH levels of 1.5 mUI/L. After discussing with the patient and a multidisciplinary team, she underwent a right lobectomy and isthmectomy. The surgery went well, with no complications. Pathology report showed a 1.4 cm classic papillary thyroid carcinoma limited to the thyroid gland and a normal, 0.2 cm, parathyroid lymph node (pT1b N0 Mx).

Assessment and Literature Review

The prevalence of differentiated thyroid cancer (DTC) has been increasing considerably worldwide. It is currently the fourth most frequent malignant neoplasm among Brazilian women, disregarding non-melanoma skin carcinomas [1]. In 2018, the National Cancer Institute – INCa – estimated an incidence of 11.2 cases per 100,000 women and 2.78 cases per 100,000 men of thyroid cancer in Rio de Janeiro [1], 90% of which are differentiated carcinomas. In addition to this, the indolent nature of the disease and the high survival rate contribute to this increasing

F. Vaisman (✉)
Department of Endocrinology, National cancer Institute- INCa, Universidade Federal do Rio de Janeiro- Medical School, Rio de Janeiro, RJ, Brazil

M. V. Cohen
Department of Endocrinology, Universidade Federal do Rio de Janeiro- Medical School, Rio de Janeiro, RJ, Brazil

G. Grani et al. (eds.), *Thyroid Cancer*,
https://doi.org/10.1007/978-3-030-61919-0_13

prevalence. Thus, ensuring a good quality of life for these patients becomes even more important.

Despite the low mortality, there is a high recurrence and persistence rate, which is estimated at 20–30% [2]. Based on this, the American Thyroid Association (ATA), as well as other organizations (European Thyroid Association [ETA] and the Latin American Thyroid Society [LATS]), began to classify DTCs according to their risk of recurrence and persistence by analyzing some postoperative characteristics. Therefore, it is defined as low risk: papillary or follicular thyroid carcinoma with no evidence of local or distant metastasis; no macroscopic signs of remnant tumor; no extrathyroidal invasion; no aggressive histological characteristics; no vascular invasion (if papillary carcinoma); up to five affected cervical lymph nodes, measuring less than 0.2 cm in diameter; no radioactive iodine (RAI)-avid metastatic foci outside the thyroid bed on the first posttreatment whole-body RAI scan; follicular thyroid carcinoma with vascular invasion of up to four foci; and unifocal or multifocal thyroid papillary microcarcinoma (<1 cm), even if BRAF V600E mutation is positive [3]. Studies assessing the risk of persistent or recurrent disease in different specialized centers around the world have shown that, in low-risk patients, 78–91% had no evidence of disease within 10 years after surgical treatment and RAI therapy. Other studies have confirmed these results, even when RAI therapy was not performed, detecting 1–2% of recurrent or persistent structural disease in these patients [3].

The treatment for differentiated thyroid carcinomas consists of total or partial thyroidectomy, with or without adjuvant RAI therapy. Patients with tumors smaller than 4 cm, no extrathyroidal extension, no lymph node or distant metastasis (apparent on preoperative imaging), no history of neck radiation, no family history of thyroid cancer in first-degree relatives, and without contralateral disease may be submitted to lobectomy since they have a high probability of being low-risk tumors. In such cases, adjuvant therapy is not routinely indicated [3]. As a result, these patients may not require thyroid hormone replacement. Both factors, RAI therapy and thyroid hormone replacement, when applied, can affect the patient's quality of life in a negative way.

The choice of how extensive the surgery should be on low-risk DTC patients has been a subject of great discussion in recent years. The advantages of total thyroidectomy in these cases include easier follow-up with biochemical markers and ultrasound as well as less uncertainty about the therapeutic response and disease-free status. However, there are some disadvantages. In addition to the complications inherent in any surgery of these proportions (anesthetic risk, poor healing with unfavorable aesthetic outcomes, and infection), vocal changes, hypoparathyroidism (transient or permanent), and possible respiratory failure due to bilateral recurrent laryngeal nerve injury have greater risk in this type of surgery than in a less extensive one. Also, patients undergoing this surgery will need thyroid hormone replacement therapy for life [2]. It is true that the decision to perform the lobectomy harbors the possibility of a complementation of the surgery if high-risk histopathological characteristics in the surgical piece are found. On the other hand, in most cases (around 80%), there is no need for postoperative hormone replacement with levothyroxine, the risks inherent to surgery are lower, and the cost of the treatment is also favorable [2, 4]. Several studies have shown that, for low-risk DTC, the prognosis, among patients undergoing total thyroidectomy or lobectomy, is similar [2, 5–9]. This way, it is up to the medical team, along with the patient, to decide what is the best surgery for them. Thus, the assessment of the patient's quality of life in face of this decision becomes crucial and can be pivotal for this choice.

Numerous studies have assessed the quality of life in DTC survivors, reporting a global fall in the parameters evaluated, with the neuropsychometric assessments being the most relevant [10, 11]. Some of these studies even showed inferior results for survivors of DTC compared to other tumors with worse prognosis and more aggressive treatment [10, 11]. Factors that have been associated with risk of poorer quality of life include younger age, female gender, and lower educational level [10]. Still, there is an instability in the quality of life of these patients, especially in the first 5 years after treatment [10]. After this period, or even earlier, a plateau can be reached and then improved back to pre-treatment levels [10, 12]. However, there are conflicting results in previous research in that some studies have supported a normalization of the quality of life, while others have demonstrated that, although improving over the years, it does not completely normalize [10–13].

The problem that arises from this treatment approach is: how should these patients be followed? Periodic clinical examination of the neck is essential, but whole-body scan using 131I (WBS) is not valuable because there is known residual thyroid tissue that will show up in imaging. A major change in the follow-up of patients with papillary thyroid cancer has been the use of neck ultrasound and serum thyroglobulin (Tg) levels, which have replaced the routine use of radioactive iodine WBS. Ultrasound is a very useful tool to follow patients who underwent lobectomies for their first surgical approach. In patients who have had thyroid ablation, serum Tg, measured while the patient is taking L-thyroxine, is a suitable "cancer" marker with high sensitivity and specificity [14]. Because Tg is produced by all thyroid tissue, normal and abnormal, it is stated that it has less value in the follow-up of patients with residual thyroid tissue [15–17].

Momesso et al. showed that the same concept of risk-adapted approach and response evaluation to the initial therapy can be applied for patients who underwent partial thyroidectomy with a very good correlation with major outcomes, such as mortality and structural recurrence [18]. Thus, it is possible to follow those patients the same way as the ones who underwent total thyroidectomy: with ultrasound (that in this scenario is crucial) and non-stimulated thyroglobulin, especially its over-time trend.

Finally, as these are low-risk patients, the ATA guidelines [3] do not recommend TSH suppressive therapy. In these cases, serum TSH levels should be between 0.5 and 2.0 mUI/L.

Back to the Patient

This is a young woman with a low-risk DTC. She has an entirely normal contralateral lobe, no auto-immune disease, and a normal thyroid function before surgery. In this case, lobectomy is the preferable approach as the complication rates are lower and the outcomes regarding recurrence and mortality are the same as total thyroidectomy. In both methods those are expected to be very low. In the long term, she should be followed up with ultrasound and non-stimulated thyroglobulin, and her goals of serum TSH levels should be less than 2.0 mUI/L.

Clinical Pearls/Pitfalls

- Low-risk unifocal thyroid cancer can be safely managed with lobectomy
- Complication rates are much lower with lobectomy than with total. thyroidectomy even in experienced hands.
- Maybe quality of life is better with lobectomy, but this needs more studies to be proven.
- Most patients will not need thyroxin replacement as they do not need TSH suppression.

References

1. http://www1.inca.gov.br/vigilancia/incidencia.asp
2. Haymart MR, et al. Controversies in the management of low risk differentiated thyroid cancer. Endocr Rev. 2017;38(4):351–78.
3. Haugen BR, et al. American Thyroid Association management guidelines for adult patients with thyroid nodules and differentiated thyroid cancer. Thyroid. 2016;26:1):1–133.
4. Lang BH, et al. Lobectomy is a more cost-effective option than total thyroidectomy for 1-4cm papillary thyroid carcinoma that do not possess clinical recognizable high-risk features. Ann Surg Oncol. 2016;23(11):3641–52.
5. Kwon H, et al. Comparison of lobectomy and total thyroidectomy in patients with papillary thyroid microcarcinoma – a retrospective individual risk factor-matches cohort study. Eur J Endocrinol. 2017;176(4):371–8.
6. Vaisman F, Momesso D, Bulzico DA, Pessoa CH, da Cruz MD, Dias F, Corbo R, Vaisman M, Tuttle RM. Thyroid lobectomy is associated with excellent clinical outcomes in properly selected differentiated thyroid cancer patients with primary tumors greater than 1 cm. J Thyroid Res. 2013;2013:398194.
7. Momesso DP, Vaisman F, Caminha LS, Pessoa CH, Corbo R, Vaisman M. Surgical approach and radioactive iodine therapy for small well-differentiated thyroid cancer. J Endocrinol Investig. 2014;37(1):57–64.
8. Aschebrook-Kilfoy B, et al. Risk factors for decreased quality of life in thyroid cancer survivors: initial findings from the North American thyroid cancer survivorship study. Thyroid. 2015;25(12):1313–21.
9. Zambeli-Ljepović A, Wang F, Dinan MA, Hyslop T, Roman SA, Sosa JA, Scheri RP. Low-risk thyroid cancer in elderly: total thyroidectomy/RAI predominates but lacks survival advantage. J Surg Res. 2019;243:189–97.

10. Zambeli-Ljepović A, Wang F, Dinan MA, Hyslop T, Stang MT, Roman SA, Sosa JA, Scheri RP. Extent of surgery for low-risk thyroid cancer in the elderly: equipoise in survival but not in short-term outcome. Surgery. 2019;166(5):895–900.
11. Schultz PN, et al. Health profiles and quality of life of 518 survivors of thyroid cancer. Head Neck. 2003;25(5):349–56.
12. Lubitz CC, et al. Measurement and variation in estimation of quality of life effects of patients undergoing treatment for papillary thyroid carcinoma. Thyroid. 2017;27(2):197–206.
13. Juxiang Gou MS, et al. Health-related quality of life assessment in surgical patients with papillary thyroid carcinoma – a single center analysis from mainland China. Medicine (Baltimore). 2017;96(38):e8070.
14. Bayer MF, McDougall IR. Differences in radioimmunoassay results for thyroglobulin that effect management of patients with thyroid cancer. Clin Chem. 1984;30:81–6.
15. Baskin HJ. Effect of postoperative 131I treatment on thy roglobulin measurements in the follow-up of patients with thyroid cancer. Thyroid. 1994;4:239–42.
16. Van Herle AJ. Serum thyroglobulin measurement in the diagnosis and management of thyroid disease. Thyroid Today. 1981;4:1–5.
17. Mazzaferri EL. Treating high thyroglobulin with radioiodine: a magic bullet or a shot in the dark. J Clin Endocrinol Metab. 1995;80:1485–7.
18. Momesso DP, Vaisman F, Yang SP, Bulzico DA, Corbo R, Vaisman M, Tuttle RM. Dynamic risk stratification in patients with differentiated thyroid cancer treated without radioactive iodine. J Clin Endocrinol Metab. 2016;101(7):2692–700.

Chapter 14
A Patient with Papillary Thyroid Carcinoma and Biochemical Evidence of Disease at Follow-Up Visits and Increasing Serum Tg Values at Follow-Up Assessments

Yasuhiro Ito and Akira Miyauchi

Case Presentation

A 70-year-old Japanese woman was referred to Kuma Hospital for the evaluation of a thyroid mass detected through an ultrasound examination for the purpose of screening for carotid atherosclerosis in August 2001. She had undergone surgery for colon cancer 3 years earlier and had no other notable medical history. She had no family history of thyroid cancer. Ultrasound examination at Kuma Hospital revealed a solid tumor measuring 32 × 24 mm in the right lobe of her thyroid and lymph nodes suspicious for metastasis in both lateral compartments (level IV). She had no hoarseness or other compressive symptoms. Laryngotracheal fiberscopy showed that her bilateral vocal cords were functioning and that the tumor in the right lobe protruded into the tracheal mucosa (approx. one-third of the circumference of the trachea) and bled easily when the tip of the fiberscope touched it. No pulmonary metastases were detected on the preoperative chest CT scan.

In November 2001, we performed a total thyroidectomy with bilateral modified radical neck dissection. A window resection of the trachea (26 × 15 mm) was performed due to the tracheal invasion, and an airtight tracheocutaneostomy was created [1], which was closed using a local skin flap in March 2002. We were able to preserve the bilateral recurrent laryngeal nerves. The pathological diagnosis was papillary thyroid carcinoma with an area of poorly differentiated thyroid carcinoma

Y. Ito
Department of Clinical Trial Management, Kuma Hospital, Center for Excellence in Thyroid Care, Kobe, Japan

Department of Surgery, Kuma Hospital, Center for Excellence in Thyroid Care, Kobe, Japan

A. Miyauchi (✉)
Department of Surgery, Kuma Hospital, Center for Excellence in Thyroid Care, Kobe, Japan
e-mail: miyauchi@kuma-h.or.jp

G. Grani et al. (eds.), *Thyroid Cancer*,
https://doi.org/10.1007/978-3-030-61919-0_14

with a solid growth pattern with invasion into the tracheal mucosa. The cranial margin of the tracheal resection was positive on the final pathology report. Only 1, 2, and 1 lymph node metastases were detected at right level VI, right level IV, and left level IV, respectively. All of the nodal metastases were smaller than 3 cm, and no extranodal extension was observed based on intraoperative and pathological findings. There were no metastases in levels II or III on either side.

Postoperative ablation using 100 mCi of radioactive iodine (RAI) was performed in April 2002, but only thyroid bed uptake was seen on the posttreatment scan. The stimulated Tg was 59.4 ng/ml. Since the margin of the tracheal resection was positive, external beam radiotherapy (50 Gy) was also performed from April to May 2002. The patient was followed with thyroid-stimulating hormone (TSH) suppression (<0.1 mU/L) because of the possible residual tumor at the tracheal resection site and detectable serum Tg levels.

The patient's non-stimulated Tg levels gradually increased from 2.8 to 11.4 ng/ml between June 2002 and August 2007 (Fig. 14.1), with no structural evidence of disease. Her anti-Tg antibody test results were always negative. In November 2007, several lung metastases were detected on chest CT image; the sizes of the largest metastases were 9.3 × 6.7 mm and 8.4 × 4.3 mm on the left and right sides, respectively (Fig. 14.2). In June 2008, RAI therapy (100 mCi) was performed, but no uptake was detected in the metastatic lesions. The patient was maintained on TSH suppressive therapy. Her serum Tg levels continued to gradually increase (Fig. 14.1).

In November 2012, an ultrasound examination detected suspicious lymph nodes measuring 11 mm and 9 mm in her right level II. However, fine-needle aspiration biopsy was not performed, since performing a reoperation for such small nodal metastases would be unlikely to improve her prognosis because of the presence of multiple lung metastases. Lung metastases had enlarged to 16.6 × 11.4 mm and 14.3 × 7.0 mm on the left and right sides, respectively, in December 2013 (Fig. 14.3), although the size of the suspicious nodes was unchanged.

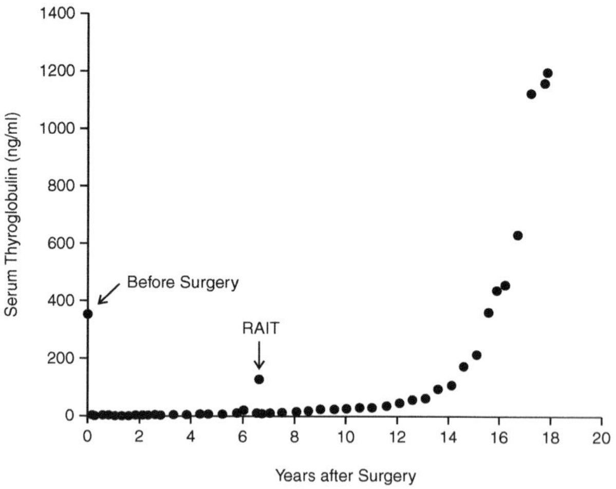

Fig. 14.1 Changes in serum non-stimulated thyroglobulin levels in the patient, a 70-year-old Japanese woman. *RAIT* radioactive iodine treatment

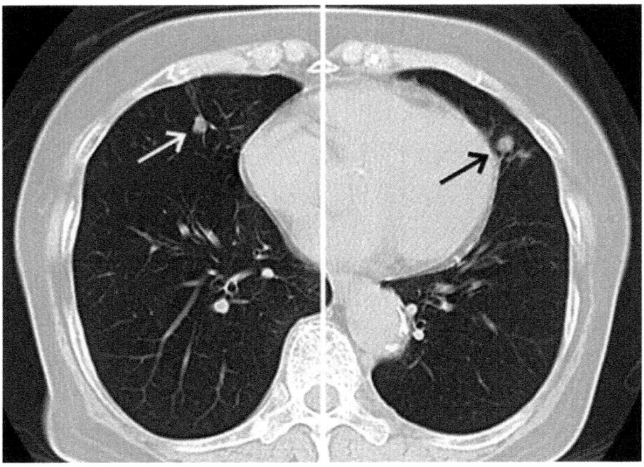

Fig. 14.2 November 2007 chest CT scan showing pulmonary metastases

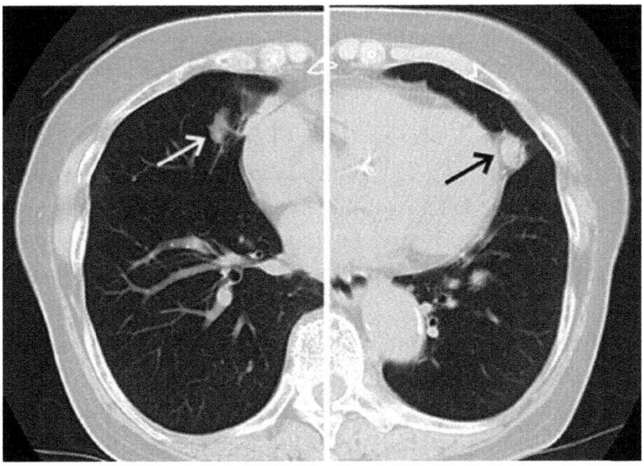

Fig. 14.3 December 2013 chest CT scan showing that the pulmonary metastases had slightly increased in size

As of June 2014, the patient was 83 years old with no symptoms of metastases, and her serum Tg level was 58.8 ng/ml (Fig. 14.1). Although she had been on prolonged TSH suppressive therapy, her bone density did not change between September 2005 and December 2012. Her TSH was suppressed to around 0.01 mIU/L.

The changes in the patient's serum non-stimulated Tg levels showed a gradual and exponential increase over time (Fig. 14.1). When we used a log scale for the vertical axis of the graph of the patient's Tg values, the change was basically linear, and the slope of the regression line did not change between before and after the RAI therapy (Fig. 14.4). We calculated the Tg-doubling time (DT) from the slope of the regression line, as we reported for the calcitonin DT in patients with medullary thyroid carcinoma [2]. A regression line, $\log y = \log a + bx$, was computed by non-linear least square regression (x, years after surgery; y, Tg level), and

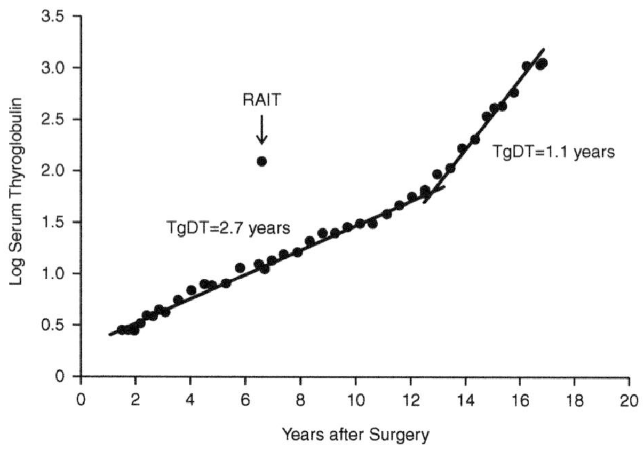

Fig. 14.4 Semilogarithmic graph showing the linear change in the patient's serum non-stimulated thyroglobulin levels. The *vertical axis* is shown in log scale for serum thyroglobulin levels. Looking at the figure carefully, one can see the slope changed to more steep after 2014. The *straight lines* represent the regression lines for the periods before and after 2014. The thyroglobulin-doubling times were calculated from the slopes of the regression lines. The Tg-DT before 2014 was 2.7 years, while the Tg-DT after 2014 was 1.1 years. *RAIT* radioactive iodine treatment

thyroglobulin-doubling time (Tg-DT) was given as (log2)/b. The thyroglobulin-doubling time (Tg-DT) calculated in June 2014 was 2.7 years. We also calculated tumor volume DTs from the sizes of the pulmonary metastatic lesions on CT images in November 2007 and December 2013. The values were 2.6 and 2.8 years for the left and right metastatic lesions, respectively. These values were very similar to the Tg-DT.

The trend in serum thyroglobulin levels over time showed exponential increase (Fig. 14.1). When we took a log scale for the vertical axis, we found that the slope became steeper after 2014 (Fig. 14.4). The Tg-DT after 2014 became shorter, at 1.1 years, although the tumor volume DTs in the same period were stable at 2.9 years and 3.8 years for the left and right metastatic lesions, respectively. The Tg value reached 1196 ng/ml in September 2019 at her age of 88 years. Although she had no specific symptoms, we performed positron emission tomography/computed tomography (PET-CT) to investigate whether any metastatic lesions other than the lung were present. Then, metastases to the sacral bone (Fig. 14.5a, b) were detected. At present, she had no symptoms, including pain and paralysis, for metastatic lesion, but we are planning external beam radiotherapy and denosumab injection every 4 weeks. We will compare the Tg levels before and after the radiotherapy to evaluate the effectiveness of external beam radiotherapy and will closely examine the change in Tg levels (Tg-DT) after radiotherapy and the structural response to decide the timing to initiate molecular-targeted therapy.

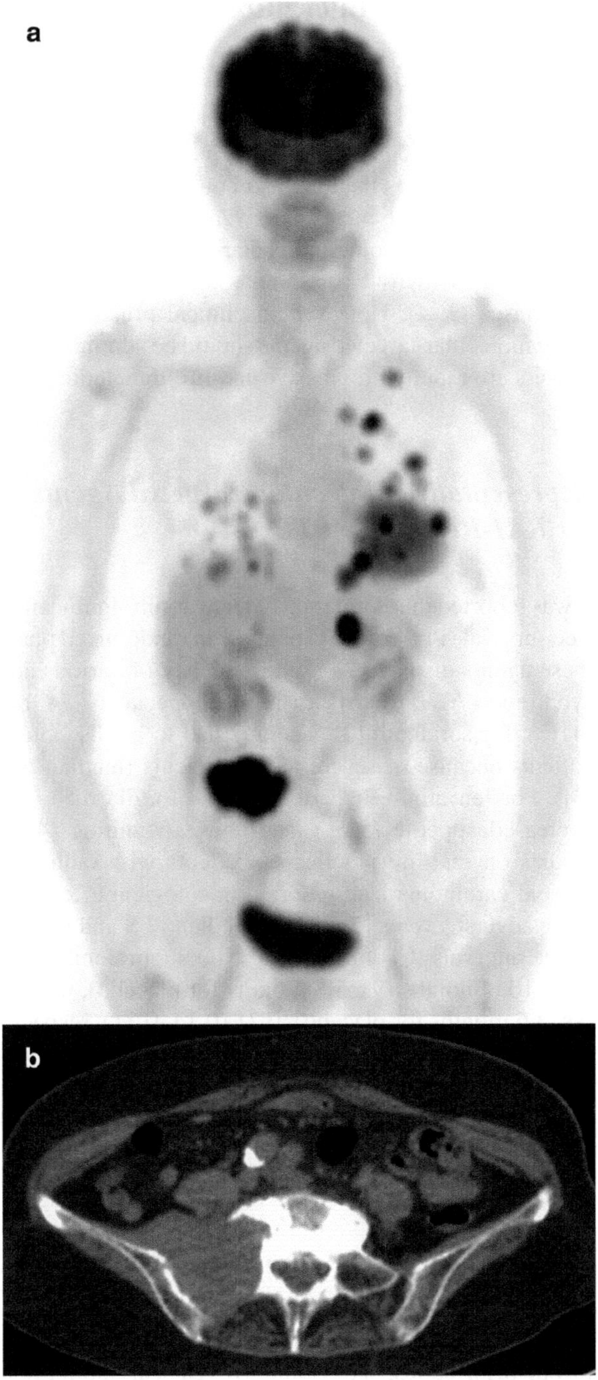

Fig. 14.5 PET-CT detected sacral bone metastasis in addition to known pulmonary metastases in September 2019 (Fig. 14.5a). CT scan of the lower abdomen showing sacral bone metastasis (Fig. 14.5b)

Assessment and Literature Review

Therapies for Metastatic PTC

Papillary thyroid carcinoma (PTC) metastasizes not only to lymph nodes but also to distant sites such as the lung and bone, for which RAI therapy is the first-line treatment. However, the metastases were RAI-refractory, so she was treated with TSH suppression only. Some molecular-targeted agents are reported to be effective for differentiated thyroid carcinomas (DTCs), including PTCs, with RAI-refractory metastases [3, 4]. However, in clinical practice, it remains unclear whether and when molecular-targeted agents should be administered, since not all RAI-refractory cancers are rapidly progressive and life-threatening.

Representative Molecular-Targeted Agents for RAI-Refractory PTC

It was reported that sorafenib and lenvatinib significantly prolonged the progression-free survival (PFS) of DTC patients in randomized phase III studies [3, 4]. However, these agents displayed a high frequency of various adverse events, e.g., hand-foot syndrome (76%), diarrhea (69%), alopecia (67%), rash (50%), and hypertension (41%), for sorafenib [3]. Therapy had to be discontinued in as many as 18.8% of patients because of severe adverse events (median treatment period 10.6 months; [3]). For lenvatinib, hypertension (68%), diarrhea (60%), fatigue/asthenia (59%), decreased appetite (50%), and nausea/vomiting (46%) were reported [4]. Other studies on real-life practice of patients with radioiodine refractory differentiated thyroid carcinoma also reported oncological effectiveness and high incidences of these adverse events [5–7]. The median PFS and hazard ratio (HR) with 95% confidence intervals (CI) of the DECISION (sorafenib) and SELECT (lenvatinib) trials were 10.8 months (vs. 5.8 months for placebo), 0.59 (0.45–0.76) and 18.3 months (vs. 3.6 months for placebo), 0.21 (0.14–0.31), respectively [3, 4]. These agents are very costly, and since these trials were crossover studies, it was not conclusively proved that they prolong overall survival of patients. Clinicians must therefore carefully weigh the advantages and disadvantages of using these agents for individual patients.

Prognosis of DTC Patients with RAI-Refractory Metastases

Not all RAI-refractory metastases are progressive or immediately life-threatening. In our prior series, the 5- and 10-year carcinoma-related death rates of 74 DTC patients with RAI-refractory metastases (metastases without RAI uptake from the time of the initial treatment) were 5% and 30%, respectively [8]. Therefore, these data suggest that not all patients with RAI-refractory thyroid cancer require immediate treatment with systemic agents. Without appropriate selection, many of these patients would likely suffer various adverse events without clear improvement in quality of life or survival.

We also demonstrated by a multivariate analysis that older age (≥60 years) was an independent prognostic factor for cancer-specific survival (CSS) [9], indicating that RAI-refractory metastases are more progressive in elderly patients. Therefore, molecular-targeted agents are more likely to be administered to elderly patients, who more often have comorbidities such as hypertension, liver and renal dysfunctions, diabetes mellitus, and lower immune resistance than younger patients.

Thyroglobulin-Doubling Time

The change in serum Tg levels is an important prognostic factor for thyroglobulin antibody (TgAb)-negative patients who have undergone a total thyroidectomy for PTC. We reported that a short Tg-DT (<1 year) after total thyroidectomy strongly predicted a poor disease-free survival (DFS) and CSS (Table 14.1) and that the Tg-DT shorter than 1 year was a very strong predictor of disease recurrence and carcinoma-related death: HR with 95% CIs for locoregional recurrence was 2.38 (1.20–4.71), for distant recurrence was 4.20 (1.73–10.21), and for carcinoma-related death was 47.06 (5.47–405.13), superior to other conventional prognostic factors in a multivariate analysis [10]. We also found that the incidence of persistent disease was significantly higher in young (<40 years) and old (≥60 years) patients than in middle-aged patients (40–59 years), whereas short Tg-DT was more frequently observed in old patients than others [11].

These findings were consistent with the evidence that younger and older patients were likely to show recurrence, but only older patients were more likely to die of carcinoma, as reported by Mazzaferri and Jhiang [12] and our group [9]. In addition, Tg-DT significantly reflects cell proliferative activity because of the inverse

Table 14.1 Relationship between cause-specific survival (CSS), distant (DRS) and locoregional recurrence-free survival rate (RFS), and Tg-DT/(first four data)

	CSS		DRS		RFS	
	5 years (%)	10 years (%)	5 years (%)	10 years (%)	5 years (%)	10 years (%)
Tg-DT						
<1 year	90	60	72	31	63	38
1–3 years	95	95	90	63	84	58
≥3 years	100	100	92	64	71	54

Tg-DT/(first four data): thyroglobulin-doubling time was calculated using the first four available data

Miyauchi et al. [10]

relationship between Tg-DT and the Ki 67 labeling index [13]. These findings indicate that Tg-DT might allow a quantified prediction of the prognosis for PTC patients. Therefore, it is suggested that Tg-DT is a useful support to predict disease progression and thus to determine the optimal time for initiating treatment such as tyrosine kinase inhibitors, although imaging confirmation of disease progression and tumor burden is needed.

Tumor-Doubling Time

After confirmation of structural disease, an estimation of disease progression may be performed using tumor-doubling time. The average tumor volume doubling time of lung metastases appears to be a good predictor of overall survival in patients with metastatic thyroid cancer. Patients with tumor-doubling time 1 year or shorter had significantly worse overall survival than those with tumor-doubling time >1 year [14]. It can be used to evaluate eligibility for systemic therapy.

A calculator of both thyroglobulin- and tumor-doubling time is available at the Kuma Hospital website (https://www.kuma-h.or.jp/english/about/doubling-time-progression-calculator/).

Management of the Case

Initial Management After Surgery

Older age, clinical lymph node metastases, and significant extrathyroid extension (corresponding to T4 in the UICC TNM classification; [15]) are representative conventional predictors of a poor prognosis for disease-free and CSS [16, 17]. We therefore speculated that our patient was likely to develop a recurrence, even though macroscopically curative surgery was performed. We therefore added RAI ablation and external beam radiotherapy because of the positive pathological margin, in order to prevent local recurrence [1]. She did not develop local recurrence, especially at the resection margin of the trachea. But, her serum Tg remained detectable and increased gradually over time. This indicated that she would likely develop a clinically apparent recurrence in the future; unfortunately this was the case.

Management After Detection of RAI-Refractory Recurrences

Eleven years after her surgery, our patient's PTC recurred at the lung, and the metastases were RAI-refractory. It is debatable whether and when molecular-targeted agents should be prescribed for her.

The metastatic foci in her lung did not accumulate RAI, and her Tg-DT also did not change following the RAI therapy. During the follow-up with TSH suppressive therapy, the RAI-refractory pulmonary metastatic lesions gradually increased in size.

The tumor DTs calculated from the sizes of the metastatic foci on CT images were 2.6 and 2.8 years for the left and right sides, respectively. These were very close to the Tg-DT (2.7 years). A tumor with a DT of 2.7 years will grow to a volume 16 times the original volume after four doublings (10.8 years later in this case). When the present patient becomes 95 years old, the metastatic tumor of the left lung would become 42 × 29 mm in size. Furthermore, the site of lung target lesions was not risky, unlike adjacent lesion to the trachea and hilar area. Based on this calculation and metastatic sites, this patient is unlikely to die of lung metastases. We therefore did not think that molecular-targeted agents were indicated for her at that time.

We showed that a Tg-DT <1 year accurately reflects carcinoma recurrence and carcinoma-related death, regardless of the patient's background and clinicopathological features [10]. Patients with a Tg-DT >2 years were very unlikely to die of PTC [10]. Molecular-targeted agents are costly and produce various adverse events, which may be even life-threatening. These agents should thus be administered to patients only when they are truly required. RAI-refractory thyroid cancer with rapid growth should be the indication for these agents. We propose a short Tg-DT (<1 year) as a convenient criterion of rapid tumor growth and a possible criterion for consideration of the use of these agents together with the findings of imaging studies.

After December 2014, however, the situation of this patient has changed. Her Tg-DT became shorter, at 1.1 years, between December 2014 and September 2019, although tumor volume DTs for lung metastases were stable. Also, her Tg level reached very high value, 1196 ng/ml, which is discrepant with the tumor burden of lung metastases. As a result of whole-body investigation, a new metastasis to the sacral bone was detected. One may think that molecular-targeted agents should be immediately administrated. Indeed, a previous study showed that lenvatinib significantly affected bone metastasis of DTC patients, including PTC [18]. However, we normally prioritize the control of local lesions by external beam radiotherapy. If required and feasible, local control therapies should be performed before systemic therapy.

In conclusion, our patient has RAI-refractory pulmonary and sacral metastases. We do not think that the currently available molecular-targeted agents are indicated at present, because of a moderately long tumor-DT or Tg-DT. Watchful follow-up under TSH suppression is recommended. When Tg-DT became shorter but tumor DT was stable, systemic investigation is desirable. However, therapy for local control should be prioritized, and Tg level, Tg-DT, and structural response should be re-evaluated. If Tg-DT remains short and structural disease progresses, molecular-targeted agent administration will be considered.

Clinical Pearls

- Molecular-targeted agents have been proven to be effective for DTC patients with RAI-refractory metastases, but these agents can cause severe adverse events, damaging the patients' quality of life.
- To evaluate when and whether molecular-targeted agents should be administered to patients, we propose a short Tg-DT (<1 year) as a convenient criterion of rapid tumor growth as a possible reason to consider the indication for these agents together with the findings of imaging studies.
- Molecular-targeted agents should be used only after carefully weighing their advantages and disadvantages.
- Before the initiation of molecular-targeted agents, therapies for local lesions such as external beam radiotherapy should be performed if required and feasible.

References

1. Ito Y, Miyauchi A, Kihara M, Higashiyama T, Kobayashi K, Miya A. Airtight tracheocutaneostomy after window resection of the trachea for invasive papillary thyroid carcinoma: experience of 109 cases. World J Surg. 2014;38:660–6.
2. Miyauchi A, Onishi T, Morimoto S, Takai S, Matsuzuka F, Kuma K, Maeda M, Kumahara Y. Relation of doubling time of plasma calcitonin levels to prognosis and recurrence of medullary thyroid carcinoma. Ann Surg. 1984;199:461–6.
3. Brose M, Nutting C, Jarzab B, Elisei R, Sieno S, et al. Sorafenib in radioactive iodine-refractory, locally advanced or metastatic differentiated thyroid cancer: a randomized, double-blind phase 3 trial. Lancet. 2014;384:319–28.
4. Schlumberger M, Tahara M, Wirth LJ, Robinson B, Brose MS, Elisei R, et al. Lenvatinib versus placebo in radioiodine-refractory thyroid cancer. N Engl J Med. 2015;372:621–30.
5. Berdelou A, Borget I, Godbert Y, Nguyen T, Garcia ME, Chougnet CN, et al. Lenvatinib for the treatment of radioiodine-refractory thyroid cancer in real-life practice. Thyroid. 2018;28(1):72–8.
6. Locati LD, Piovesan A, Durante C, Bregni M, Castagna MG, Zovato S, et al. Real-world efficacy and safety of lenvatinib: data from a compassionate use in the treatment of radioactive iodine-refractory differentiated thyroid cancer patients in Italy. Eur J Cancer. 2019;118:35–40.
7. Balmelli C, Railic N, Siano M, Feuerlein K, Cathomas R, Cristina V, et al. Lenvatinib in advanced radioiodine-refractory thyroid cancer - a retrospective analysis of the Swiss lenvatinib named patient program. J Cancer. 2018;9:250–5.
8. Ito Y, Miyauchi A, Ito M, Yabuta T, Masuoka H, Higashiyama T, et al. Prognosis and prognostic factors of differentiated thyroid carcinoma after the appearance of metastasis refractory to radioactive iodine therapy. Endocr J. 2014;61:821–4.
9. Ito Y, Miyauchi A, Kihara M, Higashiyama T, Kobayashi K, Miya A. Prognostic significance of young age in papillary thyroid carcinoma: analysis of 5733 patients with 150 months' median follow-up. Endocr J. 2014;61:491–7.
10. Miyauchi A, Kudo T, Miya A, Kobayashi K, Ito Y, Takamura Y, et al. Prognostic impact of serum thyroglobulin doubling-time under thyrotropin suppression in patients with papillary thyroid carcinoma who underwent total thyroidectomy. Thyroid. 2011;21:707–16.

11. Miyauchi A, Kudo T, Kihara M, Higashiyama T, Ito Y, Kobayashi K, et al. Relationship of biochemically persistent disease and thyroglobulin-doubling time to age at surgery in patients with papillary thyroid carcinoma. Endocr J. 2013;60:415–21.
12. Mazzaferri EL, Jhiang SM. Long-term impact of initial surgical and medical therapy on papillary and follicular thyroid cancer. Am J Med. 1994;97:418–28.
13. Miyauchi A, Kudo T, Hirokawa M, Ito Y, Kihara M, Higashiyama T, et al. Ki-67 labeling index is a predictor of postoperative persistent disease and cancer growth and a prognostic indicator in papillary thyroid carcinoma. Eur Thyroid J. 2013;2:57–64.
14. Sabra MM, Sherman EJ, Tuttle RM. Tumor volume doubling time of pulmonary metastases predicts overall survival and can guide the initiation of multikinase inhibitor therapy in patients with metastatic, follicular cell-derived thyroid carcinoma. Cancer. 2017;123:2955–64.
15. Tuttle M, Morris L, Haugen B, Shah J, Sosa J, Rohren E, et al. Thyroid-differentiated and anaplastic carcinoma (Chapter 73). In: Amin MB, Edge SB, Greene F, Byrd D, Brookland RK, Washington MK, Gershenwald JE, Compton CC, Hess KR, Sullivan DC, Jessup JM, Brierley J, Gaspar LE, Schilsky RL, Balch CM, Winchester DP, Asare EA, Madera M, Gress DM, Meyer LR, editors. AJCC cancer staging manual. 8th ed. New York: Springer International Publishing; 2017.
16. Ito M, Miyauchi A, Morita S, Kudo T, Nishihara E, Kihara M, Takamura Y, Ito Y, Kobayashi K, Miya A, Kubota S, Amino N. TSH-suppressive doses of levothyroxine are required to achieve preoperative native serum triiodothyronine levels in patients who have undergone total thyroidectomy. Eur J Endocrinol. 2012;167:373–8.
17. Ito Y, Kudo T, Kobayashi K, Miya A, Ichihara K, Miyauchi A. Prognostic factors for recurrence of papillary thyroid carcinoma in the lymph nodes, lung, and bone: analysis of 5768 patients with average 10-year follow-up. World J Surg. 2012;36:1274–8.
18. Robinson B, Schlumberger M, Wirth LJ, Dutcus CE, Song J, Taylor MH, et al. Characterization of tumor size changes over time from the phase 3 study of lenvatinib in thyroid cancer. J Clin Endocrinol Metab. 2016;101:4103–9.

Chapter 15
A Young Patient with Recurrent Lymph Node Involvement: Imaging, Cytology, and Thyroglobulin Washout

Valeria Ramundo, Sebastiano Filetti, and Cosimo Durante

Case Presentation

A 34-year-old woman was referred to our center for a small, firm mass in the left anterior neck, discovered by her general practitioner during a physical examination. Thyroid and neck ultrasound (US) revealed a 2.0 cm solid, hypoechoic left thyroid nodule, with regular margins, without extrathyroidal extension. No suspicious lymph nodes were observed. The patient was euthyroid (serum TSH level of 1.8 mU/L). Fine-needle aspiration biopsy (FNAB) revealed cytological findings consistent with papillary thyroid cancer (PTC) (Bethesda class VI) [1]. The patient underwent total thyroidectomy with central neck dissection prompted by intraoperative detection of suspicious lymph nodes. The surgical pathology showed an intracapsular PTC measuring 1.8 cm in the greatest dimension in the left thyroid lobe, without evidence of extrathyroidal extension or vascular invasion. Six out of ten central lymph nodes removed showed micro-metastatic involvement (all metastatic foci were less than 3 mm in greatest dimension), without evidence of extranodal extension. Tumor was classified as pT1b, N1a – stage 1, according to the AJCC/TNM VIII Edition [2]. According to the 2015 ATA initial risk stratification system, the patient's disease was considered to be at intermediate risk for recurrence (about 20%) [3].

Radioiodine remnant ablation (RRA) with 30 mCi activity was performed after stimulation with recombinant human TSH (rhTSH). At the time of the ablation, the stimulated serum thyroglobulin (Tg) level was 10.6 ng/mL (reference range < 10 ng/

V. Ramundo · S. Filetti · C. Durante (✉)
Department of Translational and Precision Medicine, Sapienza University of Rome, Rome, Italy
e-mail: cosimo.durante@uniroma1.it

G. Grani et al. (eds.), *Thyroid Cancer*,
https://doi.org/10.1007/978-3-030-61919-0_15

mL) with negative antithyroglobulin antibodies (TgAb). The posttreatment whole-body scan (WBS) showed radioiodine uptake only in the thyroid bed.

One year later, the rhTSH-stimulated serum Tg level dropped to 3.2 ng/mL, and TgAb levels were still undetectable. Neck US revealed a round (12.5 × 11.2 × 11.6 mm) lymph node in the left lateral neck (level III) without evidence of a fatty hilum.

Literature Review

Cervical nodes are the most common sites of persistent/recurrent disease in patients with PTC, and disease of this type occurs in 5–50% of all patients, depending on their baseline risk level and response to initial therapy [3]. Several diagnostic tools can be used to identify structural disease in the neck during the posttreatment follow-up, each with specific limitations and strengths.

Radioiodine WBS displays an overall accuracy of 90–92% in this setting, with excellent specificity (up to 100%) but much more limited sensitivity (51–55%) [4]. In 25–50% of patients, single photon emission computed tomography (SPECT)/CT can provide more precise anatomic localization of radioiodine-avid lesions, and it can affect therapy decision-making and patient management [5–8]. Neither of these methods is capable of differentiating neoplastic lesions from normal residual tissue in the central compartment [4–7], and both are ineffective for detecting radioiodine-refractory metastases [9].

Ultrasonography is considered the most sensitive tool for exploring the thyroid bed and cervical lymph node compartments, to evaluate for persistent or recurrent PTC in the neck. International guidelines concur in recommending periodic sonography after the primary treatment. The frequency of sonographic surveillance will be dictated by the initial individual risk for recurrence and the results of serum Tg assays [3, 10, 11]. There are no validated US criteria for distinguishing malignant and benign lesions of the thyroid bed (e.g., tumor recurrence compared to postoperative fibrosis or suture granulomas), but US is much more helpful for classifying cervical lymph nodes [10, 12]. As shown in Table 15.1, foci of punctate hyperechogenicity (reflecting microcalcifications), cystic features, peripheral or diffuse increases in vascularity, and the presence of hyperechoic "thyroid-like" tissue are all strongly suggestive of malignancy [10]. The presence of more than one of these features should reinforce the suspicion, but the sole presence of hyperechoic microfoci or cystic features has a positive predictive value for PTC involvement that approaches 100% [12]. The presence of neoplastic involvement is virtually excluded by visualization of the echogenic lymph node "fatty" hilum, which can be achieved with either standard grayscale or color Doppler imaging. Nonvisualization of the hilum and other features, such as a rounded shape, are highly sensitive markers of lymph node malignancy, but they are relatively nonspecific. Therefore, in the absence of other suspicious features, these findings are considered "indeterminate."

Table 15.1 Accuracy of ultrasound features in diagnosing malignant involvement of cervical lymph nodes

Features	Sensitivity (%)	Specificity (%)	NPV (%)	PPV (%)	Accuracy (%)	Prevalence (%) in normal LN
Suspicious for malignancy						
Punctate hyperechogenicity	5–69	93–100	33–60	88–100	56–72	0
Cystic aspect	10–34	91–100	30–66	77–100	48–65	0
Peripheral/diffuse vascularization	40–86	57–93	31–70	77–80	54–71	1–18
"Thyroid-like" hyperechogenicity	30–87	43–95	38–84	66–96	56–90	4–17
Indeterminate						
Round shape	37	70	45	63	–	4–36
Hilum absent	90.4–100	29–40	67.3	75.9	–	–
Normal						
Hilum present	0.5	–	–	–	–	29–48
Vascularization absent	0	–	–	–	–	33–36

Adapted from Leboulleux et al. [12] and Leenhardt et al. [10]
NPV negative predictive value, *PPV* positive predictive value, *LN* lymph node

About two-thirds of cervical lymph nodes classified as indeterminate will disappear spontaneously with time [13]. Furthermore, frequent US examinations are more likely to identify false-positive abnormalities than clinically significant structural disease recurrence [14]. The location of a suspicious node can also be informative: positive nodes are most commonly found in neck compartments III, IV, and VI [12]. Nodal metastases are also much more likely in patients whose risk of recurrence has been classified as intermediate to high and in those with abnormal serum Tg values [3]. In the presence of indeterminate findings on ultrasound (especially when they persist over time), either of these factors is usually an indication for second-line testing to determine whether or not the node is indeed malignant.

Cytological assessment of an FNAB specimen is the most common method for confirming metastatic involvement of lymph nodes with indeterminate or suspicious sonographic features. However, this is not mandatory for all structurally identifiable neck disease: lesion size (generally ≥0.8–1 cm in maximal dimension), rate of growth, proximity to vital structures, symptoms, and patient preference should determine whether a lesion represents an "actionable" finding. The FNAB should be offered only if the results will have a real impact on patient management [3]. Confirmation of locoregional metastatic involvement is often followed by further treatment, but if this course of action is already precluded by factors like advanced age, comorbidities, or patient preferences, an FNAB serves little purpose.

The aspiration should be performed under US guidance by an experienced operator, defined by the European Thyroid Association (ETA) as one who performs at least 150 procedures per year and maintains an inadequate sampling rate below 10% [10]. Material is collected with 24- to 27-gauge needles (two or more passes) and smeared on slides or suspended in liquid phase for cytological examination. False-negative results occur in 6–8% of all cases (due to sampling error), and up to 10% of samples prove to be inadequate for diagnosis. When cytological and sonographic findings conflict (i.e., normal cytology versus suspicious sonographic features) or the FNAB sample is inadequate, further diagnostic testing can be undertaken.

The diagnostic yield of an FNAB can be enhanced by assaying Tg levels and/or thyroid-specific gene transcripts in washout fluid from the needle used to collect the cytology aspirate [15] or by another dedicated pass for Tg or genetic analysis. For the Tg assay, the needle is generally flushed with 1 cc of normal saline solution. The washout is analyzed using an immunometric assay with a functional sensitivity between 0.1 and 1 mcg/L [10] that has been precalibrated in line with the CRM 457 standard. The results are expressed in nanograms per milliliter, and normal cutoffs vary. The ETA regards levels below 1 ng/mL as normal and those above 10 ng/mL as compatible with thyroid cancer metastasis in a thyroidectomized patient [10]. Values between 1 and 10 ng/mL should be interpreted together with cytology results [10].

Immunometric Tg assays can produce falsely low results in the presence of high Tg concentrations if the excess antigen saturates the binding capacity of the antibodies in the solid-phase support. This so-called hook effect can be excluded by assaying serial dilutions of the sample [16]. The reported sensitivity of washout fluid Tg levels for identifying thyroid cancer lymph node metastases ranges from 88% to 100% with a specificity from 69% to 100% [15–18]. This assay can be informative even in the presence of TgAb [19, 20], although false-negative results can also occur in this setting [21]. False negatives are also possible in the presence of anaplastic or poorly differentiated thyroid cancer metastases. False-positive results have also been reported, mainly when a remnant of normal thyroid is mistakenly identified as a suspicious level VI lymph node [15].

When cytology and washout fluid Tg levels are both noninformative, assaying a sample of the FNAB washout for mRNA for thyroid-specific genes (e.g., TSH receptor, Tg) may be useful. The washout in this case is performed with an RNA stabilization solution and the sample frozen for later assay. With polymerase chain reaction amplification, this approach can correctly identify the presence of metastatic tissue, even when the washout fluid contains only a few cells [17]. However, this assay is probably available only in tertiary care centers.

Once the presence of metastatic lymph node involvement has been established, the most effective therapy [22] and the first-line approach recommended by the ATA Practice Guidelines [3] is surgery. The first reoperation is often (50–70% of patients) successful in eradicating the disease [22–24]. However, reoperation carries an increased risk of permanent complications [25–27], including nerve resection (e.g., recurrent laryngeal, spinal accessory, and phrenic nerves), hypoparathyroidism, and tracheal or esophageal damage. A careful risk-benefit analysis, based on thorough analysis of costs, benefits, and patient preferences, should guide surgical decision, particularly in patients with risk factors for incomplete response [28]. The actual risk of complications depends in part on the skill and experience of the surgeon, so the availability of surgeons specifically trained in neck revision procedures is a critical factor to consider. The proximity of the metastatic node to vital structures in the neck should also be fully taken into account.

The ATA recommends that surgery should be considered for central neck nodes measuring >8 mm and lateral neck nodes measuring >10 mm in the greatest dimension. For smaller nodes or those that remain stable over time, conservative management based on active surveillance is more appropriate [3]. Only 20% of all suspicious lymph nodes exhibit volume increases over time [29]. Those posing no threat to vital structures that show no signs of growth can be safely and effectively monitored with periodic (every 6–12 months) US examinations [3, 10]. Thermal [30, 31] and ethanol [32] ablation has also been proposed as a less invasive treatment for patient refusing or with contraindications to surgery. These alternative therapies are most often used to treat lymph node disease in the lateral, rather than the central, neck. The patient's wishes and preferences have to be weighed and addressed in all decisions.

Back to the Patient

At the 1-year follow-up visit, the patient presented an indeterminate response, according to ATA guidelines [3], and a sonographically indeterminate left lateral neck lymph node (see Table 15.1).

With a small child to care for and a promising new job, the young woman was clearly disconcerted by the possibility (however uncertain) that the disease had spread in spite of the previous treatment and the prospect of a second operation. An FNAB was promptly obtained, and as routinely performed in our center, aliquots of the needle washout were also collected and retained for Tg levels and thyroid-specific gene expression assays. The aspirate itself proved to be inadequate for cytological analysis, and also the Tg level in the needle washout fluid was in the indeterminate range (10 ng/mL). However, the presence of metastatic PTC in the aspirated node was confirmed by the presence of mRNA for the TSH receptor and Tg genes in the washout fluid. The pros and cons of a second operation were reviewed in light of this diagnosis, and the patient decided to undergo a selective left lateral neck dissection. The operation was uneventful, and the surgical pathology confirmed metastatic PTC in 2 out of 15 lymph nodes removed. Six months later, the rhTSH-stimulated serum Tg level was below the detection limit, TgAb were negative, and no suspicious findings were detected on neck US. Five years have passed since the second operation, and the patient has remained disease-free. She continues to work and care for her family.

Clinical Pearls/Pitfalls

- US is the most accurate tool for identifying metastatic spread to cervical lymph nodes.
- Nodes displaying punctate hyperechogenicity, cystic features, diffuse or peripheral increases in vascularity, or hyperechoic “thyroid-like” tissue on neck US should raise a strong suspicion of malignancy.
- When the suspicious features are limited to a round rather than oval shape and/or the absence of a fatty hilum, the nature of node is indeterminate.
- FNAB for cytology is indicated for most suspicious lymph nodes, only if a subsequent treatment is planned.
- The diagnostic yield of the FNAB for identification of lymph node metastases can be increased by measuring Tg levels in the FNAB needle washout fluid. PCR-based assays can document even low levels of thyroid-specific gene mRNA in the FNAB washout fluid.
- The first reoperation for persistent/recurrent PTC in the neck is successful in about 50–70% of cases but carries an increased risk of permanent complications.
- Nonthreatening lymph node metastases that remain stable in size over time can be safely and effectively monitored with periodic (6–12 months) US examinations.

References

1. Cibas ES, Ali SZ. The 2017 Bethesda system for reporting thyroid cytopathology. Thyroid. 2017;27(11):1341–6.
2. Tuttle M, Morris L, Haugen B, Shah J, Sosa J, Rohren E, et al. Thyroid-differentiated and anaplastic carcinoma (Chapter 73). In: AJCC cancer staging manual. New York: Springer International Publishing; 2017.
3. Haugen BR, Alexander EK, Bible KC, Doherty GM, Mandel SJ, Nikiforov YE, et al. 2015 American Thyroid Association management guidelines for adult patients with thyroid nodules and differentiated thyroid cancer: the American Thyroid Association guidelines task force on thyroid nodules and differentiated thyroid cancer. Thyroid. 2016;26(1):1–133.
4. Franceschi M, Kusic Z, Franceschi D, Lukinac L, Roncevic S. Thyroglobulin determination, neck ultrasonography and iodine-131 whole-body scintigraphy in differentiated thyroid carcinoma. J Nucl Med. 1996;37(3):446–51.
5. Tharp K, Israel O, Hausmann J, Bettman L, Martin WH, Daitzchman M, et al. Impact of 131I-SPECT/CT images obtained with an integrated system in the follow-up of patients with thyroid carcinoma. Eur J Nucl Med Mol Imaging. 2004;31(10):1435–42.
6. Schmidt D, Szikszai A, Linke R, Bautz W, Kuwert T. Impact of 131I SPECT/spiral CT on nodal staging of differentiated thyroid carcinoma at the first radioablation. J Nucl Med. 2009;50(1):18–23.
7. Grewal RK, Tuttle RM, Fox J, Borkar S, Chou JF, Gonen M, et al. The effect of posttherapy 131I SPECT/CT on risk classification and management of patients with differentiated thyroid cancer. J Nucl Med. 2010;51(9):1361–7.

8. Zilioli V, Peli A, Panarotto MB, Magri G, Alkraisheh A, Wiefels C, et al. Differentiated thyroid carcinoma: incremental diagnostic value of (131)I SPECT/CT over planar whole body scan after radioiodine therapy. Endocrine. 2017;56(3):551–9.
9. Lamartina L, Grani G, Durante C, Borget I, Filetti S, Schlumberger M. Follow-up of differentiated thyroid cancer – what should (and what should not) be done. Nat Rev Endocrinol. 2018;14(9):538–51.
10. Leenhardt L, Erdogan MF, Hegedus L, Mandel SJ, Paschke R, Rago T, et al. 2013 European thyroid association guidelines for cervical ultrasound scan and ultrasound-guided techniques in the postoperative management of patients with thyroid cancer. Eur Thyroid J. 2013;2(3):147–59.
11. Grani G, Ramundo V, Falcone R, Lamartina L, Montesano T, Biffoni M, et al. Thyroid cancer patients with no evidence of disease: the need for repeat neck ultrasound. J Clin Endocrinol Metab. 2019;104(11):4981–9.
12. Leboulleux S, Girard E, Rose M, Travagli JP, Sabbah N, Caillou B, et al. Ultrasound criteria of malignancy for cervical lymph nodes in patients followed up for differentiated thyroid cancer. J Clin Endocrinol Metab. 2007;92(9):3590–4.
13. Lamartina L, Grani G, Biffoni M, Giacomelli L, Costante G, Lupo S, et al. Risk stratification of neck lesions detected sonographically during the follow-up of differentiated thyroid cancer. J Clin Endocrinol Metab. 2016;101(8):3036–44.
14. Peiling Yang S, Bach AM, Tuttle RM, Fish SA. Frequent screening with serial neck ultrasound is more likely to identify false-positive abnormalities than clinically significant disease in the surveillance of intermediate risk papillary thyroid cancer patients without suspicious findings on follow-up ultrasound evaluation. J Clin Endocrinol Metab. 2015;100(4):1561–7.
15. Grani G, Fumarola A. Thyroglobulin in lymph node fine-needle aspiration washout: a systematic review and meta-analysis of diagnostic accuracy. J Clin Endocrinol Metab. 2014;99(6):1970–82.
16. Giovanella L, Ceriani L, Suriano S, Crippa S. Thyroglobulin measurement on fine-needle washout fluids: influence of sample collection methods. Diagn Cytopathol. 2009;37(1):42–4.
17. Arturi F, Russo D, Giuffrida D, Ippolito A, Perrotti N, Vigneri R, et al. Early diagnosis by genetic analysis of differentiated thyroid cancer metastases in small lymph nodes. J Clin Endocrinol Metab. 1997;82(5):1638–41.
18. Xu Y, Wu D, Wu W, Jiang J, Xi C, Ye N, et al. Diagnostic value of cytology, thyroglobulin, and combination of them in fine-needle aspiration of metastatic lymph nodes in patients with differentiated thyroid cancer: a systematic review and network meta-analysis. Medicine (Baltimore). 2019;98(45):e17859.
19. Boi F, Baghino G, Atzeni F, Lai ML, Faa G, Mariotti S. The diagnostic value for differentiated thyroid carcinoma metastases of thyroglobulin (Tg) measurement in washout fluid from fine-needle aspiration biopsy of neck lymph nodes is maintained in the presence of circulating anti-Tg antibodies. J Clin Endocrinol Metab. 2006;91(4):1364–9.
20. Latrofa F, Ricci D, Montanelli L, Rocchi R, Piaggi P, Sisti E, et al. Thyroglobulin autoantibodies in patients with papillary thyroid carcinoma: comparison of different assays and evaluation of causes of discrepancies. J Clin Endocrinol Metab. 2012;97(11):3974–82.
21. Jeon MJ, Park JW, Han JM, Yim JH, Song DE, Gong G, et al. Serum antithyroglobulin antibodies interfere with thyroglobulin detection in fine-needle aspirates of metastatic neck nodes in papillary thyroid carcinoma. J Clin Endocrinol Metab. 2013;98(1):153–60.
22. Yim JH, Kim WB, Kim EY, Kim WG, Kim TY, Ryu JS, et al. The outcomes of first reoperation for locoregionally recurrent/persistent papillary thyroid carcinoma in patients who initially underwent total thyroidectomy and remnant ablation. J Clin Endocrinol Metab. 2011;96(7):2049–56.
23. Uruno T, Miyauchi A, Shimizu K, Nakano K, Takamura Y, Ito Y, et al. Prognosis after reoperation for local recurrence of papillary thyroid carcinoma. Surg Today. 2004;34(11):891–5.

24. Hughes DT, Laird AM, Miller BS, Gauger PG, Doherty GM. Reoperative lymph node dissection for recurrent papillary thyroid cancer and effect on serum thyroglobulin. Ann Surg Oncol. 2012;19(9):2951–7.
25. Roh JL, Kim JM, Park CI. Central compartment reoperation for recurrent/persistent differentiated thyroid cancer: patterns of recurrence, morbidity, and prediction of postoperative hypocalcemia. Ann Surg Oncol. 2011;18(5):1312–8.
26. Lang BH, Lee GC, Ng CP, Wong KP, Wan KY, Lo CY. Evaluating the morbidity and efficacy of reoperative surgery in the central compartment for persistent/recurrent papillary thyroid carcinoma. World J Surg. 2013;37(12):2853–9.
27. Wierzbicka M, Gurgul E, Wasniewska-Okupniak E, Gryczynska M, Piorunek T, Ruchala M. The feasibility and efficacy of secondary neck dissections in thyroid cancer metastases. Eur Arch Otorhinolaryngol. 2014;271(4):795–9.
28. Lamartina L, Borget I, Mirghani H, Al Ghuzlan A, Berdelou A, Bidault F, et al. Surgery for neck recurrence of differentiated thyroid cancer: outcomes and risk factors. J Clin Endocrinol Metab. 2017;102(3):1020–31.
29. Robenshtok E, Fish S, Bach A, Dominguez JM, Shaha A, Tuttle RM. Suspicious cervical lymph nodes detected after thyroidectomy for papillary thyroid cancer usually remain stable over years in properly selected patients. J Clin Endocrinol Metab. 2012;97(8):2706–13.
30. Mauri G, Cova L, Tondolo T, Ierace T, Baroli A, Di Mauro E, et al. Percutaneous laser ablation of metastatic lymph nodes in the neck from papillary thyroid carcinoma: preliminary results. J Clin Endocrinol Metab. 2013;98(7):E1203–7.
31. Teng D, Ding L, Wang Y, Liu C, Xia Y, Wang H. Safety and efficiency of ultrasound-guided low power microwave ablation in the treatment of cervical metastatic lymph node from papillary thyroid carcinoma: a mean of 32 months follow-up study. Endocrine. 2018;62(3):648–54.
32. Fontenot TE, Deniwar A, Bhatia P, Al-Qurayshi Z, Randolph GW, Kandil E. Percutaneous ethanol injection vs reoperation for locally recurrent papillary thyroid cancer: a systematic review and pooled analysis. JAMA Otolaryngol Head Neck Surg. 2015;141(6):512–8.

Part III
Differentiated Thyroid Cancer: Special Issues

Chapter 16
Papillary Thyroid Carcinoma Diagnosed During Pregnancy

Zachary Simons and David S. Cooper

Case Presentation

A 46-year-old pregnant female was referred for management of a recently diagnosed papillary thyroid carcinoma. During her initial prenatal visit at 11 weeks of gestation, a nurse midwife detected a right thyroid nodule. Her TSH was normal at 0.96 mU/L. Her primary care doctor arranged for a diagnostic ultrasound that revealed a 4.6 cm right thyroid nodule. She returned the following week for an ultrasound-guided fine-needle aspiration biopsy. The cytology was suspicious for a papillary thyroid carcinoma (Bethesda class V). She was referred for management options. At the time of the endocrine consultation, the patient was para 5 gravida 4 and 19 weeks pregnant. She did not have any other medical conditions. She had no history of head and neck radiation. She had no family history of thyroid disease, including thyroid cancer. She denied neck pressure, voice change, or dysphagia.

An office ultrasound of the thyroid nodule and cervical neck node survey was performed to estimate her stage and direct the extent of surgery. The ultrasound exam revealed a 4.6 × 2.1 × 2 cm solid, hypoechoic, taller-than-wide (anteroposterior/transverse diameter ratio >1) nodule in the upper right thyroid lobe (high-suspicion appearance according to the American Thyroid Association [ATA] guidelines [1], Fig. 16.1). The nodule contained microcalcifications. An ultrasound node survey of the central and lateral neck revealed two abnormal 1 and 1.5 cm partially cystic, hypervascular nodes inferior to the lower pole of the right thyroid lobe (Fig. 16.2). FNA of the nodule and one of the central neck nodes were biopsied and were positive for papillary thyroid cancer.

Z. Simons · D. S. Cooper (✉)
Division of Endocrinology, Diabetes, and Metabolism, The Johns Hopkins University School of Medicine, Baltimore, MD, USA
e-mail: dscooper@jhmi.edu

G. Grani et al. (eds.), *Thyroid Cancer*,
https://doi.org/10.1007/978-3-030-61919-0_16

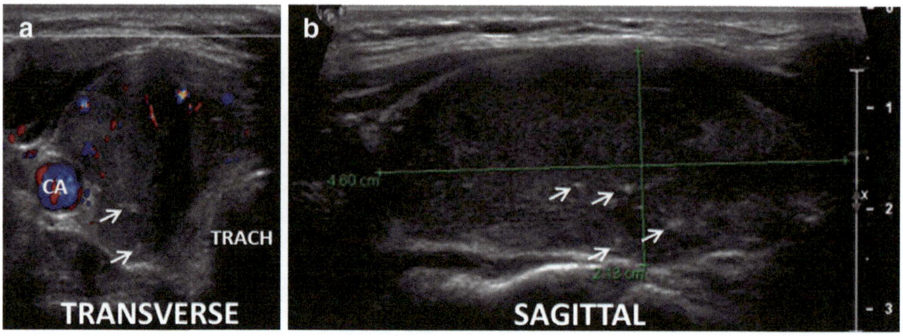

Fig. 16.1 Thyroid ultrasound of the right thyroid lobe shows a 4.6 × 2.1 × 2 cm (sagittal × antero-posterior × transverse) solid, hypoechoic nodule. This nodule is hypoechoic with taller-than-wide (anterioposterior/transverse diameter ratio >1) dimensions with microcalcification (white arrows) and low intranodular vascular flow by Doppler analysis (grade 3). (**a**) Thyroid transverse view with Doppler. (**b**) Thyroid sagittal view. CA carotid artery, TRACH trachea

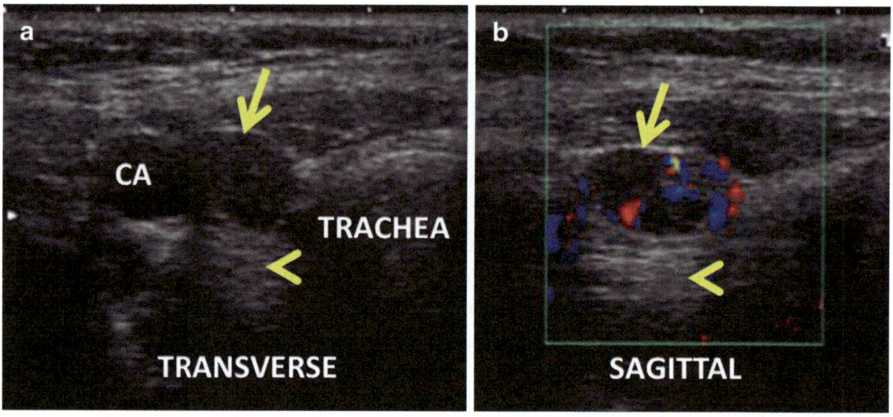

Fig. 16.2 Cervical node ultrasound. A 1.5 × 0.8 × 1 cm node (arrow) is located inferior to the thyroid in the right thyroid bed, cervical node level VI, between the carotid artery (CA) and the trachea. The node is partially cystic with post-cyst enhancement (arrowhead) and peripheral vascular flow in the solid component of the node. (**a**) Node transverse view. (**b**) Node sagittal view with Doppler analysis

Assessment and Literature Review

While thyroid cancer in general is uncommon in pregnancy (25 cases per 100,000 pregnancies), it is the second most frequent cancer to be diagnosed in pregnancy, following breast cancer, tending to occur more often in older pregnant women and in the postpartum period [2]. It is recommended that thyroid nodules in pregnant women with euthyroidism and hypothyroidism be evaluated and biopsied with the same criteria as nonpregnant adults [1, 3].

AJCC/TNM staging is a universal method of communicating extent of disease and correlates with risk of death. A young female with a >4 cm papillary thyroid carcinoma with >1 cm metastatic level 6 nodes would be a stage 1 patient in the AJCC/TNM classification scheme with a mortality risk of 0%. Given the size of the tumor and the presence of large nodal metastases, the risk of recurrence according to the ATA Risk Stratification System is in the 10–20% range [1]. Thus, the decision for surgery during pregnancy requires assessment of the risk of death and recurrence of the differentiated thyroid cancer balanced against the potential harm to the fetus.

There is no consensus to whether surgery for papillary thyroid carcinoma should be performed during pregnancy or postpartum. Most retrospective analyses have suggested that delaying surgery does not affect outcomes. In one of the original studies investigating PTC diagnosed in pregnancy, Moosa et al. compared thyroid cancer in 61 pregnant women to nonpregnant controls and showed no difference in risk of recurrence or survival [4]. Recent studies involving more rigorous biochemical and imaging follow-up have shown similar results [5, 6]. While some retrospective studies have indicated higher rates of persistent disease in the postpartum period and larger tumors with higher rates of lymph node involvement [7–9], these studies do not provide definitive evidence that delaying treatment until the postpartum period results in changes in clinical outcomes.

On the contrary, in one recent report from Memorial Sloan Kettering Cancer Center, 197 patients who had had an excellent, indeterminate, or biochemically incomplete response to therapy continued to show no evidence of structurally identifiable disease. A few (8%) had increases in basal Tg during pregnancy. In 38 women with a structural incomplete response to therapy prior to pregnancy, structural progression (≥3mm increase in the size of known disease or identification of new metastatic foci) was identified after delivery in 29% (11/38). However, additional therapy was recommended during the first postpartum years in only 8% (3/38) of those patients [10]. Thus, even though structural disease progression was seen in almost a third of the patients with known structural disease prior to pregnancy, only a minority of these patients had changes sufficient to warrant additional therapy. In two prospective studies in which pregnant women with small thyroid cancers were monitored sonographically during pregnancy, only a small minority showed an increase in size, and no patient developed nodal metastases [11, 12].

The mechanisms by which pregnancy may exert an influence on tumor progression are unknown. Some studies have suggested that hormonal changes during pregnancy may trigger thyroid cancer growth. Vannucchi et al. showed that differentiated thyroid cancers diagnosed during pregnancy or in the first year postpartum had higher likelihood of estrogen receptor alpha expression [7]. However, this could not be verified in another study [9]. A third study showed that hCG interacts with recombinant hTSH receptors transfected into human thyroid cancer cells [13], suggesting a role for hCG in stimulating thyroid cancer growth. However, there is no evidence that papillary thyroid cancer occurring in pregnancy has a more aggressive phenotype compared to cancers occurring in nonpregnant women [6].

One large study showed that thyroid surgery performed during pregnancy had greater risk of complications (hypoparathyroidism and recurrent nerve injury) and longer hospital stays [14], but did not provide data on fetal loss. Other smaller retrospective studies have shown that thyroid surgery is safe during pregnancy, with no adverse fetal or maternal outcomes [15, 16]. These studies, which report on fewer than 100 pregnant women, also show no difference in tumor stage (TNM), recurrence rate, complications of pregnancy, or adverse fetal outcome regardless of whether surgery is performed during or after pregnancy. Current ATA guidelines recommend avoiding surgery during pregnancy unless the tumor grows substantially before 24–26 weeks gestation or if malignant cervical lymph nodes are present, in which case thyroidectomy should be considered, preferably during the second trimester of pregnancy [3].

Back to the Patient

During this patient's 23rd week of pregnancy, she had an uncomplicated total thyroidectomy and bilateral central neck dissection (level 6). This was done because of the large size of the mass and the presence of nodal metastases. Her pathology showed a 4 cm partially encapsulated papillary thyroid carcinoma with 9 of 11 nodes containing metastatic papillary thyroid carcinoma. Six weeks after surgery, her thyroglobulin was 0.8 ng/mL with a TSH 0.1 mU/L on levothyroxine therapy. Radioactive iodine therapy was postponed for 1 year to allow her to breastfeed her baby (see Chap. 26). During the first year after surgery, she was followed with multiple assessments of thyroglobulin levels that were stable and did not rise and neck ultrasound examinations that did not show evidence of residual or recurrent disease.

Clinical Pearls/Pitfalls

- Thyroid cancer diagnosed during pregnancy has an indolent course of differentiated thyroid cancer typical of what is generally seen in young adults.
- Thyroid cancer without sonographic evidence of capsular invasion or metastatic nodes may be followed by ultrasound without surgery.
- More advanced disease in a pregnant woman, progression of disease demonstrated by growth of the primary tumor, evidence of invasion, and the development metastatic nodes are indications for thyroidectomy during pregnancy.
- Thyroidectomy during pregnancy is generally safe but is preferably done during the second trimester.

References

1. Haugen BR, Alexander EK, Bible KC, Doherty GM, Mandel SJ, Nikiforov YE, Pacini F, Randolph GW, Sawka AM, Schlumberger M, Schuff KG, Sherman SI, Sosa JA, Steward DL, Tuttle RM, Wartofsky L. 2015 American Thyroid Association management guidelines for adult patients with thyroid nodules and differentiated thyroid cancer: the American Thyroid Association guidelines task force on thyroid nodules and differentiated thyroid cancer. Thyroid. 2016;26:1–133.
2. Cottreau CM, Dashevsky I, Andrade SE, Li DK, Nekhlyudov L, Raebel MA, Ritzwoller DP, Partridge AH, Pawloski PA, Toh S. Pregnancy-associated cancer: a U.S. population-based study. J Womens Health. 2018;28:250–7.
3. Alexander E, Pearce E, Brent G, Brown R, Chen H, Dosiou C, Grobman W, Laurberg P, Lazarus J, Mandel S, Peeters R, Sullivan S. 2017 guidelines of the American Thyroid Association for the diagnosis and management of thyroid disease during pregnancy and the postpartum. Thyroid. 2017;27:315–89.
4. Moosa M, Mazzaferri E. Outcome of differentiated thyroid cancer diagnosed in pregnant women. J Clin Endocrinol Metab. 1997;82:2862–6.
5. Yasmeen S, Cress R, Romano PS, Xing G, Berger-Chen S, Danielsen B, Smith LH. Thyroid cancer in pregnancy. Int J Gynecol Obstet. 2005;91:15–20.
6. Chen A, Livhits M, Du L, Wu J, Kuo E, Yeh M, Leung A. Recent pregnancy is not associated with high-risk pathological features of well-differentiated thyroid cancer. Thyroid. 2018;28:68–71.
7. Vannucchi G, Perrino M, Rossi S, Colombo C, Vicentini L, Dazzi D, Beck-Peccoz P, Fugazzola L. Clinical and molecular features of differentiated thyroid cancer diagnosed during pregnancy. Eur J Endocrinol. 2010;162:145–51.
8. Lee J, Zhao J, Clifton-Bligh R, Gill A, Gundara J, Ip J, Sywak M, Delbridge L, Robinson B, Sidhu S. Papillary thyroid carcinoma in pregnancy: a variant of the disease? Ann Surg Oncol. 2012;19:4210–6.
9. Messuti I, Corvisieri S, Bardesono F, Rapa I, Giorcelli J, Pellerito R, Volante M, Orlandi F. Impact of pregnancy on prognosis of differentiated thyroid cancer: clinical and molecular features. Eur J Endocrinol. 2014;170:659–66.
10. Rakhlin L, Fish S, Tuttle R. Response to therapy status is an excellent predictor of pregnancy-associated structural disease progression in patients previously treated for differentiated thyroid cancer. Thyroid. 2017;27:396–401.
11. Ito Y, Miyauchi A, Kudo T, Ota H, Yoshioka K, Oda H, Sasai H, Nakayama A, Yabuta T, Masuoka H, Fukushima M, Higashiyama T, Kihara M, Kobayashi K, Miya A. Effects of pregnancy on papillary microcarcinomas of the thyroid re-evaluated in the entire patient series at Kuma Hospital. Thyroid. 2016;26:156–60.
12. Oh H, Kim W, Park S, Kim M, Kwon H, Jeon M, Lee J, Baek J, Song D, Kim T, Shong Y, Kim W. Serial neck ultrasonographic evaluation of changes in papillary thyroid carcinoma during pregnancy. Thyroid. 2017;27:773–7.
13. Yoshimura M, Hershman JM. Thyrotropic action of human chorionic gonadotropin. Thyroid. 1995;5:425–34.
14. Kuy S, Roman SA, Desai R, Sosa JA. Outcomes following thyroid and parathyroid surgery in pregnant women. Arch Surg. 2009;144:399–406.
15. Herzon FS, Morris DM, Segal MN, Rauch G, Parnell T. Coexistent thyroid cancer and pregnancy. Arch Otolaryngol Head Neck Surg. 1994;120:1191–3.
16. Uruno T, Shibuya H, Kitagawa W, Nagahama M, Sugino K, Ito K. Optimal timing of surgery for differentiated thyroid cancer in pregnant women. World J Surg. 2014;38:704–8.

Chapter 17
Risks of Thyroid Hormone Suppression for Differentiated Thyroid Cancer in the Elderly

Swaytha Yalamanchi and David S. Cooper

Case Presentation

A 91-year-old woman presents for management of papillary thyroid carcinoma (PTC). She underwent a total thyroidectomy six years previously. Pathology demonstrated a 1.3 cm focus of PTC with focal tall cell features and metastases in one of four central and two of five left lateral lymph nodes. She was treated with 75 mCi of I-131 and her posttreatment scan showed two foci of radiotracer localization in the thyroid bed and three foci in the anterior lower thorax. The patient underwent resection of a level VI lymph node 4 years later. Pathology showed a 1.5 cm lymph node replaced by PTC and extensive skeletal muscle involvement. Chest CT scan showed multiple pulmonary nodules suspicious for metastatic disease, none of which were iodine-avid on subsequent I-123 scan. The patient also has a history of osteoporosis with a femoral fragility fracture and is being treated with risedronate. Recent biochemical assessment includes serum thyroid-stimulating hormone (TSH) 0.68 mU/L (0.50–4.50), serum free T4 1.6 ng/dl (0.8–1.8), and basal serum thyroglobulin 120 ng/ml with negative serum thyroglobulin antibody titers.

S. Yalamanchi
Division of Endocrinology, Diabetes, and Metabolism, Palo Alto Medical Foundation, Palo Alto, CA, USA

D. S. Cooper (✉)
Division of Endocrinology, Diabetes, and Metabolism,
The Johns Hopkins University School of Medicine, Baltimore, MD, USA
e-mail: dscooper@jhmi.edu

G. Grani et al. (eds.), *Thyroid Cancer*,
https://doi.org/10.1007/978-3-030-61919-0_17

Assessment and Literature Review

PTC is associated with low rates of mortality and recurrence, particularly in patients with low-risk disease. Fully suppressive thyroxine (T4) therapy (serum TSH<0.1 mU/L) does not have a role in the long-term management of low-risk PTC, though may improve survival in patients with high-risk disease. Iatrogenic hyperthyroidism may negatively impact cardiovascular and bone health, particularly in the elderly. Individualized goals regarding T4 suppressive therapy are necessary.

Prevalence

The incidence of DTC, particularly low-risk PTC, has increased rapidly over the past 15 years [1]. Although there has been increased detection of incidental subclinical disease on imaging studies, rates of aggressive PTC and thyroid cancer-specific mortality, have also increased [2, 3].

Efficacy of Thyroid Hormone Suppression Therapy

DTC treatment has traditionally included total thyroidectomy, suppression of serum TSH to undetectable levels, and, in selected cases, radioiodine (RAI) ablation. Older studies suggested that suppressed TSH levels, regardless of the stage, may be associated with decreased rates of disease progression and recurrence and increased rates of relapse-free survival [4, 5]. Multiple studies since that time, however, have shown that aggressive thyroid hormone suppression is not beneficial in low-risk disease. A prospective study of the National Thyroid Cancer Treatment Cooperative Study Group (NTCTCSG) ($n=617$), a thyroid cancer registry in the United States, found no effect of thyroid hormone suppression in stages I and II disease with minimal effects seen in stages III and IV after adjustment by multivariate analysis [6, 7]. A subsequent study of 4,491 patients in this cohort (median follow-up six years) suggested that in all stages overall survival was improved in those with moderate TSH suppression as compared to individuals with serum TSH levels in the normal/elevated range [8]. Hovens et al. ($n=366$, mean follow-up 8.85 years) demonstrated no differences in thyroid carcinoma-related death in individuals with suppressed and unsuppressed TSH levels. However, high TSH levels were predictors of cancer-related death and recurrence: median serum TSH level >2 mU/L in patients with T1-3, M0 tumors was associated with higher rates of recurrence (HR 1.41; 95 % CI 1.03–1.95) and death (HR 2.03; 95 % CI 1.22–3.37) as compared to individuals with serum TSH <2 mU/L [9]. A non-inferiority randomized control trial of low-risk DTC Japanese patients ($n=433$, mean follow-up 6.9 years) demonstrated that disease-free survival in euthyroid patients (mean serum TSH 3.2 mU/L) was similar to those with suppressed serum TSH, even in high-risk patients. Of note, the majority of patients underwent central neck dissection and did not receive radioiodine, patterns of care that differ from North America and Europe [10]. Among individuals who undergo lobectomy for management of low-risk DTC, limited data suggest targeting a serum TSH <2 mU/L is not associated with recurrence-free survival. Again, prophylactic unilateral central neck dissection was performed in this population, and it warrants caution in extrapolation of these results [11]. Overall, patients with low- and intermediate-risk DTC have an excellent prognosis, and aggressive TSH suppression is unlikely to be beneficial. The appropriate degree of TSH suppression by thyroid hormone suppression therapy in more aggressive disease remains unknown.

Recommendations for Serum TSH Suppression Goals

The 2015 American Thyroid Association (ATA) guidelines recommend initial serum TSH suppression goals for high- and intermediate-risk thyroid cancer patients of <0.1 mU/L and 0.1–0.5 mU/L, respectively. The recommended serum TSH level for low-risk patients with detectable serum thyroglobulin regardless of remnant ablation status is 0.1–0.5 mU/L. Low-risk patients with undetectable serum thyroglobulin levels regardless of whether they have undergone remnant ablation may have serum TSH maintained at 0.5–2 mU/L [12]. Serum TSH goals at the time of initial assessment should be based on comorbidities [12]. TSH targets in the long-term follow-up of DTC depend on comorbidities, the risk of recurrence, and response to treatment (Table 17.1) [12].

Adverse Effects Associated with Suppressive T4 Therapy in the Elderly

While T4 suppressive therapy may reduce recurrence and mortality rates in individuals with high-risk DTC, there are inherent risks (e.g., cardiovascular disease and decreased bone health) associated with iatrogenic thyrotoxicosis, particularly in the elderly. Suppressive thyroxine therapy may negatively impact quality of life [13].

It is unclear if endogenous hyperthyroidism and exogenous thyrotoxicosis cause similar adverse events. Serum free T4 levels are high normal or elevated in both situations; it is uncommon for serum T3 levels to be high normal/elevated in iatrogenic thyrotoxicosis, as compared to endogenous hyperthyroidism. This difference in serum T4/T3 ratios may be associated with different end-organ effects [14].

Table 17.1 Suggested long-term serum TSH targets in patients with DTC. (Table from 2015 ATA guidelines [12])

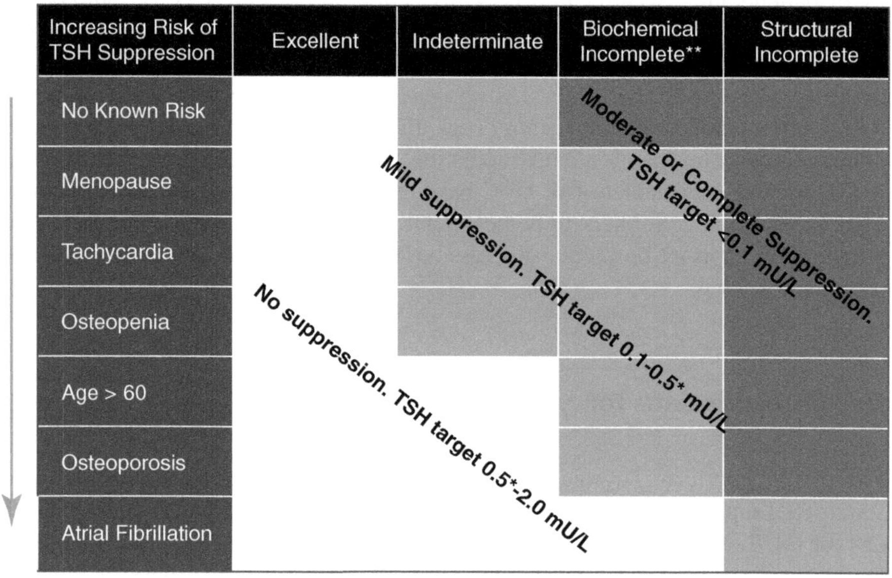

* 0.5 mU/L represents the lower limit od the reference range for the TSH assay which can be 0.3-0.5 mU/L depending on the specific assay

** TSH target for patient wich a biochemical incomplete response can be quite different based on original ATA risk, Tg level, Tg trend over time and risk of TSH suppression

- No suppression. TSH target 0.5*-2.0 mU/L
- Mild suppression. TSH target 0.1-0.5* mU/L
- Moderate or Complete suppression. TSH target <0.1 mU/L

Cardiovascular Disease

Dysrhythmias

Elderly individuals with iatrogenic thyrotoxicosis are at increased risk of cardiovascular (CV) disease and dysrhythmias. Studies have reported adverse CV effects including systolic and diastolic dysfunction, decreased arterial elasticity, and prothrombotic effects [15–18]. Adverse cardiac function may be more common in individuals treated with long-term suppressive therapy (>6 months)[19]. The elderly tend to be less symptomatic and thus warrant heightened clinical suspicion [20].

The prevalence of atrial fibrillation (AF) in DTC patients ≥60 years has been estimated to be as high as 17.5 %, with paroxysmal AF more common than persistent AF [21]. A Scottish observational study including 17,684 patients (females 85.9 % with mean age of 60.3 years; males, mean age of 61.8 years; median follow-up

4.5 years) on levothyroxine for ≥6 months demonstrated that individuals with serum TSH levels of <0.03 mU/L were at increased risk for CV disease (adjusted HR 1.37; 95 % CI 1.17–1.60) and dysrhythmias (adjusted HR 1.6; 95 % CI 1.10–2.33) after adjustment for age, sex, previous thyroid condition, socioeconomic status, and history of diabetes mellitus. The subset of patients with low but non-suppressed serum TSH levels (0.04 to 0.4 mU/L) did not have an increased risk of cardiac events [22]. In a retrospective cohort study using the Korean National Health Insurance data, patients with thyroid cancer had an elevated risk of coronary heart disease (HR 1.15, 95% CI, 1.10–1.22) and ischemic stroke (HR 1.15, 95% CI 1.09–1.22); the risk of atrial fibrillation was dose dependent with T4 therapy and felt to account for 4.4% of ischemic stroke incidence (n=128/2914) [23]. Similar data were reported in study from Finland [23]. Not all data demonstrate an association of degree of TSH suppression with atrial fibrillation [24].

RAI has been hypothesized to have an adverse CV effect as the sodium iodide symporter is expressed in cardiac tissue, potentially impacting cardiac inflammation, oxidative stress, and fibrosis [25, 26].

Cardiovascular Mortality

There are conflicting data regarding whether exogenous hyperthyroidism results in increased cardiovascular mortality. Some data have demonstrated a reduction in CV mortality [23]. Bauer et al. found no difference in mortality rates between women on long-term thyroxine therapy and nonusers (relative hazard 1.11, 95 % CI 0.98–1.24, $p \leq 0.09$), even when stratified by serum TSH (<0.5 mU/L vs. >5 mU/L). A prior history of hyperthyroidism, however, was associated with a small increase in all-cause and cardiovascular mortality [27]. In contrast, a population-based observational study (mean age 49 ± 14 years, median follow-up 8.5 years) demonstrated an increase in CV mortality and all-cause mortality by 3.3- and 4.4-fold, respectively, in patients with DTC independent of age, sex, and CV risk factors. Each tenfold decrease in geometric mean serum TSH was associated with a 3.1-fold increase in CV mortality [28]. Yang et al. similarly observed that among thyroid cancer patients, cardiac disease and cerebrovascular disease were the most frequent causes of non-cancer mortality [29]. The mechanism for increased CV mortality is unclear, but is postulated to be related to an increased risk of AF, impaired diastolic function, and increased left ventricular mass, leading to increased risk of stroke, heart failure, and myocardial infarction, respectively [30].

Bone Mineral Density and Fracture Risk

Data regarding the effect of iatrogenic hyperthyroidism on bone mineral density (BMD) are conflicting, but largely suggestive of a decrease in BMD and increase in fracture risk in postmenopausal women. Multiple factors including, but not limited to, low body mass index may adversely impact bone density, while factors such as hypoparathyroidism may be associated with increased bone density in the postmenopausal population [31, 32]. The majority of data have not shown compelling evidence of a significant change in bone health in premenopausal women or men treated with T4 suppressive therapy, as compared to postmenopausal women [33–43].

Wang et al. demonstrated that among individuals with low- and intermediate-risk DTC (n=791 with 569 women, mean age 48±14 years; median follow-up 6.5 years), the risk of postoperative osteoporosis was increased among women with TSH level <0.4 mU/L vs. >0.4 mU/L (HR 3.5, p=0.023, 95% CI 1.2–10.2). No associated risk was observed at a median serum TSH level of approximately 1 mU/L [44]. Similarly, a study including elderly individuals (n=87; median age 80 years) showed significant increases in rates of osteoporosis with more suppressed TSH levels (0.1–0.3 mU/L and <0.1 mU/L vs. 0.3–0.5 mU/L) [45].

Bauer et al. prospectively followed 686 women ≥ 65 years of age with subclinical thyrotoxicosis (exogenous and endogenous) and demonstrated that women with a serum TSH level ≤0.1 mU/L had a threefold increased risk of hip fracture (relative hazard, 3.6 [95 % CI, 1.0–12.9]) and a fourfold increased risk of vertebral fracture (odds ratio 4.5, 95 % CI 1.3–15.6) as compared to controls (serum TSH 0.5–5.5 mU/L) [46]. The Thyroid Epidemiology Audit and Research Study (TEARS) also demonstrated an increased risk of fractures in both individuals with suppressed serum TSH (<0.03 mU/L) (adjusted HR 2.02, 95 % CI 1.55–2.62) and elevated serum TSH (>4.0 mU/L) (adjusted HR 1.83, 95 % CI 1.41–2.37). Elevated serum TSH levels in the latter group were considered to be a marker for poor compliance with medical therapy. Similar to the pattern seen in cardiovascular events as previously described, individuals with low but non-suppressed serum TSH levels (0.04–0.4 mU/L) did not have an increased risk of fracture [22]. Shin et al. also showed a J-shaped association between TSH suppression and fracture risk with both higher and lower doses of T4 therapy associated with increased risk [47]. A cross-sectional study including 178 postmenopausal women demonstrated higher vertebral fracture prevalence among women with serum TSH <0.5 mU/L as compared to those with higher levels. In the entire cohort, vertebral fractures were independently associated with TSH level <1.0 mU/L, diagnosis of osteoporosis by densitometry, age, and duration of levothyroxine therapy [41].

A meta-analysis including five population-based prospective studies demonstrated a nonsignificant increase in the risk of hip fractures (HR 1.38 [CI, 0.92–2.07]) and non-spine fractures when patients with endogenous and exogenous subclinical thyrotoxicosis were pooled. The strength of the relationship between subclinical thyrotoxicosis and fractures appeared stronger in the setting of a suppressed serum TSH (<0.1 mU/L), but only two studies provided such data [48]. These findings are in keeping with meta-analyses by Faber et al. and Uzzan et al. suggesting that T4 suppressive therapy results in bone loss at an annual rate of 1 % in postmenopausal women [49, 50]. Differences in studies may be partially explained by varying rates of thyroid hormone suppression and calcium intake in the studies [35]. Data from two additional meta-analyses suggest that TSH suppression is associated with a lower BMD of the total hip and spine in postmenopausal woman and possible risk of osteoporotic fracture [39, 51].

Treatment

Calcium and bisphosphonates are useful in managing bone health in iatrogenic hyperthyroidism. Kung et al. demonstrated that calcium monotherapy (1000 mg/day) was effective in mitigating bone loss, while intranasal calcitonin offered little further benefit [52]. Postmenopausal women on suppressive levothyroxine not receiving calcium and vitamin D supplementation have higher rates of bone loss [43]. Bisphosphonates are effective in increasing BMD in the lumbar spine and femoral neck in postmenopausal women receiving T4 suppressive therapy in the short term [53].

Management of the Patient

Our patient has recurrent stage IVc PTC with likely pulmonary metastases. Given her persistent high-risk disease, she qualifies for moderate to complete suppressive thyroxine therapy by the 2015 ATA guidelines. However, the patient is postmenopausal with known osteoporosis; due to age, she is at an increased risk of AF and may have underlying cardiac disease that could increase her risk of CV mortality. In weighing the benefits and risks of suppressive therapy, the patient's goal serum TSH is in the mildly suppressed range (0.1–0.50 mU/L). Given the proximity to the goal TSH in the low-normal range, the patient's dose of levothyroxine was not adjusted.

Clinical Pearls/Pitfalls

- T4 suppressive therapy does not improve survival in patients with low-risk DTC though it may be beneficial in high-risk patients.
- Serum TSH targets in the long-term follow-up of individuals with DTC depends on the risk of recurrence, evidence of disease, and comorbidities.
- The elderly are at the high risk of developing complications from T4 suppressive therapy, particularly atrial fibrillation and osteoporosis.
- Calcium and bisphosphonates may be useful in mitigating the risk of bone loss in postmenopausal women on suppressive doses of T4.
- The potential risks of adverse cardiovascular and skeletal effects are minimized by targeting subnormal, rather than fully suppressed serum TSH levels (Table 17.1).

References

1. SEER cancer statistics review, 1975–2011, National Cancer Institute. Bethesda, MD. Based on November 2013 SEER data submission, released April 2014. http://seer.cancer.gov/csr/1975_2011/.
2. McLeod DS, Sawka AM, Cooper DS. Controversies in primary treatment of low-risk papillary thyroid cancer. Lancet. 2013;381(9871):1046–57.
3. Lim H, Devesa SS, Sosa JA, Check D, Kitahara CM. Trends in Thyroid Cancer Incidence and Mortality in the United States, 1974-2013. JAMA. 2017;317(13):1338–48.
4. Pujol P, Daures JP, Nsakala N, Baldet L, Bringer J, Jaffiol C. Degree of thyrotropin suppression as a prognostic determinant in differentiated thyroid cancer. J Clin Endocrinol Metab. 1996;81(12):4318–23.
5. McGriff NJ, Csako G, Gourgiotis L, Lori CG, Pucino F, Sarlis NJ. Effects of thyroid hormone suppression therapy on adverse clinical outcomes in thyroid cancer. Ann Med. 2002;34(7–8):554–64.
6. Cooper DS, Specker B, Ho M, et al. Thyrotropin suppression and disease progression in patients with differentiated thyroid cancer: results from the national thyroid cancer treatment cooperative registry. Thyroid. 1998;8(9):737–44.
7. Jonklaas J, Sarlis NJ, Litofsky D, et al. Outcomes of patients with differentiated thyroid carcinoma following initial therapy. Thyroid. 2006;16(12):1229–42.
8. Carhill AA, Litofsky DR, Ross DS, Jonklaas J, Cooper DS, Brierley JD, Ladenson PW, Ain KB, Fein HG, Haugen BR, Magner J, Skarulis MC, Steward DL, Xing M, Maxon HR, Sherman SI. Long-term outcomes following therapy in differentiated thyroid carcinoma: NTCTCS registry analysis 1987-2012. J Clin Endocrinol Metab. 2015;100(9):3270–9.
9. Hovens GC, Stokkel MP, Kievit J, et al. Associations of serum thyrotropin concentrations with recurrence and death in differentiated thyroid cancer. J Clin Endocrinol Metab. 2007;92(7):2610–5.
10. Sugitani I, Fujimoto Y. Does postoperative thyrotropin suppression therapy truly decrease recurrence in papillary thyroid carcinoma? A randomized controlled trial. J Clin Endocrinol Metab. 2010;95(10):4576–83.
11. Park S, Kim WG, Han M, Jeon MJ, Kwon H, Kim M, Sung TY, Kim TY, Kim WB, Hong SJ, Shong YK. Thyrotropin suppressive therapy for low-risk small thyroid cancer: a propensity score-matched cohort study. Thyroid. 2017;27(9):1164–70.
12. Haugen BR, Alexander EK, Bible KC, Doherty GM, Mandel SJ, Nikiforov YE, Pacini F, Randolph GW, Sawka AM, Schlumberger M, Schuff KG, Sherman SI, Sosa JA, Steward DL, Tuttle RM, Wartofsky L. American Thyroid Association Management Guidelines for patients with thyroid nodules and differentiated thyroid cancer. Thyroid. 2016;26:1):1–133.
13. Giusti M, Melle G, Fenocchio M, et al. Five-year longitudinal evaluation of quality of life in a cohort of patients with differentiated thyroid carcinoma. J Zhejiang Univ Sci B. 2011;12(3):163–73.
14. Biondi B, Cooper DS. Benefits of thyrotropin suppression versus the risks of adverse effects in differentiated thyroid cancer. Thyroid. 2010;20(2):135–46.
15. Smit JW, Eustatia-Rutten CF, Corssmit EP, Pereira AM, Frölich M, Bleeker GB, Holman ER, van der Wall EE, Romijn JA, Bax JJ. Reversible diastolic dysfunction after long-term exogenous subclinical hyperthyroidism: a randomized, placebo-controlled study. J Clin Endocrinol Metab. 2005;90(11):6041–7.
16. Abdulrahman RM, Delgado V, Hoftijzer HC, Ng AC, Ewe SH, Marsan NA, Holman ER, Hovens GC, Corssmit EP, Romijn JA, Bax JJ, Smit JW. Both exogenous subclinical hyperthyroidism and short-term overt hypothyroidism affect myocardial strain in patients with differentiated thyroid carcinoma. Thyroid. 2011;21(5):471–6.
17. Shargorodsky M, Serov S, Gavish D, Leibovitz E, Harpaz D, Zimlichman R. Long-term thyrotropin-suppressive therapy with levothyroxine impairs small and large artery elasticity and increases left ventricular mass in patients with thyroid carcinoma. Thyroid. 2006;16(4):381–6.

18. Abdulrahman RM, Delgado V, Ng AC, Ewe SH, Bertini M, Holman ER, Hovens GC, Pereira AM, Romijn JA, Bax JJ, Smit JW. Abnormal cardiac contractility in long-term exogenous subclinical hyperthyroid patients as demonstrated by two-dimensional echocardiography speckle tracking imaging. Eur J Endocrinol. 2010;163(3):435–41.
19. Wang R, Yang L, Jin S, Han X, Liu B. Thyroid stimulating hormone suppression time on cardiac function of patients with differentiated thyroid carcinoma. Cancer Cell Int. 2018;18:189.
20. Boelaert K, Torlinska B, Holder RL, Franklyn JA. Older subjects with hyperthyroidism present with a paucity of symptoms and signs: a large cross-sectional study. J Clin Endocrinol Metab. 2010;95(6):2715–26.
21. Abonowara A, Quraishi A, Sapp JL, et al. Prevalence of atrial fibrillation in patients taking TSH suppression therapy for management of thyroid cancer. Clin Invest Med. 2012;35(3):E152–6.
22. Flynn RW, Bonellie SR, Jung RT, MacDonald TM, Morris AD, Leese GP. Serum thyroid-stimulating hormone concentration and morbidity from cardiovascular disease and fractures in patients on long-term thyroxine therapy. J Clin Endocrinol Metab. 2010;95(1):186–93.
23. Pajamäki N, Metso S, Hakala T, Ebeling T, Huhtala H, Ryödi E, Sand J, Jukkola-Vuorinen A, Kellokumpu-Lehtinen PL, Jaatinen P. Long-term cardiovascular morbidity and mortality in patients treated for differentiated thyroid cancer. Clin Endocrinol (Oxf). 2018;88(2):303–10.
24. Klein Hesselink EN, Lefrandt JD, Schuurmans EP, Burgerhof JG, Groen B, Gansevoort RT, van der Horst-Schrivers AN, Dullaart RP, Van Gelder IC, Brouwers AH, Rienstra M, Links TP. Increased risk of atrial fibrillation after treatment for differentiated thyroid carcinoma. J Clin Endocrinol Metab. 2015;100(12):4563–9.
25. Spitzweg C, Joba W, Eisenmenger W, Heufelder AE. Analysis of human sodium iodide symporter gene expression in extrathyroidal tissues and cloning of its complementary deoxyribonucleic acids from salivary gland, mammary gland, and gastric mucosa. J Clin Endocrinol Metab. 1998;83(5):1746–51.
26. Biondi B, Cooper DS. Thyroid hormone suppression therapy. Endocrinol Metab Clin North Am. 2019;48(1):227–37.
27. Suh B, Shin DW, Park Y, Lim H, Yun JM, Song SO, Park JH, Cho B, Guallar E. Increased cardiovascular risk in thyroid cancer patients taking levothyroxine: a nationwide cohort study in Korea. Eur J Endocrinol. 2019;180(1):11–20.
28. Bauer DC, Rodondi N, Stone KL, Hillier TA, Study of Osteoporotic Fractures Research Group: Universities of California (San Francisco), Pittsburgh, Minnesota (Minneapolis), Kaiser Permanente Center for Health Research, Portland. Thyroid hormone use, hyperthyroidism and mortality in older women. Am J Med. 2007;120(4):343–9.
29. Klein Hesselink EN, Klein Hesselink MS, de Bock GH, et al. Long-term cardiovascular mortality in patients with differentiated thyroid carcinoma: an observational study. J Clin Oncol. 2013;31(32):4046–53.
30. Yang L, Shen W, Sakamoto N. Population-based study evaluating and predicting the probability of death resulting from thyroid cancer and other causes among patients with thyroid cancer. J Clin Oncol. 2013;31(4):468–74.
31. de Melo TG, da Assumpção LV, Santos Ade O, Zantut-Wittmann DE. Low BMI and low TSH value as risk factors related to lower bone mineral density in postmenopausal women under levothyroxine therapy for differentiated thyroid carcinoma. Thyroid Res. 2015;8:7.
32. Kim CW, Hong S, Oh SH, Lee JJ, Han JY, Hong S, Kim SH, Nam M, Kim YS. Change of Bone Mineral Density and Biochemical Markers of Bone Turnover in Patients on Suppressive Levothyroxine Therapy for Differentiated Thyroid Carcinoma. J Bone Metab. 2015;22(3):135–41.
33. Heemstra KA, Hamdy NA, Romijn JA, Smit JW. The effects of thyrotropin-suppressive therapy on bone metabolism in patients with well-differentiated thyroid carcinoma. Thyroid. 2006;16(6):583–91.

34. Waring AC, Harrison S, Fink HA, et al. A prospective study of thyroid function, bone loss, and fractures in older men: the MrOS study. J Bone Miner Res. 2013;28(3):472–9.
35. Quan ML, Pasieka JL, Rorstad O. Bone mineral density in well-differentiated thyroid cancer patients treated with suppressive thyroxine: a systematic overview of the literature. J Surg Oncol. 2002;79(1):62–9. discussion 69–70
36. Notsu M, Yamauchi M, Morita M, Nawata K, Sugimoto T. Papillary thyroid carcinoma is a risk factor for severe osteoporosis. J Bone Miner Metab 2020;38(2):264–70.
37. Papaleontiou M, Banerjee M, Reyes-Gastelum D, Hawley ST, Haymart MR. Risk of Osteoporosis and Fractures in Patients with Thyroid Cancer: A Case-Control Study in U.S. Veterans. Oncologist. 2019;24(9):1166–73.
38. Soydal Ç, Özkan E, Nak D, Elhan AH, Küçük NÖ, Kır MK. Risk Factors for Predicting Osteoporosis in Patients Who Receive Thyrotropin Suppressive Levothyroxine Treatment for Differentiated Thyroid Carcinoma. Mol Imaging Radionucl Ther. 2019;28(2):69–75.
39. Yoon BH, Lee Y, Oh HJ, Kim SH, Lee YK. Influence of Thyroid-stimulating Hormone Suppression Therapy on Bone Mineral Density in Patients with Differentiated Thyroid Cancer: A Meta-analysis. J Bone Metab. 2019;26(1):51–60.
40. De Mingo Dominguez ML, Guadalix Iglesias S, Martin-Arriscado Arroba C, López Alvarez B, Martínez Diaz-Guerra G, Martinez-Pueyo JI, Ferrero Herrero E, Hawkins Carranza F. Low trabecular bone score in postmenopausal women with differentiated thyroid carcinoma after long-term TSH suppressive therapy. Endocrine. 2018;62(1):166–73.
41. Mazziotti G, Formenti AM, Frara S, Olivetti R, Banfi G, Memo M, Maroldi R, Giubbini R, Giustina A. High prevalence of radiological vertebral fractures in women on thyroid-stimulating hormone-suppressive therapy for thyroid carcinoma. J Clin Endocrinol Metab. 2018;103(3):956–64.
42. Mendonça Monteiro de Barros G, Madeira M, Vieira Neto L, de Paula Paranhos Neto F, Carvalho Mendonça LM, Corrêa Barbosa Lima I, Corbo R, Fleiuss Farias ML. Bone mineral density and bone microarchitecture after long-term suppressive levothyroxine treatment of differentiated thyroid carcinoma in young adult patients. J Bone Miner Metab. 2016;34(4):417–21.
43. Kim MK, Yun KJ, Kim MH, Lim DJ, Kwon HS, Song KH, Kang MI, Baek KH. The effects of thyrotropin-suppressing therapy on bone metabolism in patients with well-differentiated thyroid carcinoma. Bone. 2015;71:101–5.
44. Wang LY, Smith AW, Palmer FL, Tuttle RM, Mahrous A, Nixon IJ, Patel SG, Ganly I, Fagin JA, Boucai L. Thyrotropin suppression increases the risk of osteoporosis without decreasing recurrence in ATA low-and intermediate-risk patients with differentiated thyroid carcinoma. Thyroid. 2015;25(3):300–7.
45. Xia Q, Dong S, Bian PD, Wang J, Li CJ. Effects of endocrine therapy on the prognosis of elderly patients after surgery for papillary thyroid carcinoma. Eur Arch Otorhinolaryngol. 2016;273(4):1037–43.
46. Bauer DC, Ettinger B, Nevitt MC, Stone KL, Study of Osteoporotic Fractures Research Group. Risk for fracture in women with low serum levels of thyroid-stimulating hormone. Ann Intern Med. 2001;134(7):561–8.
47. Shin DW, Suh B, Lim H, Yun JM, Song SO, Park Y. J-shaped association between postoperative levothyroxine dosage and fracture risk in thyroid cancer patients: a retrospective cohort study. J Bone Miner Res. 2018;33(6):1037–43.
48. Wirth CD, Blum MR, da Costa BR, et al. Subclinical thyroid dysfunction and the risk for fractures: a systematic review and meta-analysis. Ann Intern Med. 2014;161(3):189–99.
49. Faber J, Galloe AM. Changes in bone mass during prolonged subclinical hyperthyroidism due to L-thyroxine treatment: a meta-analysis. Eur J Endocrinol. 1994;130(4):350–6.
50. Uzzan B, Campos J, Cucherat M, Nony P, Boissel JP, Perret GY. Effects on bone mass of long term treatment with thyroid hormones: a meta-analysis. J Clin Endocrinol Metab. 1996;81(12):4278–89.

51. Lee Y, Yoon BH, Lee S, Chung YK, Lee YK. Risk of osteoporotic fractures after thyroid-stimulating hormone suppression therapy in patients with thyroid cancer. J Bone Metab. 2019;26(1):45–50.
52. Kung AW, Yeung SS. Prevention of bone loss induced by thyroxine suppressive therapy in postmenopausal women: the effect of calcium and calcitonin. J Clin Endocrinol Metab. 1996;81(3):1232–6.
53. Panico A, Lupoli GA, Fonderico F, et al. Osteoporosis and thyrotropin-suppressive therapy: reduced effectiveness of alendronate. Thyroid. 2009;19(5):437–42.

Chapter 18
A Case with Postsurgical Hypoparathyroidism: Treatment Options

Jessica Pepe and Salvatore Minisola

Case Presentation

A 59-year-old woman complaining of perioral and digital numbness/tingling was referred to our outpatient Mineral Metabolism Unit. One year before, she had a thyroidectomy for benign multinodular goiter. According to the pathology report, the surgical procedure resulted in the accidental removal of three parathyroid glands. After the thyroidectomy, the patient complained of mild paresthesias and tingling; her serum calcium level was 1.96 mmol/L (normal range 2.2–2.6 mmol/L). The patient was started on intravenous calcium gluconate, which provided relief from the symptoms. Two days after surgery, the patient was discharged with a calcium level of 2.20 mmol/L while on oral calcium (1 g/day) and calcitriol (0.50 mcg twice a day) therapy. After discharge from the hospital, the patient suffered diarrhea and experienced dyspepsia due to a previously diagnosed irritable bowel syndrome. To avoid the symptoms of hypocalcemia and dyspepsia, the general practitioner tried frequent modifications of both the calcium supplement and the calcitriol dosage. However, during the following six months, she had acute symptoms of hypocalcemia which brought her twice to the emergency room. Intravenous calcium gluconate was administered to relieve symptoms and achieve serum calcium levels of 2.0 mmol/l. She was following her last prescription of calcitriol (1 mcg twice a day) and calcium carbonate 2000 mg per day when she came to our unit with symptoms of mild paresthesia. The thyroid function was well controlled on oral thyroxine.

As an outpatient, her initial laboratory tests were as follows: calcium 1.83 mmol/L, phosphorus 2.41 mmol/L (normal range 0.8–1.45 mmol/L), parathyroid hormone (PTH) 5 ng/L (normal range 14–72 ng/L), and 24-h urinary calcium 14

J. Pepe (✉) · S. Minisola
Department of Clinical, Internal, Anesthesiological and Cardiovascular Sciences, "Sapienza" University of Rome, Rome, Italy
e-mail: jessica.pepe@uniroma1.it

G. Grani et al. (eds.), *Thyroid Cancer*,
https://doi.org/10.1007/978-3-030-61919-0_18

mmol (normal range 1.25–10 mmol/24 h). On physical examination, she had no pathological signs, except both a positive Trousseau and Chvostek sign, which are signs of latent tetany. Indeed, tapping her facial nerve in front of the ear, just below the zygomatic arch, elicited the Chvostek sign, which is a momentary abnormal contraction of the ipsilateral facial muscles. By inflating the sphygmomanometer to a pressure higher than the systolic blood pressure and holding it in place for three minutes, we caused the Trousseau sign, which includes wrist flexion, interphalangeal joint extension, and thumb adduction. These clinical data were indicative of symptomatic postsurgical hypoparathyroidism which required an adjustment of therapy.

Assessment and Literature Review

Since 2015, new data on the management of hypoparathyroidism has been published [1–4] which has led to the creation of new statement on this topic by the American Thyroid Association (ATA) [5], new guidelines by the European Society of Endocrinology [6] and by a consensus of experts in the First International Conference on the management of hypoparathyroidism [7]. The interest on this topic has grown because patients are not always adequately treated, as shown by a recent survey on chronic hypoparathyroidism, which unveiled that 44% of patients were hospitalized at least once for hypocalcemia and 16% for hypercalcemia [8]. The majority of the patients in this study (87%) felt that an emergency card would be highly needed or useful [8].

Definition and Prevalence

Hypocalcemia and absent or low levels of parathyroid hormone (PTH) are the major biochemical features of hypoparathyroidism. An increased renal calcium excretion and serum hyperphosphatemia as a result of the lack of PTH, which physiologically enhances renal tubular calcium reabsorption and increases phosphate excretion, are also present. Postsurgical hypoparathyroidism may occur after any type of neck surgery for several indications, but it occurs most frequently after a total thyroidectomy [9]. When postsurgical hypoparathyroidism persists six months or more after the surgery, it is considered as a case of chronic hypoparathyroidism.

A recent systematic review investigated how hypoparathyroidism is defined and whether different definitions and selected thresholds for hypocalcemia affect the incidence: it confirmed that the incidence of hypoparathyroidism ranged from 0.0% to 20.2% due to the different definitions [10]. Overall, postsurgical hypocalcemia is clearly recognized as a very common medical problem worldwide, with little difference in epidemiological data across geographical areas, as recently reported in the USA [11], Denmark [12], Norway [13], Scotland [14], and Italy [15, 16].

Predictors of Post-thyroidectomy Hypocalcemia

Recently there has been a great deal of interest in identifying perioperative factors that can predict hypocalcemia in order to reduce hospitalization length.

No single factor may predict the occurrence of hypocalcemia, but a high-volume surgeon (who has performed more than 100 thyroidectomies) is likely to have a reduction in the number of cases of postsurgical hypoparathyroidism [17]. Also, the indication and extent of surgery is important: the central neck lymph node dissection is more frequently associated with hypoparathyroidism development, as well as intervention for Graves' disease [18]. Autotransplantation of the parathyroid gland is an option, but data on the real effectiveness to reduce hypocalcemia are conflicting [5, 18].

Measurement of PTH 4 hours after surgery is a good predictor of subsequent hypoparathyroidism, but no consensus on the threshold of the PTH level is currently available. Indeed, some studies proposed a cutoff for PTH of 10 pg/ml [19], while others 3.75 pg/ml for transient and 2.48 pg/ml for permanent hypoparathyroidism [20].

A recent retrospective chart review study of 429 patients, who underwent total thyroidectomy, showed that the rate of drop in serum calcium and the postoperative serum calcium level remained the only significant predictors of symptom development, after adjustment for other significant covariates. Using a receiver operating characteristics curve, a rate of calcium drop >0.083 mg/dl/h, that is, 1 mg/dl over 12 h, has a sensitivity of 71% and specificity of 73% for detecting hypocalcemic symptoms [21].

Vitamin D deficiency is another independent predictor of hypocalcemia [22], and preoperative vitamin D supplementation can reduce its occurrence [23].

Therapy

The conventional therapy is based on calcium supplements and the active form of vitamin D (calcitriol), with the primary purpose of achieving a serum calcium level of 2 mmol/l and the absence of hypocalcemic symptoms [24]. Effective absorption of calcium carbonate, which is usually prescribed at a daily dose of 1000 mg subdivided into two doses, requires an acidic environment. Alternatives that do not require a low gastric pH (such as calcium citrate) are recommended for persons taking acid-blocking therapy.

In the case of hypomagnesemia, a magnesium supplement should be administered because magnesium regulates PTH secretion [7].

A recent meta-analysis of ten randomized controlled trials showed that calcium supplementation after surgery decreased the risk of transient postoperative hypocalcemia (OR 0.48 [95% CI, 0.31–0.74]; P<.001) but did not decrease the demand for intravenous supplementation or the rate of permanent hypocalcemia compared to no treatment [25]. Another recent meta-analysis evaluated the effectiveness of routine postoperative administration of calcium with or without vitamin D3 compared with treatment based on serum calcium levels to prevent postoperative symptomatic and biochemical hypocalcemia after thyroidectomy [26]. Routine supplementation with calcium plus vitamin D3 reduced the risk of symptomatic and biochemical hypocalcemia (risk difference (RD) -0.25, 95% CI -0.32 to -0.18) compared to treatment based on the measurement of calcium levels [26].

Although routine treatment of hypoparathyroidism with oral calcium and calcitriol (from 0.25 mcg to 2 mcg subdivided into two doses daily) increases serum calcium, in the long term, it may be associated with ectopic calcification and hypercalciuria, as the lack of PTH increases renal leak of calcium [4].

An advance in the chronic management of hypoparathyroidism is the administration of PTH peptides. Before the approval by the FDA in 2015 of PTH 1-84 (injected subcutaneously once daily) for hypoparathyroidism, teriparatide was utilized in hypoparathyroid patients not responding to conventional therapy [4]. Teriparatide (PTH 1-34) is a PTH analog produced by recombinant technology, and it is usually prescribed for osteoporosis treatment at a dosage of 20 mcg injected subcutaneously daily for a maximum period of two years [4].

A systematic review of nine randomized controlled trials and two cohort studies demonstrated that recombinant PTH was effective for correcting serum calcium levels and significantly reduced the daily requirements of calcium and active vitamin D supplements compared to placebo. Urinary calcium excretion was reduced with PTH 1-34 compared to conventional calcium and vitamin D supplements, but unchanged with PTH 1-84 [27].

A retrospective analysis of patients treated for 10 years with PTH 1-84 showed a stable restoration of the calcium parameters, with an approximate 50% reduction of the needed calcium supplement and a 75% reduction of the needed calcitriol [28]. A new sustained-release prodrug of PTH (1-34) was tested in phase I trial and phase II trial is ongoing [29].

Due to the high cost of PTH 1-84 therapy, only a subset of patients would benefit from this treatment. An international consensus of experts, in 2016, suggested that this therapy should only be prescribed to patients with well-established, chronic hypoparathyroidism, with variable and inconstant control of the serum calcium with frequent episodes of hypo- and hypercalcemia [7]. Patients with renal complications such as nephrolithiasis, nephrocalcinosis, or reduced creatinine clearance (eGFR < 60 mL/min); hypercalciuria and/or other biochemical indices of kidney stone risk are also considered appropriate candidates. Moreover, persistently elevated serum phosphate and/or calcium phosphate product (higher than 55 mg^2/dL^2 or 4.4 $mmol^2/L^2$) is considered an indication. Other indications are excessive amounts of oral medications required to control symptoms such as >2.5 g of calcium and/or > 1.5 mcg of active vitamin D daily, or both, and a gastrointestinal tract disorder that might lead to variable calcium and vitamin D absorption.

A recent European Society of Endocrinology guideline advised the use of active vitamin D and calcium supplements as the primary treatment for long-term hypoparathyroidism [6]. The routine use of recombinant PTH in long-term hypoparathyroidism was not recommended due to the potential risk of osteosarcoma, as reported in rat studies. ATA statement suggested to use it only in specific cases of unresponsiveness to treatment [5].

Long-Term Follow-Up

Patients with permanent hypoparathyroidism should receive appropriate follow-up care to monitor for long-term complications. Based on the international consensus of experts, biochemical evaluation of serum calcium and phosphorus should be performed every six months in order to keep albumin-adjusted calcium in the lower range and avoid hyperphosphatemia. Renal function should be monitored annually with creatinine assessment together with 24-hour urinary calcium [7].

Biochemical surveillance is essential because a recent case-control study reported a positive association between a relatively high plasma phosphate level and/or a high calcium phosphate product and mortality, as well as risk of renal diseases and infections [30]. Despite biochemical evaluation, some complications such as renal impairment appeared to be related to conventional therapy. Recently, in a cohort of hypoparathyroid patients with a maximum follow-up of 12 years, a multivariate linear regression model showed a statistically significant ($p=0.027$) relationship between the duration of calcitriol treatment and renal function decline at a rate of 1.06 ml/min/1.73 m^2 per year of calcitriol therapy, while correcting for the mean calcium phosphate product and age [31].

Moreover, in a population study of 5000 patients who had undergone thyroidectomy for benign diseases, followed for approximately 4.5 years, hypoparathyroid patients had an increased risk for renal insufficiency (hazard ratio, HR 4.88; 95% CI 2.00–11.95) and any malignancy (HR 2.15; 95% CI 1.08–4.27). Those hypoparathyroid patients who already had cardiovascular disease at the time of thyroidectomy had an increased risk for cardiovascular events during follow-up (HR 1.88; 95% CI 1.02–3.47) [32].

Management of the Case

The patient exhibited symptoms and biochemical features of permanent postsurgical hypoparathyroidism, unresponsive to the prescribed therapy.

Hypocalcemic symptoms are uncommon unless serum calcium level is below 2.0 mmol/L (8.0 mg/dL) [4], although it is not known which calcium concentrations will trigger symptoms in any given person and whether the knowledge of this concentration is of clinical importance [4]. Symptoms probably depend on the degree and rapidity of onset of the hypocalcemia, ranging from mild paresthesias and tingling to more severe cramps, tetany, seizures, laryngospasm, congestive heart failure, and arrhythmias due to prolonged QT intervals.

It is important to exclude other potential causes of hypocalcemia that might be potential causes of unsuccessful treatment. These include poor adherence, which was the case of the patient due to dyspepsia, which brought her to a seldom self-reduction of calcium supplements or the concomitant use of medication reducing calcium absorption (excluded in this particular case). Malabsorption is another potential cause, but tests for celiac disease, usually performed to clarify long-lasting hypocalcemia, unresponsive to therapy, were negative in this case as well as lactose intolerance test. Her previous diagnosis of irritable bowel syndrome was made based on her symptoms and negative upper and lower tract endoscopy. Hypomagnesemia was excluded. In some cases, treatment failure might also be due to the so-called hungry bone syndrome. This is caused by a rapid influx of calcium into the bones due to high bone turnover; it is a recognized cause of hypocalcemia following thyroidectomy for thyrotoxicosis; however, the patient had a preoperative TSH level of 1.27 mUI/L, thus excluding this possibility.

Due to the symptoms the patient experienced, she complained of a reduced quality of life; her poor adherence was unlikely to be corrected.

In fact, irritable bowel syndrome results in alternating episodes of diarrhea and constipation, together with dyspepsia; calcium supplements exacerbate these symptoms.

She was initially taking 2 grams of calcium and 2 mcg of calcitriol: her serum calcium level was 1.9 mmol/L. She could not tolerate a higher dosage of calcium supplements. A new regimen with PTH 1-84 (50 mcg) once daily was started. Simultaneously, the dose of calcium was reduced by 50%. The serum calcium concentration was monitored within the first week of initiation and increased to 2.1 mmol/L. At the second week's evaluation, calcitriol was reduced to 1.5 mcg daily. Her 24-hour urinary calcium was 14 mmol/24 hour (normal range 1.25–10 mmol/24 h). She was already on a low-salt diet, and we tried to add hydrochlorothiazide 12.5 daily to avoid hypercalciuria, but the patient, who was normotensive, complained of hypotension. A further reduction of calcitriol to 0.50, twice daily, was proposed. Her serum magnesium was within the normal range.

After 4 weeks, laboratory evaluation showed a calcium level of 2.1 mmol/L and hypercalciuria with a 24 h urinary calcium of 11 mmol/24 h (normal range 1.25–10 mmol/24 h).

After other 4 weeks, the biochemical parameters were satisfactory [serum calcium, 2.20 mmol/L; serum phosphorus, 1.55 mmol/L (normal range, 0.75–1.45); 24-h urinary calcium, 10 mmol (normal range 1.25-10 mmol/24 hours)].The patient was free of symptoms of hypocalcemia and physical examination showed negative Chvostek and Trousseau signs. Her quality of life, as reported by the patient, was improved.

Clinical Pearls/Pitfalls

- The prevalence of postsurgical hypoparathyroidism varies from 0% to 20% according to how it is defined; thus a universal definition, in the literature, is needed.
- Prediction of post-thyroidectomy hypocalcemia remains a challenge, but 4-hour-postoperative PTH, preoperative vitamin D, and postoperative changes in calcium of 1 mg/dl in 12 hours should be considered predictors of post-thyroidectomy hypocalcemia.
- Treatment with calcium and calcitriol aims to keep the level of albumin-adjusted calcium at the lower end of the normal range, to reduce the risk of hypercalcemia and hypercalciuria.
- Long-term complications such as renal insufficiency should be monitored.
- PTH (1-84) therapy may be another therapeutic option for cases of permanent hypoparathyroidism with poor response to conventional therapy, renal impairment, or malabsorption.

References

1. Gafni RI, Collins MT. Hypoparathyroidism. N Engl J Med. 2019;380(18):1738–47.
2. Kakava K, Tournis S, Papadakis G, Karelas I, Stampouloglou P, Kassi E, et al. Postsurgical hypoparathyroidism: a systematic review. In Vivo. 2016;30(3):171–9.
3. Hakami Y, Khan A. Hypoparathyroidism. Front Horm Res. 2019;51:109–26.
4. Cusano NE, Bilezikian JP. Update on hypoparathyroidism. Curr Opin Rheumatol. 2019;31(4):381–7.
5. Orloff LA, Wiseman SM, Bernet VJ, Fahey TJ 3rd, Shaha AR, Shindo ML, et al. American Thyroid Association statement on postoperative hypoparathyroidism: diagnosis, prevention, and management in adults. Thyroid. 2018;28:830–41.
6. Bollerslev J, Rejnmark L, Marcocci C, Shoback DM, Sitges-Serra A, van Biesen W, et al. European Society of Endocrinology clinical guideline: treatment of chronic hypoparathyroidism in adults. Eur J Endocrinol. 2015;173(2):1–20.
7. Brandi ML, Bilezikian JP, Shoback D, et al. Management of hypoparathyroidism: summary statement and guidelines. J Clin Endocrinol Metab. 2016;101:2273–83.
8. Astor MC, Zhu W, Björnsdottir S, Bollerslev J, Kämpe O, Husebye ES. Is there a need for an emergency card in hypoparathyroidism? J Intern Med. 2019;285(4):429–35.
9. Clarke BL, Brown EM, Collins MT, Jüppner H, Lakatos P, Levine MA, et al. Epidemiology and diagnosis of hypoparathyroidism. J Clin Endocrinol Metab. 2016;101(6):2284–99.
10. Harsløf T, Rolighed L, Rejnmark L. Huge variations in definition and reported incidence of postsurgical hypoparathyroidism: a systematic review. Endocrine. 2019;64(1):176–83.
11. Powers J, Joy K, Ruscio A, Lagast H. Prevalence and incidence of hypoparathyroidism in the United States using a large claims database. J Bone Miner Res. 2013;28:2570–6.
12. Underbjerg L, Sikjaer T, Mosekilde L, Rejnmark L. Post-surgical hypoparathyroidism – risk of fractures, psychiatric diseases, cancer, cataract, and infections. J Bone Miner Res. 2014;29:2504–10.
13. Astor MC, Løvås K, Debowska A, Eriksen EF, Evang JA, Fossum C, et al. Epidemiology and health-related quality of life in hypoparathyroidism in Norway. J Clin Endocrinol Metab. 2016;101(8):3045–53.

14. Vadiveloo T, Donnan PT, Leese GP. A population-based study of the epidemiology of chronic hypoparathyroidism. J Bone Miner Res. 2018;33(3):478–85.
15. Cipriani C, Pepe J, Biamonte F, Manai R, Biondi P, Nieddu L, et al. The epidemiology of hypoparathyroidism in Italy: An 8-Year Register-Based Study. Calcif Tissue Int. 2017;100(3):278–85.
16. Cianferotti L, Parri S, Gronchi G, Marcucci G, Cipriani C, Pepe J, et al. Prevalence of chronic hypoparathyroidism in a mediterranean region as estimated by the analysis of anonymous healthcare database. Calcif Tissue Int. 2018;103(2):144–50.
17. Cianferotti L, Marcucci G, Brandi ML. Causes and pathophysiology of hypoparathyroidism. Best Pract Res Clin Endocrinol Metab. 2018;32(6):909–25.
18. Păduraru DN, Ion D, Carsote M, Andronic O, Bolocan A. Post-thyroidectomy hypocalcemia - risk factors and management. Chirurgia (Bucur). 2019;114(5):564–70.
19. Raffaelli M, De Crea C, D'Amato G, Moscato U, Bellantone C, Carrozza C, et al. Post-thyroidectomy hypocalcemia is related to parathyroid dysfunction even in patients with normal parathyroid hormone concentrations early after surgery. Surgery. 2016;159(1):78–84.
20. Chang JW, Park KW, Jung SN, Liu L, Kim SM, Koo BS. The most reliable time point for intact parathyroid hormone measurement to predict hypoparathyroidism after total thyroidectomy with central neck dissection to treat papillary thyroid carcinoma: a prospective cohort study. Eur Arch Otorhinolaryngol. 2019; https://doi.org/10.1007/s00405-019-05693-1. [Epub ahead of print]
21. Saad RK, Boueiz NG, Akiki VC, Fuleihan GAE. Rate of drop in serum calcium as a predictor of hypocalcemic symptoms post total thyroidectomy. Osteoporos Int. 2019;30(12):2495–504.
22. Al-Khatib T, Althubaiti AM, Althubaiti A, Mosli HH, Alwasiah RO, Badawood LM. Severe vitamin D deficiency: a significant predictor of early hypocalcemia after total thyroidectomy. Otolaryngol Head Neck Surg. 2015;152:424–31.
23. Khan Bhettani M, Rehman M, Ahmed M, Altaf HN, Choudry UK, Khan KH. Role of pre-operative vitamin D supplementation to reduce post-thyroidectomy hypocalcemia; Cohort study. Int J Surg. 2019;71:85–90.
24. Edafe O, Mech CE, Balasubramanian SP. Calcium, vitamin D or recombinant parathyroid hormone for managing post-thyroidectomy hypoparathyroidism. Cochrane Database Syst Rev. 2019;5:CD012845.
25. Xing T, Hu Y, Wang B, Zhu J. Role of oral calcium supplementation alone or with vitamin D in preventing post-thyroidectomy hypocalcaemia: A meta-analysis. Medicine (Baltimore). 2019;98(8):e1445.
26. Sanabria A, Rojas A, Arevalo J. Meta-analysis of routine calcium/vitamin D3 supplementation versus serum calcium level-based strategy to prevent postoperative hypocalcaemia after thyroidectomy. Br J Surg. 2019;106(9):1126–37.
27. Ramakrishnan Y, Cocks HC. Impact of recombinant PTH on management of hypoparathyroidism: a systematic review. Eur Arch Otorhinolaryngol. 2016;273(4):827–35.
28. Tay YD, Tabacco G, Cusano NE, Williams J, Omeragic B, Majeed R, et al. Therapy of hypoparathyroidism With rhPTH(1-84): a prospective, 8-Year investigation of efficacy and safety. J Clin Endocrinol Metab. 2019;104(11):5601–10.
29. Holten-Andersen L, Pihl S, Rasmussen CE, Zettler J, Maitro G, Baron J, et al. Design and preclinical development of TransCon PTH, an investigational sustained-release PTH replacement therapy for hypoparathyroidism. J Bone Miner Res. 2019;34(11):2075–86.
30. Underbjerg L, Sikjaer T, Rejnmark L. Long-term complications in patients with hypoparathyroidism evaluated by biochemical findings: a case-control study. J Bone Miner Res. 2018;33(5):822–31.
31. Coudenys E, Van Meerhaeghe T, Unuane D, Buyl R, Bravenboer B. Long-term treatment with calcitriol in postsurgical hypoparathyroidism leads to renal function decline. Horm Metab Res. 2019;51(6):362–6.
32. Bergenfelz A, Nordenström E, Almquist M. Morbidity in patients with permanent hypoparathyroidism after total thyroidectomy. Surgery. 2020;167(1):124–8.

Chapter 19
A Patient with Postsurgical Recurrent Laryngeal Nerve Damage and Nerve Monitoring

David L. Steward and Adam D. Goodale

Case Presentation

A 54-year-old female was referred for evaluation of an asymptomatic multinodular goiter with a 4 cm left-sided nodule that was cytologically suspicious for papillary carcinoma. She had no prior history of radiation exposure nor a family history of thyroid cancer. Thyroid function tests were normal. An ultrasound showed a large goiter with a dominant 4 cm left-sided nodule with mild left substernal extension without suspicious lymph nodes. A flexible laryngeal exam was performed which revealed symmetric, mobile vocal cords bilaterally. The patient desired a total thyroidectomy for treatment due to the size of the suspicious nodule and the presence of bilateral nodules. The risks of postoperative hypocalcemia, bleeding, and vocal cord paralysis were explained, and she was scheduled for surgery.

Several weeks later, the patient underwent a total thyroidectomy. Intraoperative nerve monitoring (IONM) was performed using an endotracheal tube-based electrode. Her goiter was largest on the left and this was the initial side of surgery. The nerve stimulator was used to assist in confirming identification of the recurrent laryngeal nerve. After removal of the left lobe, the nerve stimulator confirmed the integrity of the recurrent laryngeal nerve. The right lobe was then dissected in a similar fashion. The nerve stimulator had a positive signal at the beginning of dissection; however, after the thyroid was removed, there was a loss of nerve signal. The position of the endotracheal tube was checked as well as the setup of the

D. L. Steward (✉)
Department of Otolaryngology – Head & Neck Surgery, University of Cincinnati College of Medicine, Cincinnati, OH, USA
e-mail: steward@uc.edu

A. D. Goodale
The Christ Hospital Physicians – Ear, Nose & Throat, Liberty Township, OH, USA
e-mail: goodale@uc.edu

G. Grani et al. (eds.), *Thyroid Cancer*,
https://doi.org/10.1007/978-3-030-61919-0_19

remainder of the system. Despite troubleshooting, the nerve signal from the right recurrent laryngeal nerve (RLN) remained absent. Visually the nerve was grossly intact; however, palpation of the arytenoid failed to confirm nerve integrity with stimulation. The surgery was concluded and the patient was discharged home. She had no obvious voice disturbance immediately following surgery.

Assessment and Literature Review

RLN damage is a potential complication following thyroid surgery. Despite advances in surgical technique, anatomical knowledge, and intraoperative nerve monitoring, the rate of RLN injury remains relatively high. A recent systematic review reported an incidence of temporary RLN palsy in 9.8% of thyroidectomies and permanent RLN injury in 2.3% [1]. Injury rates are even higher for cases of revision thyroidectomy, substernal goiter, and thyroid malignancy [2–5]. Surgeon experience has been shown to influence nerve injury with high-volume thyroid surgeons (those performing more than 100 thyroidectomies a year) having significantly lower nerve injury rates than lower-volume surgeons [6]. Vocal cord paralysis is known to negatively affect both quality of life and work activity with symptoms of breathy dysphonia and dysphagia with unilateral injury, and stridor and airway obstruction with bilateral injury.

To accurately assess RLN function, a preoperative laryngeal exam is essential. Although some physicians reserve laryngeal exam for symptomatic patients, studies have shown a poor correlation between voice changes and vocal cord paralysis [7, 8]. Often patients will develop progressive paralysis over time with adequate contralateral vocal cord compensation to limit noticeable voice changes. In one study in particular, the authors performed routine laryngeal exam prior to thyroidectomy and noted that one-third of patients with preoperative vocal fold motion impairment was asymptomatic [7]. Thus, to accurately determine the presence of iatrogenic vocal cord paralysis, a preoperative baseline exam is necessary. In cases of thyroid malignancy, preoperative RLN paralysis is highly predictive of invasive disease and thus alters surgical management and patient counseling [9]. Although there is variation among physician practices, an accurate assessment of preoperative laryngeal function is beneficial for both planning the extent of surgery and managing patients postoperatively [10].

Mechanism of Nerve Injury

The intimate relationship between the thyroid and RLN places the nerve at risk for injury during surgical removal. The majority of RLN injuries are secondary to compression, traction, devascularization, or thermal damage during thyroid removal, wherein the structural integrity of the nerve remains intact but with damage of its underlying neural elements. The RLN innervates the intrinsic muscles of the larynx and consists of a complement of nerve fibers for both abduction and adduction of the vocal folds. Coordinated laryngeal function is highly dependent on each axon innervating its specific motor unit. When the RLN is damaged, the ultimate effect on laryngeal function, as well as prognosis for recovery, is dependent on the degree of nerve injury which has been categorized by Sunderland [11]. Neuropraxic injuries are the least severe and are characterized by focal myelin damage without disruption of the axon leading to partial or temporary blockage of nerve conduction with a good prognosis for recovery. More severe damage results in disruption of the nerve axons, or axonotmesis, which leads to significant disruption of nerve conduction; however, the perineurium remains intact which improves the potential for functional recovery. Transection of the nerve, or neurotmesis, results in disruption of the axons, perineurium, and epineurium which is the most severe form of injury and carries the worst prognosis for recovery. The mechanism and extent of injury is important when considering prognosis for recovery and postoperative management.

The superior laryngeal nerve and branches of the RLN must be considered during thyroidectomy. The external branch of the superior laryngeal nerve (EBSLN) traverses in an anteroinferior direction along the inferior constrictor muscle to innervate the cricothyroid muscle. Commonly the EBSLN is closely associated with the blood supply to the superior pole of the thyroid placing it at risk for injury during ligation of these vessels. Damage to the EBSLN often limits the ability to achieve higher pitches as well as increased vocal fatigue. Patients with injury to the EBSLN typically have normal laryngeal exams which limit accurate determination of the incidence of nerve damage. Few studies, all with limited patient populations, have utilized EMG to evaluate postoperative cricothyroid function with incidence of EBSLN injury ranging from 5% to 58% [12, 13] (Figs. 19.1 and 19.2).

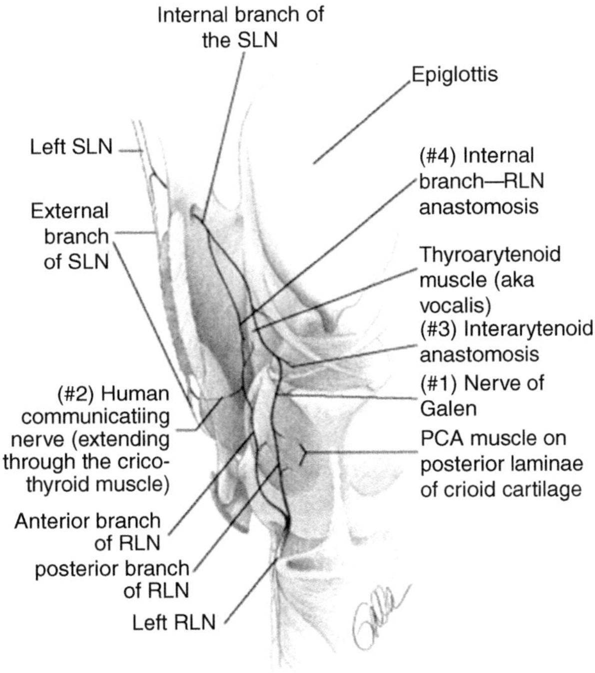

Fig. 19.1 Ant post RLN caption: Posterior view of the left hemilarynx, detailing the complexity of the superior (SLN) and recurrent (RLN) laryngeal nerves and their anastomotic regions (Reprinted from Ref. [33], Copyright 2021 with permission from Elsevier)

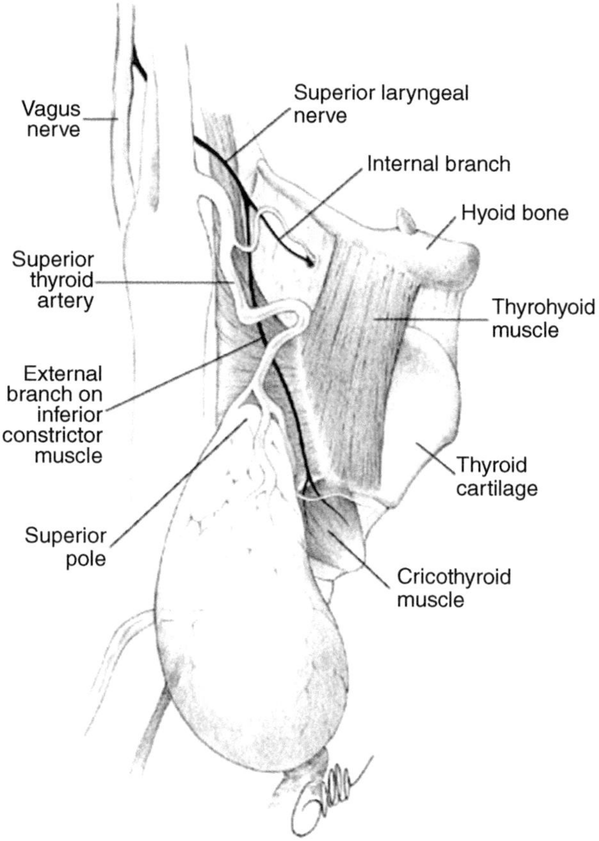

Fig. 19.2 EBSLN caption: The anatomical relationship between the external branch of the superior laryngeal nerve (EBSLN) innervation of the cricothyroid muscle near the superior pole of the thyroid gland and the superior thyroid artery (Reprinted from Ref. [33], Copyright 2021 with permission from Elsevier)

Branches of the RLN prior to entering the larynx are also subject to inadvertent injury. Typically these consist of an anterior and posterior branch and are present in 20–30% of patients [14, 15]. The anterior branch is primarily responsible for laryngeal muscle function, while the posterior branch contains mainly sensory nerve fibers but may occasionally innervate the posterior cricoarytenoid muscle. If branching is not identified, the posterior branch may be mistaken for the primary RLN with inadvertent transection of the anterior branch resulting in vocal cord paralysis. When present, the branches typically occur distally and are often identifiable at the level of Berry's ligament; however, variation does exist. The presence of these extralaryngeal branches doubles the likelihood of postoperative vocal cord paralysis and should be identified and preserved when present [16]. Branches of the RLN to the esophagus and inferior constrictor may also be present and when injured can impair swallowing postoperatively. Thus, surgeons must maintain a sound knowledge of anatomical variations to limit inadvertent injury to the various nerves in close approximation with the thyroid.

Evaluating Recurrent Laryngeal Nerve Function Intraoperatively

Injury to the RLN is often difficult to assess intraoperatively. The nerve may appear intact to visual inspection, while there can be significant functional damage. Given the inability to assess nerve function, surgeons poorly predict postoperative RLN function with one study reporting as few as 10% of damaged nerves correctly identified intraoperatively [17, 18]. IONM with nerve stimulation has several key benefits, but its most notable is the ability to assess neural integrity in the operating room and better predict postoperative laryngeal function [19]. Most commonly, IONM is performed using an endotracheal tube-based surface electrode to continuously monitor RLN integrity during thyroidectomy. Manipulation or electrical stimulation of the RLN is recorded by either an audio only system or a system with both audio and visual waveform data to notify the surgeon of evoked neural activity. While continuous nerve monitoring can be useful, nerve stimulation has shown the most promise to improve surgical outcomes. Positive nerve stimulation is very sensitive for intact RLN function. However, a loss of signal is less specific for nerve damage, as this may be secondary to either technical issues or actual nerve damage. Efficient troubleshooting is necessary to limit inappropriate loss of signal. When used by surgeons familiar with IONM, high specificity has been shown to be obtainable [19]. This is particularly valuable when planning a total thyroidectomy to limit the frequency of bilateral RLN paralysis and its associated complications. When the RLN signal is lost on the initial side of surgery during a total thyroidectomy, some surgeons have started to postpone removal of the contralateral lobe. This change in surgical management resulted in a decrease in bilateral RLN paralysis from 17% to 0% when the initial side of dissection resulted in a loss of RLN signal [20]. Since most RLN injuries are temporary in nature, a completion thyroidectomy can be performed, if necessary, once nerve function returns.

Although nerve stimulation is a useful tool to protect RLN integrity [21], visual nerve identification remains the gold standard for nerve protection [3, 22]. One of the main hopes for IONM was to further limit the frequency of RLN injury; however, this has yet to be clearly proven. Numerous studies have been published with varying results. A recent meta-analysis of 44 studies showed no statistical difference in RLN injury rates when comparing visual identification of the RLN to IONM [23]. Dralle et al. published a review of approximately 30,000 nerves at risk comparing visual identification versus nerve monitoring with no statistical decrease in RLN injury rates [2]. The only randomized clinical trial evaluating RLN injury rates and IONM did show a statistical benefit for ESBLN [24]. Other studies have shown benefit using IONM in more complex cases. Chan et al. showed decreased laryngeal nerve injury rates when using IONM for revision thyroidectomy and thyroidectomy for malignancy [4].

Despite the lack of evidence to support improved patient outcomes, the use of IONM has become increasingly popular over the past two decades. A recent survey of endocrine surgeons showed that approximately 40% routinely use IONM, and this was most prevalent among high-volume surgeons (greater than 100 cases per year) and younger surgeons (age 35–44) [25]. Cost considerations are minimal given that nerve integrity monitoring endotracheal tubes cost approximately $200.

Clinical Manifestations

A large majority of patients report voice and swallowing complaints after thyroidectomy regardless of RLN function. One study reported that 80% of patients demonstrated hoarseness and 54% reported dysphagia 1 week post-thyroidectomy despite normal RLN function [26]. These symptoms typically resolve over the first month postoperatively and are thought secondary to localized swelling, intubation trauma, or muscle injury. On the other hand, patients with RLN injury may not experience voice changes in the immediate postoperative period. Acute laryngeal edema from intubation trauma may create enough bulk for normal voice production; however, once swelling resolves, voice changes will become evident and often present as a "breathy" voice due to insufficient glottal closure. In contrast, bilateral RLN paralysis is often apparent in the immediate postoperative period with acute onset stridor and airway obstruction. Dysphagia is more common in elderly patients with a few experiencing severe aspiration. Given the variety of symptoms, a routine laryngeal exam is required to definitively assess RLN function. This is typically performed between 1 and 8 weeks postoperatively and can be done by indirect mirror exam, flexible fiber-optic laryngeal exam, or video laryngoscopy. There can be large variability in laryngeal findings in the setting of RLN injury. Some patients may have persistent voice changes in the setting of normal vocal cord mobility, while other patients will have a flaccid hemilarynx with significant glottic incompetence. The degree of dysfunction is often related to the extent of nerve damage. The use of intraoperative corticosteroids has shown mild benefit in postoperative voice outcomes [27, 28]. In particular, using corticosteroids resulted in a shorter recovery time for temporary RLN paralysis when compared to placebo. The frequency of temporary RLN paralysis was also lower with intraoperative corticosteroids; however, this was not statistically significant. Intraoperative findings should be correlated with laryngeal exam to assist with postoperative management, prognosis, and patient expectations.

Management

The management of RLN injury is dependent on both the nature of injury and the severity of the patient's symptoms. The majority of nerve damage is temporary with approximately 80–90% of patients experiencing full recovery within 6 months after surgery [2, 20, 29]. Limited improvement in function is expected after that time and more definitive treatment may be necessary. Treatment options of unilateral RLN injury include voice and swallowing therapy, injection laryngoplasty, and laryngeal framework surgery. When the nerve is transected, management begins intraoperatively. For patients with bilateral RLN, paralysis management focuses on maintaining a patent airway, most commonly with a tracheostomy. The appropriate treatment option should be individualized for each patient.

As with all peripheral nerves, the RLN has the ability for regeneration after injury. Post-injury laryngeal function is dependent upon reestablishing pre-injury innervation patterns. Misdirected nerve regeneration results in synkinesis or uncoordinated muscle contractions, leading to impaired laryngeal function. The degree of synkinesis is dependent upon the severity of injury and will dictate the expected return of function. Neuropraxic injuries maintain the integrity of each nerve axon allowing for similar post-injury innervation patterns. With more severe damage, as with axonotmesis and neurotmesis, newly created axons will likely reinnervate motor units dissimilar from pre-injury targets leading to varying degrees of synkinesis. Since laryngeal function and vocal cord motion are dependent upon a highly coordinated series of muscle contractions, synkinesis typically results in absent vocal fold motion. However, due to the predominance of adduction nerve fibers within the RLN, nerve fiber regeneration typically results in medialization of the larynx over time. This results in improved phonation and explains why many patients experience symptomatic improvement without intervention.

Voice and Swallowing Therapy

Patients found to have unilateral vocal cord hypomotility or immotility should be referred to an otolaryngologist or speech pathologist for further evaluation and treatment. Video laryngoscopy can be performed to better characterize vocal cord motility, laryngeal muscle tone, and glottic closure. This initial assessment will establish an objective baseline to evaluate for improvement with various treatment options. In the setting of aspiration, speech pathologist can perform a modified barium swallow (MBS) study or a fiber-optic endoscopic evaluation of swallowing (FEES) to accurately assess the degree of aspiration. Furthermore, these studies can be used to determine an appropriate diet for patients and educate them on certain swallowing maneuvers to limit aspiration. Patients often benefit from swallowing with their head turned toward the affected side to improve glottic closure or tightly holding their breath while swallowing to encourage supraglottic closure and limit aspiration. Patients with persistent aspiration despite swallowing therapy may require additional intervention. When symptoms are limited to voice disturbance, patients should initially be managed conservatively with voice therapy. The goal of voice therapy is to improve glottic closure while avoiding unfavorable compensatory maneuvers, such as supraglottic phonation. Voice therapy is most effective for patients with mild to moderate dysfunction and has been shown to decrease the need for surgical voice intervention [30]. Patients with severe dysfunction are more likely to require surgical intervention; however, voice therapy can still be beneficial. Patients can expect improvement in voice as long as 6 months after surgery; after that time, surgical intervention may be required to further improve voice outcomes.

Surgical Management

Surgical options for unilateral RLN paralysis consist primarily of injection laryngoplasty and laryngeal framework surgery. The goal of surgical augmentation is to improve phonation and glottic closure by medializing the paralyzed vocal cord to abut the contralateral functioning vocal cord during phonation and deglutition. Injection laryngoplasty is a useful tool for voice improvement and has become increasingly popular in the outpatient setting after recent advancements in fiberoptic laryngeal technology and improved injectable materials. Flexible transnasal laryngoscopy with distal chip cameras allows for high-definition laryngeal visualization to ensure accurate injection. There are numerous injectable materials on the market, each with various benefits. Often, the choice of material is based on the desired duration of effect and surgeon preference. Commonly used materials include the following: carboxymethylcellulose (Radiesse Voice Gel), hyaluronic acid, collagen, calcium hydroxyapatite (Radiesse Voice), micronized dermis (Cymetra), and autologous fat. Injection laryngoplasty was previously reserved for patients who failed conservative voice therapy. However, recent studies have shown that early injection laryngoplasty, deemed within the first year of injury, can decrease the need for future open laryngeal surgery [31]. Injection laryngoplasty remains limited by its isolated effect on the vocal fold as well as its temporary duration of effect – lasting approximately 6 months – however, in numerous patient populations, its use can be highly beneficial. Injection laryngoplasty adds bulk to the paralyzed vocal fold allowing the contralateral mobile fold to make contact improving the voice. The procedure can be performed in the office under local anesthesia or in the operating room under general anesthesia. The beneficial effect usually lasts about 6 months often allowing time for the injured nerve to recover. It can be repeated or more permanent medialization performed if the nerve fails to recover and voice inadequate.

Patients with severe vocal cord dysfunction, or who fail injection laryngoplasty, can be treated with open laryngeal framework surgery. Paralysis of the RLN results in anterior, inferior, and lateral displacement of the arytenoid with associated shortening and lateralization of the vocal fold. While injection laryngoplasty is limited to modifying vocal fold volume, open procedures can modify arytenoid and vocal fold position in three dimensions which offers more predictable long-term results. In particular, these procedures can adjust vocal fold height, vocal fold tension, and arytenoid position. These procedures primarily consist of thyroplasty and arytenoid adduction. Other laryngeal framework surgeries that exist, including cricothyroid subluxation and adduction arytenopexy, however, are beyond the scope of this chapter. Thyroplasty is performed by creating a window within the laryngeal cartilage at the level of the vocal fold and inserting a solid material to medialize the vocal fold. Both Silastic and Gore-Tex are commonly used each with good biocompatibility. Although thyroplasty does not augment arytenoid position, it provides long-term vocal fold medialization with good stability over time. Arytenoid adduction uses a permanent suture to reposition the vocal process of the arytenoid into a more medial phonatory position. This procedure has the benefit of modifying arytenoid position in multiple dimensions to personalize the procedure for each variation in vocal cord position.

Management of a transected recurrent laryngeal nerve, either secondary to iatrogenic injury or removal after malignant invasion, starts within the operating room [32]. In regard to malignant invasion, preference is given to attempted preservation of the RLN when vocal cord function is intact preoperatively and sacrifice of the RLN is necessary in the setting of preoperative vocal cord paralysis or encasement by tumor. When a transection injury is identified, reanastomosis should be attempted. Although normal vocal cord function is rare after neurorrhaphy, maintained neural input limits post-injury atrophy with increased bulk and medialization of the arytenoid for improved phonation. Typically the epineurium is reanastomosed using two or three interrupted sutures under microscopic guidance. When a segment of nerve is removed or there is significant retraction of the nerve, a local nerve transfer or cable graft may be required to limit tension at the anastomosis site. Most commonly, the ansa cervicalis is anastomosed to the distal end of the RLN for continued neural input. The ansa cervicalis is primarily active during respiration, deglutition, and phonation which is ideal for laryngeal reinnervation. The ansa cervicalis is also a good candidate for nerve transfer given its similar size to the RLN as well as the limited functional deficit when used. A cable graft can be performed using the great auricular nerve or other cervical sensory donor nerves as a bridge between the proximal and distal ends of the transected RLN. This is less commonly used as it requires two neurorrhaphies which hinder nerve regeneration. Patients with a repaired RLN after transection have the potential for good voice outcomes; however, they may require static voice augmentation procedures, such as thyroplasty, for further improvement.

Although the frequency of bilateral RLN injury is relatively low, patients with post-extubation stridor or airway distress require immediate evaluation. A flexible laryngeal exam should be performed to visually assess the vocal cords. Initial management should focus on establishing a secure airway, typically by either reintubation or tracheostomy. Management of patients with permanent bilateral RLN injury is a balance between maintaining a patent airway and limiting aspiration. Tracheostomy remains the gold standard; however, other procedures, such as arytenoidectomy, cordotomy, and vocal cord lateralization, exist and should be individualized for each patient.

Although care is taken to limit RLN injury, surgeons must be familiar with management options for patients with this operative complication. The majority of patients will experience spontaneous recovery over time and can be managed with conservative therapy. The remainder of patients may require more invasive therapy to limit aspiration and improve voice outcomes.

Back to the Patient: Outcome

One week after surgery, the patient was seen in the office for postoperative evaluation. She reported having a "breathy" voice since surgery with associated voice fatigue. She denied difficulty with swallowing. A flexible laryngeal exam showed hypomotility of the right vocal cord. The patient was referred to speech pathology for voice therapy. She was seen in follow-up 3 months later with resolution of her voice complaints. A repeat laryngeal exam at that time showed symmetric vocal cord motility with improved phonation time.

Clinical Pearls

- Intraoperative nerve stimulation is a useful tool to assess RLN function intraoperatively.
- A loss of nerve signal may be due to either technical issues or true nerve injury.
- Laryngeal exam is the only way to definitively assess RLN function both before and after surgery.
- The majority of RLN injuries are secondary to compression and traction injuries and are often temporary in duration.
- Neurorrhaphy should be performed in the event of RLN transection.
- Early injection laryngoplasty decreases the need for surgical laryngeal surgery in the setting of RLN injury.

References

1. Jeannon JP, Orabi AA, Bruch GA, Abdalsalam HA, Sima R. Diagnosis of recurrent laryngeal nerve palsy after thyroidectomy: a systematic review. Int J Clin Pract. 2009;63(4):624–9.
2. Dralle H, Sekulla C, Haerting J, Timmermann W, Neumann HJ, Kruse E, et al. Risk factors of paralysis and functional outcome after recurrent laryngeal nerve monitoring in thyroid surgery. Surgery. 2004;136(6):1310–21.
3. Jatzko GR, Lisborg PH, Muller MG, Wette VM. Recurrent nerve palsy after thyroid operations: principal nerve identification and a literature review. Surgery. 1994;115:139–44.
4. Chan W-F, Lang BH, Lo CY. The role of intraoperative neuromonitoring of recurrent laryngeal nerve during thyroidectomy: a comparative study on 1000 nerves at risk. Surgery. 2006;140:866.
5. Martensson H, Terins J. Recurrent laryngeal nerve palsy in thyroid gland surgery related to operations and nerves at risk. Arch Surg. 1985;120:475–7.
6. Sosa JA, Bowman HM, Tielsch JM, Powe NR, Udelsman R. The importance of surgeon experience for clinical and economic outcomes from thyroidectomy. Surgery. 1998;228:320–30.
7. Farrag TY, Samlan RA, Lin FR, Tufano RP. The utility of evaluating true vocal fold motion before thyroid surgery. Laryngoscope. 2006;116:235–8.
8. Steurer M, Passler C, Denk DM, Schneider B, Niederle B, Bigenzahn W. Advantages of recurrent laryngeal nerve identification in thyroidectomy and parathyroidectomy and the impor-

tance of preoperative and postoperative laryngoscopic examination in more than 1000 nerves at risk. Laryngoscope. 2002;112:124–33.
9. Randolph GW, Kamani D. The importance of preoperative laryngoscopy in patients undergoing thyroidectomy: voice, vocal cord function, and the preoperative detection of invasive thyroid malignancy. Surgery. 2006;139:357–62.
10. Sinclair CF, Bumpous JM, Haugen BR, Chala A, Meltzer D, Miller BS, Tolley NS, Shin JJ, Woodson G, Randolph GW. Laryngeal examination in thyroid and parathyroid surgery: an American head and neck society consensus statement: AHNS consensus statement. Head Neck. 2016;38(6):811–9.
11. Sunderland S. A classification of peripheral nerve injuries producing loss of function. Brain. 1951;74:491–516.
12. Barczyński M, Randolph GW, Cernea CR, Dralle H, Dionigi G, Alesina PF, Mihai R, Finck C, Lombardi D, Hartl DM, Miyauchi A, Serpell J, Snyder S, Volpi E, Woodson G, Kraimps JL, Hisham AN, International Neural Monitoring Study Group. External branch of the superior laryngeal nerve monitoring during thyroid and parathyroid surgery: international neural monitoring study group standards **guideline** statement. Laryngoscope. 2013;123(Suppl 4):S1–14.
13. Furlan JC, Cordeiro AC, Brandao LG. Study of some "intrinsic risk factors" that can enhance an iatrogenic injury of the external branch of the superior laryngeal nerve. Otolaryngol Head Neck Surg. 2003;128:396–400.
14. Jansson S, Tisell LE, Hagne I, Sanner E, Stenborg R, Svensson P. Partial laryngeal nerve lesions before and after thyroid surgery. World J Surg. 1988;12:522.
15. Serpell JW, Yeung MJ, Grodski S. The motor fibers of the recurrent laryngeal nerve are located in the anterior extralaryngeal branch. Ann Surg. 2009;249(4):648–52.
16. Casella C, Pata G, Nascimbeni R, Mittempergher F, Salerni B. Does extralaryngeal branching have an impact on the rate of postoperative transient or permanent recurrent laryngeal nerve palsy? World J Surg. 2009;33:261–5.
17. Sancho JJ, Pascual-Damieta M, Pereira JA, Carrera MJ, Fontane J, Sitges-Serra A. Risk factors for transient vocal cord palsy after thyroidectomy. Br J Surg. 2008;95:961–7.
18. Bergenfelz A, Jansson S, Kristoffersson A, Martensson H, Reihner E, Wallin G, et al. Complications to thyroid surgery: results as reported in a database from a multicenter audit comprising 3660 patients. Langenbeck's Arch Surg. 2008;393:667–73.
19. Schneider R, Randolph GW, Dionigi G, Wu CW, Barczynski M, Chiang FY, Al-Quaryshi Z, Angelos P, Brauckhoff K, Cernea CR, Chaplin J, Cheetham J, Davies L, Goretzki PE, Hartl D, Kamani D, Kandil E, Kyriazidis N, Liddy W, Orloff L, Scharpf J, Serpell J, Shin JJ, Sinclair CF, Singer MC, Snyder SK, Tolley NS, Van Slycke S, Volpi E, Witterick I, Wong RJ, Woodson G, Zafereo M, Dralle H. International neural monitoring study group guideline 2018 part I: staging bilateral thyroid surgery with monitoring loss of signal. Laryngoscope. 2018;128(Suppl 3):S1–S17.
20. Goretzki PE, Schwarz K, Brinkmann J, Wirowski D, Lammers BJ. The impact of intraoperative neuromonitoring (IONM) on surgical strategy in bilateral thyroid disease: is it worth the effort? World J Surg. 2010;34:1274–84.
21. Randolph GW, Kamani D. Intraoperative neural monitoring in thyroid cancer surgery. Langenbeck's Arch Surg. 2014;399:199–207.
22. Chandrasekhar SS, Randolph GW, Seidman MD, Rosenfeld RM, Angelos P, Barkmeier-Kraemer J, et al. Clinical practice guideline: improving voice outcomes after thyroid surgery. Otolaryngol Head Neck Surg. 2013;148:1–37.
23. Higgins TS, Gupta R, Ketcham AS, Sataloff RT, Wadsworth JT, Siancori JT. Recurrent laryngeal nerve monitoring versus identification along on post-thyroidectomy true vocal fold paralysis: a meta-analysis. Laryngoscope. 2011;1212:1009–17.
24. Barczynski M, Konturek A, Stopa M, Honowska A, Nowak W. Randomized controlled trial of visualization versus neuromonitoring of the external branch of the superior laryngeal nerve during thyroidectomy. World J Surg. 2012;36:1340–7.

25. Sturgeon C, Sturgeon T, Angelos P. Neuromonitoring in thyroid surgery: attitudes, usage patterns, and predictors of use among endocrine surgeons. World J Surg. 2009;33:417–25.
26. Lombardi CP, Raffaelli M, D'Alatri L, Marchese MR, Rigante M, Paludetti G, et al. Voice and swallowing changes after thyroidectomy in patient without inferior laryngeal nerve injuries. Surgery. 2006;140:1026–34.
27. Wang LF, Lee KW, Kuo WR, Wu CW, Lu SP, Chiang FY. The efficacy of intraoperative corticosteroids in recurrent laryngeal nerve palsy after thyroid surgery. World J Surg. 2006;30:299–303.
28. Worni M, Schudel HH, Seifert E, Inglin R, Hagemann M, Vorburger SA, Candinas D. Randomized controlled trial on single dose steroids before thyroidectomy for benign disease to improve postoperative nausea, pain, and vocal function. Ann Surg. 2008;248:1060–6.
29. Sadowski SM, Soardo P, Leuchter I, Robert JH, Triponez F. Systematic use of recurrent laryngeal nerve neuromonitoring changes the operative strategy in planned bilateral thyroidectomy. Thyroid. 2013;23:329–33.
30. Heuer RJ, Sataloff RT, Emerich K, Rulnick R, Baroody M, Spiegel JR, et al. Unilateral recurrent laryngeal nerve paralysis: the importance of "preoperative" voice therapy. J Voice. 1997;11:88–94.
31. Friedman AD, Burns JA, Heaton JT, Zeitels SM. Early versus late injection medialization for unilateral vocal cord paralysis. Laryngoscope. 2010;120:2042–6.
32. Wu CW, Dionigi G, Barczynski M, Chiang FY, Dralle H, Schneider R, Al-Quaryshi Z, Angelos P, Brauckhoff K, Brooks JA, Cernea CR, Chaplin J, Chen AY, Davies L, Diercks GR, Duh QY, Fundakowski C, Goretzki PE, Hales NW, Hartl D, Kamani D, Kandil E, Kyriazidis N, Liddy W, Miyauchi A, Orloff L, Rastatter JC, Scharpf J, Serpell J, Shin JJ, Sinclair CF, Stack BC Jr, Tolley NS, Slycke SV, Snyder SK, Urken ML, Volpi E, Witterick I, Wong RJ, Woodson G, Zafereo M, Randolph GW. International neuromonitoring study group guidelines 2018: part II: optimal recurrent laryngeal nerve management for invasive thyroid cancer-incorporation of surgical, laryngeal, and neural electrophysiologic data. Laryngoscope. 2018;128(Suppl 3):S18–27.
33. Gregory WR. Surgery of the thyroid and parathyroid glands, 3rd edition. Surgical anatomy and monitoring of the superior laryngeal nerve. 35:316–25.

Part IV
Differentiated Thyroid Cancer: Managing higher risk patients

Chapter 20
A Case of Papillary Thyroid Cancer Without Aggressive Histological Features with a Nodal Metastasis Detected During Follow-Up in a Young Patient

Lucia Brilli, Tania Pilli, Furio Pacini, and Maria Grazia Castagna

The Case

A19-year-old woman underwent a total thyroidectomy in 2014 for a suspicious nodule; final pathology described a 1.4 cm papillary cancer, classical variant, with no extrathyroidal extension. No central neck dissection was performed. After surgery, 30 mCi of radioiodine was administered. The first follow-up visit documented absence of residual disease with undetectable serum thyroglobulin (Tg) and normal neck ultrasound.

During a subsequent follow-up visit (5 years after initial treatment), neck ultrasound showed a 7×7×9 mm thyroid bed nodule suspicious for recurrent disease; fine-needle aspiration (FNA) biopsy confirmed the presence of a lymph node metastasis from papillary thyroid cancer. At that time, basal Tg was 1.1 ng/ml, rising to 3.4 ng/ml after recombinant human TSH stimulation. A second course of radioiodine was administered at a dose of 150 mCi of 131I. The post-therapy scan showed no uptake in the neck. Her endocrinologist recommended surgery in the near future, and she came to our center to discuss whether this was necessary.

L. Brilli · T. Pilli
Policlinico Santa Maria alle Scotte, Siena, Italy

F. Pacini
Department of Medical, Surgical and Neurological Sciences, University of Siena, Siena, Italy

M. G. Castagna (✉)
Policlinico Santa Maria alle Scotte, Siena, Italy

Department of Medical, Surgical and Neurological Sciences, University of Siena, Siena, Italy
e-mail: mariagraziacastagna@unisi.it

G. Grani et al. (eds.), *Thyroid Cancer*,
https://doi.org/10.1007/978-3-030-61919-0_20

Assessment and Literature Review

In differentiated thyroid cancer, structural tumor recurrences in the post-surgery follow-up occur in about 1–2% of cases with an excellent response to initial therapy regardless of their initial risk stratification [1–6].

In the case of cervical lymph node recurrences, the management may include no therapy, compartmental lymph node dissection, radioiodine therapy, ethanol injection and radiofrequency or laser ablation. The final decision should be made after discussions involving the endocrinologist, the surgeon and the patient [7].

Roughly two-thirds of neck lymph nodes classified as indeterminate on ultrasound will spontaneously disappear after several months, so watchful waiting is appropriate for small indeterminate nodes. Overall, only a small proportion of these lymph nodes will grow over time, but no complication due to size increase has been reported during follow-up [8–10].

In particular, in a retrospective review of 191 patients with at least 1 thyroid bed nodule (≤11mm) over a median follow-up of 5 years, only 9% of patients had an increase in size of at least 1 nodule, with a low rate of growth (median 1.3 mm/year) [8]. Suspicious cervical lymph nodes left untreated also revealed a low rate of growth. After a median follow-up of 3.5 years, only 9% of them (15/166) grew at least 5 mm in the longest diameter, with a rate of growth of 1.5 mm/year with no associated disease-related mortality. Among the 15 patients, 7 underwent FNA biopsy, and cytology was consistent with papillary thyroid cancer in 5 cases [9]. In the most recent series a total of 113 lesions were followed up (18 thyroid bed masses, 95 lymph nodes). During surveillance (median 3.7 y), group with indeterminate lesions only had significantly lower rates than group with one or more lesions classified as suspicious of lesion growth, defined as >3 mm in the largest diameter (8% vs. 36%, $P = .01$) and persistence (64% vs. 97%, $P = .014$) [10].

Unfortunately, no prospective and randomized trials with longer follow-up have compared the outcome of recurrent lymph node metastases treated by surgery or untreated.

Based on the most recent studies and reviews, the 2015 ATA guidelines stated that smaller lesions (<8 mm in the smallest diameter for central neck nodes and <10 mm for lateral neck nodes) probably can be best managed with active surveillance with serial ultrasound complemented by neck CT scans, reserving FNA and subsequent surgical intervention for documented structural disease progression [7].

Apart from size, other factors such as the patient's emotional status, lymph node location (near or not to vital structure), the functional status of vocal cords, the patient's comorbidities, histology of primary tumor, and Tg doubling time should be taken into account in the decision to operate. In selected cases, metastatic nodes greater than 8–10 mm in the shortest diameter may be followed without intervention, selecting for surgery those patients in whom there is disease progression during follow-up. This is probably mainly feasible in case of indeterminate rather than suspicious neck lesions, where there is the possibility of a disappearance of abnormalities during follow-up [10].

In the case of larger lymph nodes, surgery is the preferred approach. The experience of the surgeon and the risks associated with a second surgery (mostly when the lymph node is localized in a compartment previously dissected) should be taken into account. Compartmental surgery is recommended over "berry picking", due to the high risk of recurrence and higher morbidity in case of re-operative surgery. Careful neck dissection in experienced hands has been associated with short-term decreases in serum Tg levels in 60–90% of patients, while undetectable serum Tg was obtained in only 30–50% [11–13]. However, most series suggest that surgery results in the disappearance of structural disease in over 90% of patients [14]. Recently a retrospective study, analyzing efficacy, safety and prognostic factor of first neck re-operation in differentiated thyroid cancer, demonstrated that only age >45 years, aggressive histology and >10 N1 at re-operation were independent risk factors of secondary relapse [15].

Back to the Patient

The patient was reassured that her thyroid bed nodules could be closely monitored until there was evidence of progression. Serial neck ultrasound was then performed with a gradual increase in size of the thyroid bed nodule (9×11×17 mm vs. 7×7×9 mm). After 5 years, it was decided to perform a compartmental level VI dissection. Final pathology was consistent with a lymph node metastasis from a papillary thyroid cancer. Six months after the surgery, serum Tg was undetectable and neck ultrasound was negative. She was considered to be in clinical remission and has been followed with annual Tg and neck ultrasound.

Clinical Pearls

- In differentiated thyroid cancer, structural tumor recurrences in the post-surgery follow-up period occur in about 1–2% of patients with an excellent response to initial therapy regardless of their initial risk stratification.
- Suspicious central neck nodes ≥8 mm and lateral neck nodes ≥10mm in the smallest diameter should be considered for surgical removal while indeterminate neck lesions in selected cases could be managed with follow-up.
- Suspicious, but small, stable cervical lymph nodes may be followed with serial ultrasound without intervention.

References

1. Castagna MG, Maino F, Cipri C, Belardini V, Theodoropoulou A, Cevenini G, Pacini F. Delayed risk stratification, to include the response to initial treatment (surgery and radioiodine ablation), has better outcome predictivity in differentiated thyroid cancer patients. Eur J Endocrinol. 2011;165:441–6. https://doi.org/10.1530/EJE-11-0466.
2. Tuttle RM, Tala H, Shah J, Leboeuf R, Ghossein R, Gonen M, Brokhin M, Omry G, Fagin JA, Shaha A. Estimating risk of recurrence in differentiated thyroid cancer after total thyroidectomy and radioactive iodine remnant ablation: using response to therapy variables to modify the initial risk estimates predicted by the new American Thyroid Association staging system. Thyroid. 2010;20:1341–9. https://doi.org/10.1089/thy.2010.0178.
3. Lee SG, Lee WK, Lee HS, Moon J, Lee CR, Kang SW, Jeong JJ, Nam KH, Chung WY, Jo YS, Lee J. Practical performance of the 2015 American Thyroid Association guidelines for predicting tumor recurrence in patients with papillary thyroid cancer in South Korea. Thyroid. 2017;27:174–81. https://doi.org/10.1089/thy.2016.0252.
4. Park S, Kim WG, Song E, Oh HS, Kim M, Kwon H, Jeon MJ, Kim TY, Shong YK, Kim WB. Dynamic risk stratification for predicting recurrence in patients with differentiated thyroid cancer treated without radioactive iodine remnant ablation therapy. Thyroid. 2017;27:524–30. https://doi.org/10.1089/thy.2016.0477.
5. Schlumberger M, Leboulleux S, Catargi B, Deandreis D, Zerdoud S, Bardet S, Rusu D, Godbert Y, Buffet C, Schvartz C, Vera P, Morel O, Benisvy D, Bournaud C, Toubert ME, Kelly A, Benhamou E, Borget I. Outcome after ablation in patients with low-risk thyroid cancer (ESTIMABL1): 5-year follow-up results of a randomised, phase 3, equivalence trial. Lancet Diabetes Endocrinol. 2018;6:618–26. https://doi.org/10.1016/S2213-8587(18)30113-X.
6. Dehbi HM, Mallick U, Wadsley J, Newbold K, Harmer C, Hackshaw A. Recurrence after low-dose radioiodine ablation and recombinant human thyroid-stimulating hormone for differentiated thyroid cancer (HiLo): long-term results of an open-label, non-inferiority randomised controlled trial. Lancet Diabetes Endocrinol. 2019;7:44–51. https://doi.org/10.1016/S2213-8587(18)30306-1.
7. Haugen BR, Alexander EK, Bible KC, Doherty GM, Mandel SJ, Nikiforov YE, Pacini F, Randolph GW, Sawka AM, Schlumberger M, Schuff KG, Sherman SI, Sosa JA, Steward DL, Tuttle RM, Wartofsky L. 2015 American Thyroid Association Management guidelines for adult patients with thyroid nodules and differentiated thyroid cancer: The American Thyroid Association Guidelines Task Force on thyroid nodules and differentiated thyroid cancer. Thyroid. 2016;26:1–133. https://doi.org/10.1089/thy.2015.0020.
8. Rondeau G, Fish S, Hann LE, Fagin JA, Tuttle RM. Ultrasonographically detected small thyroid bed nodules identified after total thyroidectomy for differentiated thyroid cancer seldom show clinically significant structural progression. Thyroid. 2011;21:845–53. https://doi.org/10.1089/thy.2011.0011.
9. Robenshtok E, Fish S, Bach A, Domínguez JM, Shaha A, Tuttle RM. Suspicious cervical lymph nodes detected after thyroidectomy for papillary thyroid cancer usually remain stable over years in properly selected patients. J Clin Endocrinol Metab. 2012;97:2706–13. https://doi.org/10.1210/jc.2012-1553.
10. Lamartina L, Grani G, Biffoni M, Giacomelli L, Costante G, Lupo S, Maranghi M, Plasmati K, Sponziello M, Trulli F, Verrienti A, Filetti S, Durante C. Risk stratification of neck lesions detected sonographically during the follow-up of differentiated thyroid cancer. J Clin Endocrinol Metab. 2016;101:3036–44. https://doi.org/10.1210/jc.2016-1440.
11. Al-Saif O, Farrar WB, Bloomston M, Porter K, Ringel MD, Kloos RT. Long-term efficacy of lymph node reoperation for persistent papillary thyroid cancer. J Clin Endocrinol Metab. 2010;95:2187–94. https://doi.org/10.1210/jc.2010-0063.
12. Schuff KG, Weber SM, Givi B, Samuels MH, Andersen PE, Cohen JI. Efficacy of nodal dissection for treatment of persistent/recurrent papillary thyroid cancer. Laryngoscope. 2008;118:768–75. https://doi.org/10.1097/MLG.0b013e318162cae9.

13. Yim JH, Kim WB, Kim EY, Kim WG, Kim TY, Ryu JS, Gong G, Hong SJ, Shong YK. The outcomes of first reoperation for locoregionally recurrent/persistent papillary thyroid carcinoma in patients who initially underwent total thyroidectomy and remnant ablation. J Clin Endocrinol Metab. 2011;96:2049–56. https://doi.org/10.1210/jc.2010-2298.
14. Tufano RP, Clayman G, Heller KS, Inabnet WB, Kebebew E, Shaha A, Steward DL, Tuttle RM, American Thyroid Association Surgical Affairs Committee Writing Task Force. Management of recurrent/persistent nodal disease in patients with differentiated thyroid cancer: a critical review of the risks and benefits of surgical intervention versus active surveillance. Thyroid. 2015;25:15–27. https://doi.org/10.1089/thy.2014.0098.
15. Lamartina L, Borget I, Mirghani H, Al Ghuzlan A, Berdelou A, Bidault F, Deandreis D, Baudin E, Travagli JP, Schlumberger M, Hartl DM, Leboulleux S. Surgery for neck recurrence of differentiated thyroid cancer: outcomes and risk factors. J Clin Endocrinol Metab. 2017;1(102):1020–31. https://doi.org/10.1210/jc.2016-3284.

Chapter 21
A Patient with a Large Hürthle Cell Carcinoma of the Thyroid and Nodal Metastases

Leonard Wartofsky

Case

A 67-year-old man was referred to our endocrine clinic by his primary care physician for the management of a 5.6 cm thyroid nodule in the left lobe with a recent fine-needle aspiration (FNA) cytology interpreted as an indeterminate diagnosis favoring a follicular neoplasm, otherwise unspecified (Bethesda class IV). A repeat FNA was sent for mutational analysis by ThyroSeq, and a mutation in the *RAS* subfamily (*HRAS*) was found. The patient was referred for thyroidectomy. Preoperative ultrasonography confirmed the left lobe nodule which was hypoechoic with irregular margins and lacked any calcification, and there was suspicion for involved lateral neck lymph nodes. Fine-needle aspiration of the suspicious lymph node confirmed thyroid cancer, and he underwent a total thyroidectomy and central and modified left neck dissection. The surgical pathology described a 6 cm poorly encapsulated tumor with both local invasiveness with extrathyroidal extension and vascular invasion at eight identified sites. The predominant cell type was oncocytic or oxyphilic with microfollicle formation consistent with a Hürthle cell carcinoma. Extrathyroidal extension was evident with several implants of tumor ranging from 2 to 11 mm in the lateral neck; 6/12 lymph nodes from Level VI and 12/31 lymph nodes from left Levels II and III were positive for metastatic tumor [Stage IVA (T4, N1B, MX)] (Fig. 21.1).

L. Wartofsky (✉)
MedStar Health Research Institute,
MedStar Washington Hospital Center, Washington, DC, USA

Georgetown University School of Medicine, Washington, DC, USA
e-mail: Leonard.Wartofsky@medstar.net

G. Grani et al. (eds.), *Thyroid Cancer*,
https://doi.org/10.1007/978-3-030-61919-0_21

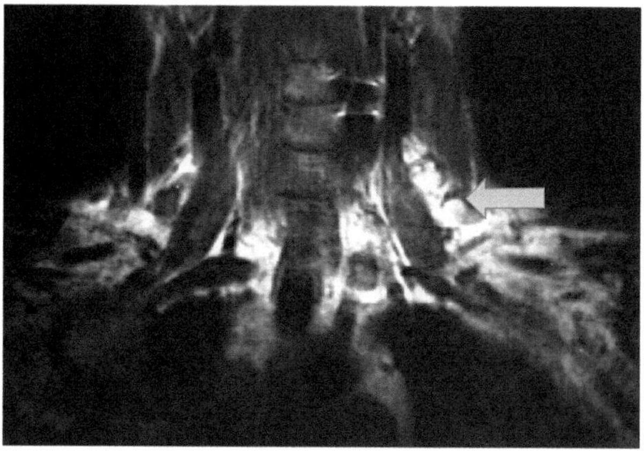

Fig. 21.1 Magnetic resonance imaging (MRI) of patient's neck demonstrating lymph node metastases in the left neck (*arrow*)

Hürthle Cell Carcinoma: Literature Review

Some thyroid tumors with predominant oncocytic cytology may be benign or so-called Hürthle cell adenomas [1]. Based upon postoperative surgical pathology, the risk of carcinoma in a nodule with FNA cytology read as Hürthle cell neoplasm ranges from 10% to 45 % in various series [2]. The likelihood that such a nodule is a carcinoma increases with nodule size [3] with approximately 50 % of tumors >4 cm and 100 % of tumors >6 cm being malignant [4]. In addition to tumor size, other factors associated with malignancy are male sex, age>65, and highly elevated serum levels of thyroglobulin (Tg) [5], but cancer is still common but less frequent when Tg levels are <500 ng/mL [6]. One recent study [7] suggests that whole-transcriptome sequencing may distinguish between benign and malignant Hürthle cell tumors with the finding that CHL 1 (Close homolog of L1) is overexpressed in these cancers.

In this patient, the finding of a RAS mutation on the fine-needle aspirated material constituted an additional motivation for proceeding to total thyroidectomy [8]. Although a reading of follicular lesion of uncertain significance (FLUS) carries a low risk of malignancy of 5–20 %, in this patient the interpretation as follicular neoplasm (FN; Bethesda class IV) carries a somewhat higher risk of 20–30 %, and the large size of the nodule implies an even higher risk [9]. In one study, 87/513 (17%) of indeterminate nodules on FNA had a positive mutation, and 70 % of these were RAS point mutations as in our patient [10]. In contrast to our patient who had a Hürthle cell carcinoma, most RAS-positive thyroid cancers are papillary thyroid cancers and tend to have a good prognosis [11]. However, other mutations could be present in this patient's tumor with the first-generation ThyroSeq analysis employed having possibly provided a false-negative result. The Afirma (Veracyte) first-generation gene expression classifier is known to provide false-positive results in Hürthle cell tumors [12].

Sonography cannot reliably predict which nodules may be carcinoma as these lesions may present a wide variety of sonographic findings [13], but typically will lack micro- or macrocalcifications. Current guidelines of the American Thyroid Association [14] do not recommend screening thyroid nodules with FDG-PET scans, but thyroid nodules found incidentally to be positive on PET scan warrant FNA cytology to rule out malignancy. Because there is a correlation between PET positivity and clinical aggressiveness of tumors, Hürthle cell carcinoma is likely to be positive on FDG-PET [15] and was recently also found to be positive on an 18-F DOPA PET scan [16].

Hürthle cells are often present in Hashimoto's thyroiditis, and the presence of a Hürthle cell lesion in a thyroid gland involved with Hashimoto's thyroiditis can present a difficult challenge [17]. A Hürthle cell variant of follicular thyroid cancer was first described in 1928 on the basis of the distinctive cellular features of oxyphilic cells with abundant cytoplasm that lack any of the typical cytologic features of papillary thyroid carcinoma such as nuclear pseudoinclusions. Earlier studies identified similarities between classic follicular thyroid carcinoma and Hürthle cell cancers and classified both as either minimally invasive with less than four foci of capsular invasion or widely invasive [18]. However, while Hürthle cell cancers previously were considered a variant of follicular thyroid carcinoma, the recent WHO classification of endocrine tumors [19] distinguishes Hürthle cell cancer as a unique entity from follicular thyroid cancer based upon both molecular differences in the tumors [20, 21] as well as their clinical behavior and response to therapy [22].

In general, both Hürthle cell and follicular thyroid cancer are more likely to metastasize to distant sites like the lung and bone via vascular invasion and hematogenous spread, than to local or regional lymph nodes as is typical of papillary thyroid cancer. But the presence of involved lymph nodes in our patient constitutes an independent predictor of reduced disease-free survival [23]. Moreover, Bishop et al. [24] noted that locoregional soft tissue metastases may be more characteristic of this tumor than lymph node metastases. A more aggressive, poorly differentiated variant of Hürthle cell cancer has been described as well in 6% of oncocytic tumors which histologically demonstrate extensive angioinvasion and coagulative tumor necrosis with a high likelihood of distant metastases [25].

Whether the prognosis of small, fully encapsulated minimally invasive Hürthle cell cancers may be excellent is controversial, with one recent study indicating significant risk of residual or recurrent disease [26]. On the other hand, the ATA guidelines [14] suggest that tumors with only capsular invasion or which demonstrate less than four foci of vascular invasion can be considered as having low risk of recurrence and therefore could be treated more conservatively and there is some support for this approach [27]. However, because Hürthle cell cancer tends to carry a poorer prognosis [28, 29], I would want to thoroughly exclude residual disease by all diagnostic means available, as well as committing to careful long-term follow-up, before abandoning treatment such as radioiodine in a patient with Hürthle cell carcinoma considered to be "low risk."

The more invasive types of Hürthle cell cancer such as the solid or trabecular subtypes are more aggressive, and their course is often marked by both locoregional and distant metastases [20, 30, 31]. Identification and classification of the degree of invasiveness is critical to the determination of how aggressively therapy is to be implemented. Unfortunately, a large proportion of Hürthle cell cancers do not trap radioiodine, and even those that may demonstrate 131-I uptake tend to be less radiosensitive than are papillary thyroid cancers. Chindris et al. [32] observed that very few patients with lung metastases demonstrated 131-I uptake and the worst outcomes were seen in males with Stage III or IV disease. Nevertheless, in contrast to the general consensus, and based on an analysis of clinical outcomes in 485 patients with follicular thyroid cancer and 73 patients with Hürthle cell cancer, Sugino et al. [33] concluded, as have other investigators [34, 35], that the Hürthle cell cancer patients may fare no worse in regard to prognosis. The belief that Hürthle cell tumors do not take up 131-I, without confirmation by performance of an 131-I scan, may explain why many patients with these tumors are not so treated. Jillard et al. [36] surveyed reports of 1909 patients and discovered that only 60.9% were treated with 131-I. In our view, radioiodine avidity should be assessed, and, when present, therapy can be associated with improved survival [36].

Management of the Patient

Postoperatively, the patient was started on levothyroxine 0.15 mg/day and placed on a low-iodine diet in preparation for diagnostic radioiodine scanning and potential remnant ablation. At 4 weeks postsurgery when his serum TSH level was 0.38, his serum Tg measured 1224 ng/mL, and after preparation with recombinant human thyrotropin (rhTSH; Thyrogen®), an iodine-123 scan indicated moderate uptake in the right thyroid bed and faint uptake in three foci in the left lateral neck and one focus in the anterior mediastinum. The scan results prompted repeat ultrasonography of the neck which indicated either nodules or suspicious lymph nodes in the left neck. Magnetic resonance imaging (MRI) [37, 38] confirmed the lesions which appeared to correlate with the foci of radioiodine uptake on the isotopic scan, and the patient was referred back to his surgeon. A repeat left lateral neck compartmental node dissection was performed with removal of 18 additional lymph nodes, 9 of which were positive for metastatic tumor. At 3 months after his original surgery, his serum Tg was 88 ng/mL with a TSH of 0.03. He was again placed on a low-iodine diet, and after 2 weeks, he was treated with an activity of 175 mCi radioiodine facilitated by rhTSH preparation. His posttreatment total body scan revealed only modest uptake of iodine-131 in the mediastinum, and it is anticipated that he may need to be treated with external radiotherapy [39] which has shown benefit in some series [40], or local interventional ablation [41, 42] should persistent locoregional disease be documented. There are no published evidence-based guidelines for the continued management of this patient, and our plan will be for monitoring serum Tg every 3 months with a rising Tg constituting the signal to employ neck ultrasound and PET/CT imaging to identify structural disease and any indication for additional intervention.

Clinical Pearls/Pitfalls

1. While the majority of Hürthle cell neoplasms based on cytologic examination may be benign, tumors larger than 4 cm and advanced patient age are worrisome for an increased likelihood of Hürthle cell carcinoma.
2. Hürthle cell carcinomas can present with locoregional lymph node or soft tissue metastasis and hence are an exception to the general teaching that follicular cancers are angioinvasive and present with distant metastases.
3. Finding four or more sites of invasion through the capsule classifies these tumors as highly invasive and associated with greater risk, thereby warranting more aggressive therapy.
4. Hürthle cell carcinoma frequently will not take up sufficient radioiodine to result in effective therapy, and external radiation or targeted chemotherapy may be required. However, assessment of radioiodine uptake and radioiodine remnant ablation is always recommended.

Acknowledgments Grant support from the Catherine Heron and Al Schneider Thyroid Cancer Fellowship Fund.

References

1. Rossi ED, Martini M, Straccia P, Raffaelli M, Pennacchia I, Marrucci E, Lombardi CP, Pontecorvi A, Fadda G. The cytologic category of oncocytic (Hürthle) cell neoplasm mostly includes low-risk lesions at histology: an institutional experience. Eur J Endocrinol. 2013;169(5):649–55.
2. Auger M. Hürthle cells in fine-needle aspirates of the thyroid: a review of their diagnostic criteria and significance. Cancer Cytopathol. 2014;122(4):241–9.
3. Lee KH, Shin JH, Ko ES, Hahn SY, Kim JS, Kim JH, Oh YL. Predictive factors of malignancy in patients with cytologically suspicious for Hürthle cell neoplasm of thyroid nodules. Int J Surg. 2013;11(9):898–902.
4. Sippel RS, Elaraj DM, Khanafshar E, Zarnegar R, Kebebew E, Duh QY, Clark OH. Tumor size predicts malignant potential in Hürthle cell neoplasms of the thyroid. World J Surg. 2008;32(5):702–7.
5. Strazisar B, Petric R, Sesek M, Zgajnar J, Hocevar M, Besic N. Predictive factors of carcinoma in 279 patients with Hürthle cell neoplasm of the thyroid gland. J Surg Oncol. 2010;101(7):582–6.
6. Suh I, Vriens MR, Guerrero MA, Griffin A, Shen WT, Duh QY, Clark OH, Kebebew E. Serum thyroglobulin is a poor diagnostic biomarker of malignancy in follicular and Hürthle-cell neoplasms of the thyroid. Am J Surg. 2010;200:41–6.

7. Li W, Xia S, Aronova A, Min IM, Verma A, Scognamiglio T, Gray KD, et al. CHL 1 expression differentiates Hürthle cell carcinoma from benign Hürthle cell nodules. J Surg Oncol. 2018;118:1042–9.
8. Yip L, Wharry LI, Armstrong MJ, Silbermann A, McCoy KL, Stang MT, et al. A clinical algorithm for fine-needle aspiration molecular testing effectively guides the appropriate extent of initial thyroidectomy. Ann Surg. 2014;260:163–7.
9. McCoy KL, Carty SE, Armstrong MJ, Seethala RR, Ohori NP, Kabaker AS, et al. Intraoperative pathologic examination in the era of molecular testing for differentiated thyroid cancer. J Am Coll Surg. 2012;215:546–54.
10. Nikiforov YE, Nikiforova MN. Molecular genetics and diagnosis of thyroid cancer. Nat Rev Endocrinol. 2011;7:569–80.
11. Gupta N, Dasyam AK, Carty SE, Nikiforova MN, Ohori NP, Armstrong M, et al. RAS mutations in thyroid FNA specimens are highly predictive of predominantly low-risk follicular pattern cancers. J Clin Endocrinol Metab. 2013;98:E914–22.
12. Parajuli S, Jug R, Ahmadi S, Jiang XS. Hürthle cell predominance impacts results of Afirma gene expression classifier and ThyroSeq molecular panel performance in indeterminate thyroid nodules. Diagn Cytopathol. 2019;47(11):1177–83. https://doi.org/10.1002/dc.24290. Epub Jul 26 2019
13. Maizlin ZV, Wiseman SM, Vora P, Kirby JM, Mason AC, Filipenko D, Brown JA. Hürthle cell neoplasms of the thyroid: sonographic appearance and histologic characteristics. J Ultrasound Med. 2008;27(5):751–7.
14. Haugen BR, Alexander EK, Bible KC, Doherty GM, Mandel SJ, Nikiforov Y, et al. American Thyroid Association Management Guidelines for patients with thyroid nodules and differentiated thyroid cancer. Thyroid. 2016;26:1–133.
15. Riemann B, Uhrhan K, Dietlein M, Schmidt D, Kuwert T, et al. Diagnostic value and therapeutic impact of (18)F-FDG-PEET-CT in differentiated thyroid cancer. Results of a German multicentre study. Nuklearmedizin. 2013;53:1–6.
16. Pauleau G, Palazzo FF, Essamet W, Sebag F, Taieb D. Hürthle cell neoplasms: a new differential diagnosis of 18F-FDOPA-avid thyroid nodules? J Clin Endocrinol Metab. 2013;98:865–6.
17. Lee J, Hasteh F. Oncocytic variant of papillary thyroid carcinoma associated with Hashimoto's thyroiditis: a case report and review of the literature. Diagn Cytopathol. 2009;37(8):600–6.
18. Mai KT, Khanna P, Yazdi HM, Perkins DG, Veinot JP, Thomas J, Lamba M, Nair BD. Differentiated thyroid carcinomas with vascular invasion: a comparative study of follicular. Hürthle cell and papillary thyroid carcinoma. Pathology. 2002;34:239–44.
19. Lloyd RV, Osamura RY, Kloppel G, Rosai J. WHO classification of tumours of endocrine organs. 4th ed. Geneva, Switzerland: WHO; 2017.
20. Ganly I, Ricarte FJ, Eng S, Ghossein R, Morris LG, Liang Y, Socci N, Kannan K, Mo Q, Fagin JA, Chan TA. Genomic dissection of Hürthle cell carcinoma reveals a unique class of thyroid malignancy. J Clin Endocrinol Metab. 2013;98:E962–72.
21. Ganly I, McFadden DG. Short Review: Genomic Alterations in Hürthle Cell Carcinoma. Thyroid. 2019;29(4):471–9. https://doi.org/10.1089/thy.2019.0088.
22. Grani G, Lamartina L, Durante C, Filetti S, Cooper DS. Follicular thyroid cancer and Hürthle cell carcinoma: challenges in diagnosis, treatment, and clinical management. Lancet Diabetes Endocrinol. 2018;6:500–14.
23. Mills SC, Haq M, Smellie WJ, Harmer C. Hürthle cell carcinoma of the thyroid: retrospective review of 62 patients treated at the Royal Marsden Hospital between 1946 and 2003. Eur J Surg Oncol. 2009;35(3):230–4.
24. Bishop JA, Wu G, Tufano RP, Westra WH. Histological patterns of locoregional recurrence in Hürthle cell carcinoma of the thyroid gland. Thyroid. 2012;22(7):690–4.
25. Bai S, Baloch ZW, Samulski TD, Montone KT, LiVolsi VA. Poorly differentiated oncocytic (Hürthle cell) follicular carcinoma: an institutional experience. Endocr Pathol. 2015;26:164–9.
26. Kuo EJ, Roman SA, Sosa JA. Patients with follicular and Hürthle cell microcarcinomas have compromised survival: a population level study of 22,738 patients. Surgery. 2013;154:1246–53.

27. Ahmadi S, Stang M, Jiang XS, Sosa JA. Hürthle cell carcinoma: current perspectives. Onco Targets Ther 2016;9:6873-6884. eCollection 2016.
28. Stojadinovic A, Hoos A, Ghossein RA, Urist MJ, Leung DH, Spiro RH, Shah JP, Brennan MF, Singh B, Shaha AR. Hürthle cell carcinoma: a 60-year experience. Ann Surg Oncol. 2002;9(2):197–203.
29. Khokar AM, Holoubek SA, Kuchta KM, Winchester DJ, Prinz RA, Moo-Young TA. Survival with follicular and Hürthle cell microcarcinoma compared to papillary thyroid microcarcinoma: A population study of 84,532 patients. World J Surg 2019; 20.https://doi.org/10.1007/s00268-019-05264-9. (E pub ahead of print).
30. Haigh PI, Urbach DR. The treatment and prognosis of Hürthle cell follicular thyroid carcinoma compared with its non-Hürthle cell counterpart. Surgery. 2005;138:1152–7.
31. Ghossein RA, Hiltzik DH, Carlson DL, Patel S, Shaha A, Shah JP, Tuttle RM, Singh B. Prognostic factors of recurrence in encapsulated Hürthle cell carcinoma of the thyroid gland: a clinicopathologic study of 50 cases. Cancer. 2006;106:1669–76.
32. Chindris A-M, Casler JD, Bernet VJ, Rivera M, Thomas C, Kachergus JM, et al. Clinical and molecular features of Hürthle cell carcinoma of the thyroid. J Clin Endocrinol Metab. 2015;100:55–62.
33. Sugino K, Kameyama K, Ito K, Nagahama M, Kitagawa W, Shibuya H, Ohkuwa K, et al. Does Hürthle cell carcinoma of the thyroid have a poorer prognosis than ordinary follicular thyroid carcinoma? Ann Surg Oncol. 2013;20(9):2944–50.
34. Wenter V, Jellinek A, Unterrainer M, Ahmaddy F, Lehner S, Albert NL, Bartenstein P, Knolel T, Spitzweg C, Ilhan H, Todica A. Long-term outcome of rare oncocytic papillary (Hürthle cell) thyroid carcinoma following (adjuvant) initial radioiodine therapy. Eur J Nucl Med Mol Imaging. 2019;46(12):2526–35. https://doi.org/10.1007/s00259-019-04456-8. E pub Aug 13, 2019.
35. Yang Q, Zhao Z, Zhong G, Jin A, Yu K. Effect of adjuvant radioactive iodine therapy on survival in rare oxyphilic subtype of thyroid cancer (Hürthle cell carcinoma). Peer J. 2019;7:e7458. https://doi.org/10.7717/peerj.7458. eCollection 2019.
36. Jillard CL, Youngwirth L, Scheri RP, Roman S, Sosa JA. Radioactive iodine treatment is associated with improved survival for patients with Hürthle cell carcinoma. Thyroid. 2016;26(7):959–64.
37. Takashima S, Sone S, Takayama F, Wang Q, Kobayashi T, Horii A, Yoshida JI. Papillary thyroid carcinoma: MR diagnosis of lymph node metastasis. AJNR Am J Neuroradiol. 1998;19:509–13.
38. Gross ND, Weissman JL, Talbot JM, Andersen PE, Wax MK, Cohen JI. MRI detection of cervical metastasis from differentiated thyroid carcinoma. Laryngoscope. 2001;111:1905–9.
39. Foote RL, Brown PD, Garces YI, McIver B, Kasperbauer JL. Is there a role for radiation therapy in the management of Hürthle cell carcinoma? Int J Radiat Oncol Biol Phys. 2003;56:1067–72.
40. Zavitsanos P, Amdur RJ, Drew PA, Cusi K, Werning JW, Morris CG. Favorable outcome of Hurthle cell carcinoma of the thyroid treated with total thyroidectomy, radioiodine, and selective use of external-beam radiotherapy. Am J Clin Oncol. 2017;40:433–7.
41. Lewis BD, Hay ID, Charboneau JW, McIver B, Reading CC, Goellner JR. Percutaneous ethanol injection for treatment of cervical lymph node metastases in patients with papillary thyroid carcinoma. Am J Roentgenol. 2002;178:699–704.
42. Dupuy DE, Monchik JM, Decrea C, Pisharodi L. Radiofrequency ablation of regional recurrence from well-differentiated thyroid malignancy. Surgery. 2001;130:971–7.

Chapter 22
A Case of a Large, Invasive PTC with Gross Residual Disease (pT4) After Surgery

Meredith Giuliani and James Brierley

Case Presentation

A 62-year-old previously healthy man presented with a slowly enlarging right neck mass associated with progressive hoarseness over a 3-month period. He denied neck pain, or difficulty swallowing or breathing. His family physician ordered a neck ultrasound that confirmed a 4 cm mass in the right thyroid lobe, and he referred the patient to a head and neck surgeon. In addition to the palpable mass, on flexible nasopharyngoscopy, he had a paralyzed right vocal cord. Computed tomography (CT) scan of the neck confirmed a 4 cm mass in the right thyroid lobe with possible extrathyroidal extension posteriorly toward the tracheoesophageal groove and several suspicious right-sided lymph nodes (Fig, 22.1a). A fine needle biopsy of the thyroid mass confirmed the diagnosis of papillary thyroid cancer (Bethesda Class VI). The patient was treated with a total thyroidectomy and right central and lateral neck dissections. The tumor involved the right cricothyroid joint, and gross disease was left in situ as it was not resectable without significant functional impairment. The final pathology was a 4.0 cm angioinvasive papillary carcinoma with extrathyroidal extension and positive margins; 4 of 51 lymph nodes were involved: 3 from level VI and 1 from level IV. The final stage was pT4a N1b. Postoperatively he received 125 mCi (4.62 GBq) of ^{131}I and was placed on suppressive doses of levothyroxine. His post-therapy radioiodine scan showed two foci of uptake in the thyroid bed, possibly representing residual disease. There was no evidence of distant disease.

M. Giuliani · J. Brierley (✉)
Department of Radiation Oncology, University of Toronto, Toronto, Canada

Department of Radiation Oncology, Princess Margaret Cancer Centre, Toronto, Canada
e-mail: James.Brierley@rmp.uhn.on.ca

G. Grani et al. (eds.), *Thyroid Cancer*,
https://doi.org/10.1007/978-3-030-61919-0_22

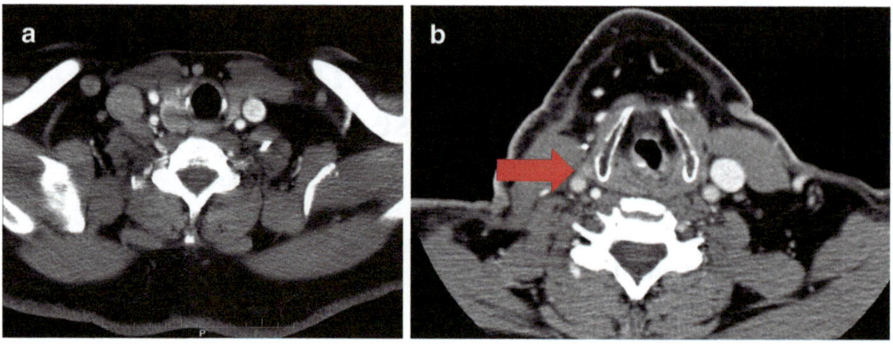

Fig. 22.1 Staging CT images. (**a**) preoperative CT, the red arrow indicates the mass in the right lobe of the thyroid; (**b**) a postoperative CT, the red arrow indicated the area of gross residual disease

Literature Review

Most patients with differentiated thyroid carcinoma (DTC) are treated by complete surgical excision (thyroidectomy or hemithyroidectomy) and, depending on the risk of recurrence, may receive postoperative radioiodine (^{131}I) combined with TSH suppressive therapy. Both of these therapies have been reported to reduce locoregional recurrence and improve disease-specific survival in higher-risk patients [1].

Locally advanced DTC with extrathyroidal extension is an uncommon clinical scenario, although more frequent in older patients, especially men. It can be a significant management challenge if it recurs, as uncontrolled cancer in the neck can be devastating with laryngeal, tracheal, and esophageal obstruction, skin ulceration and necrosis, and even carotid artery rupture. Surgery and postoperative ^{131}I may not adequately control persistent cervical disease. Consequently, additional treatment with external beam radiotherapy (EBRT) may be beneficial. However, there is a lack of evidence from randomized trials to guide its use and confirm its benefit. The only randomized trial comparing observation with EBRT was in patients with pT3/4 pN0/1 with DTC, and it closed early due to poor patient accrual with enrollment of many patients with lower-risk disease who were unlikely to benefit from EBRT [1, 2].

With the lack of data from randomized trials, institutional cohort studies have been used to inform management. One series reported a 5-year locoregional control rate with EBRT for patients with clear or microscopic margins was 89%, compared to a 69% rate of control in those with macroscopic residual or unresectable disease [3]. Our own data have shown that EBRT in older patients (age >60) with extrathyroidal extension (ETE) have a significantly improved 5-year local relapse-free rate. Pertinent to this patient, the study showed that in patients with postoperative gross residual disease treated with radiotherapy, the 10-year cause-specific survival and local recurrence-free rates were 48% and 90%, respectively. These data demonstrate clearly that even though local disease can be controlled with EBRT, patients continue to die from distant metastatic disease [4]. More recently, a retrospective cohort study of patients with T4a disease treated with RAI with or without EBRT reported worse locoregional control with RAI alone compared to RAI and EBRT. Patients with only recurrent nerve invasion did not routinely undergo EBRT, and RAI alone appeared to give good disease control. However, RAI was insufficient if there was tracheal perichondrium or esophageal muscularis involvement, and these patients appeared to benefit from EBRT [5]. It is unclear whether any of the study patients with RLN invasion had gross residual disease after surgery as did our patient. Although concurrent chemoradiation is standard therapy in the management of squamous cell cancers of the head and neck, differentiated thyroid cancer is not generally regarded as sensitive to conventional chemotherapy. Therefore, concurrent chemoradiation has not been frequently utilized in the treatment of differentiated thyroid cancer. However, in 1 report of 66 patients with advanced nonanaplastic, nonmedullary thyroid cancer, a median survival of 42 months was reported. The local relapse-free rate was 90% following chemoradiation and 73% with radiation alone. This difference was not statistically significant and the numbers small, only 21 patients having had chemoradiation. Further, the local control rate with EBRT was somewhat low compared to other studies in the pooled analysis discussed below. Therefore, more data are required before chemoradiation can be routinely recommended for these patients [6].

A larger study of 254 patients from 18 French institutions identified 254 patients who had T3 or T4 disease, nodal disease, or positive surgical margins. A propensity score analysis was performed, and EBRT resulted in reduced locoregional failure but not overall survival [7]. In a systematic literature review of the role of EBRT in differentiated thyroid cancer, 16 articles met the authors' initial criteria for review. This resulted in a pooled population of 5114 patients. In the 13 studies that reported local regional recurrence rates, the recurrence rate was 20% without EBRT but only 13% with EBRT. In a pooled quantitative analysis of 8 studies with detailed information of 2388 patients, the mean recurrence rate in patients receiving EBRT regardless of stage or residual disease status was 8%, and in those who did not receive EBRT, it was 25%, a statistically significant difference ($p = 0.03$). The authors concluded that there was an improvement in local regional control following EBRT in high-risk patients over age 45 [8].

The 2009 ATA guidelines recommend consideration of EBRT in patients older than 45 years with gross extrathyroidal extension and high likelihood of microscopic residual disease. The more recent 2016 American Thyroid Association guideline is not so specific, but comments that for tumors that invade the upper aerodigestive tract, surgery combined with additional therapy such as RAI and/or EBRT is generally advised [1, 9]. The United Kingdom guidelines recommend that EBRT should be considered in addition to RAI in patients with unresectable tumors and where there is residual disease after surgery even if the residual tumor concentrated RAI [10]. The American Head and Neck Society has stated that EBRT is recommended for patients with gross residual or unresectable locoregional disease, except for patients <45 years old with limited gross disease that is RAI-avid and that a higher age cutoff would be appropriate [11].

It is our policy to recommend EBRT in patients over age 50 with gross residual disease after surgery or with extrathyroidal extension that invades posteriorly into the tracheoesophageal groove that is unlikely to be controlled by ^{131}I and in whom salvage surgery may require an ablative surgical procedure such as laryngectomy (T4a or T4b). Patients with minimal ETE (T3) with positive margins or ETE that invades anteriorly into the strap muscles can usually be resected with clear margins and do not require EBRT. Patients with only recurrent laryngeal nerve involvement that is resected with no gross residual disease, as suggested by the report from MD Anderson discussed above [5], may not benefit from EBRT. We rarely recommend EBRT in younger patients unless they have T4b disease.

Minimizing toxicity is important. Toxicity is related to both radiation dose and the tissue volume irradiated. Larger elective target volumes have the potential to reduce recurrence, but are associated with increased toxicity. Structures of particular concern include the parotid glands, the pharyngeal constrictors, and the mandible. Our usual radiation volume includes the surgical thyroidectomy bed and nodal levels III, IV, and VI and part of level V, extending from the hyoid bone superiorly to the aortic arch inferiorly. Other centers use larger volumes which may result in fewer nodal recurrences but greater toxicity. We reported 90% local relapse-free rate in our series [7], and we do not think that target volumes need to be extended.. Intensity-modulated radiotherapy (IMRT) allows more sparing of normal tissues than 2D or 3D conformal radiation techniques. In randomized studies in squamous cell carcinomas of the head and neck, IMRT reduced side effects and improved quality of life and may confer a survival advantage [7].

It is our institutional policy to deliver 60Gy in 30 fractions to the thyroid bed and areas of surgical dissection if there is concern for microscopic residual disease and 54Gy in 30 fractions to undissected areas at risk of microscopic disease. In the case of gross residual disease, a dose of 66Gy in 33 fractions is given, plus a margin for uncertainty with 56Gy in 33 fractions to the areas at risk of microscopic disease. A preoperative CT scan with contrast is a great aid in planning any postoperative radiation therapy that may be contemplated, as well as being helpful to the surgeon in planning the operation. In our institution, surgeons routinely perform CT scans with contrast in any patient with a potential T4 tumor (a large mass, pain, or, as in the case described, hoarseness). Previously, concern has been expressed that the use of iodinated contrast may interfere with the effectiveness of ^{131}I by reducing uptake. However, with modern water-soluble contrast media, only a 1- or 2-month delay is required for the urinary iodine levels to normalized, which is not an undue delay. Although in theory EBRT could reduce the uptake and effectiveness of ^{131}I, there is no good evidence to support this. It is our preference to give ^{131}I and then perform postoperative CT scans after the post ^{131}I therapy scan and reassess the extent residual of disease using all imaging modalities. A PET scan, if available, may provide additional information. If, however, there is concern about the extent of local disease that may cause an oncological emergency without control of that disease, such as gross residual disease after spinal cord decompression, then we will give EBRT before ^{131}I therapy.

Management of the Patient

His postoperative CT scan showed a 5 mm area of likely residual disease in the right thyroid bed (Fig. 22.1b). He was treated with 66 Gy in 33 fractions of radiotherapy to the area of gross residual disease and 60Gy in 33 fractions to the thyroid bed and bilateral necks with an IMRT plan (Fig. 22.2). The patient experienced a 7% weight loss during radiotherapy as well as Radiotherapy Oncology Group (RTOG) grade 2 mucositis, esophagitis, laryngitis, and skin reactions. He was supported throughout treatment without a feeding tube. He has subsequently made a full recovery and is able to tolerate a normal diet. He does not experience xerostomia and remains free of local recurrence 5 years later. He has however developed small microscopic pulmonary nodules with a rising serum thyroglobulin and negative 5 mCi ^{131}I whole-body scan which are being followed.

Clinical Pearls/Pitfalls

- Gross residual disease following surgery for differentiated thyroid cancer is a complex clinical situation requiring multidisciplinary input and management.
- EBRT can increase locoregional control and possibly survival in older patients with extrathyroidal extension and with gross residual disease, but the risk of distant relapse remains.
- The ideal dose and treatment volumes remain uncertain.
- IMRT provides an improvement in the toxicity profile and possibly even survival.

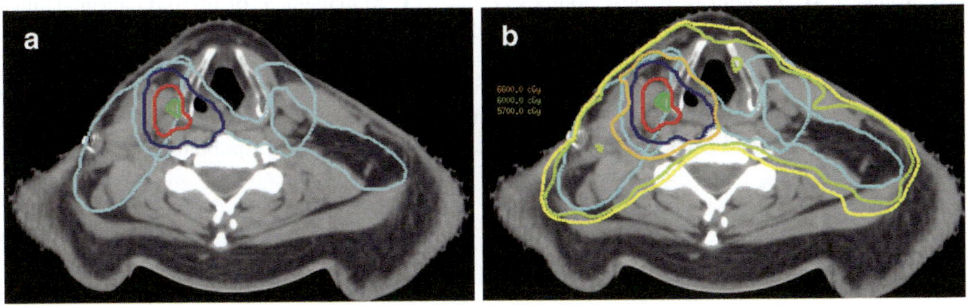

Fig. 22.2 Radiotherapy plan. (**a**) The green represents the gross tumor volume (GTV), red the high-risk tumor volume (HTV), dark blue the clinical target volume (CTV)66, and light blue the CTVs60; (**b**) the addition of the radiotherapy isodose lines 66Gy in light orange, 60Gy in green yellow, and 57Gy in yellow

References

1. Haugen BR, Alexander EK, Bible KC, Doherty GM, Mandel SJ, Nikiforov YE, et al. 2015 American Thyroid Association Management Guidelines for Adult Patients with Thyroid Nodules and Differentiated Thyroid Cancer: The American Thyroid Association Guidelines Task Force on Thyroid Nodules and Differentiated Thyroid Cancer. Thyroid: official journal of the American Thyroid Association. 2016;26:1):1–133. Epub 2015/10/16
2. Brierley JD. Update on external beam radiation therapy in thyroid cancer. The Journal of clinical endocrinology and metabolism. 2011;96(8):2289–95. Epub 2011/08/06
3. Azrif M, Slevin NJ, Sykes AJ, Swindell R, Yap BK. Patterns of relapse following radiotherapy for differentiated thyroid cancer: implication for target volume delineation. Radiother Oncol. 2008;89(1):105–13.
4. Sia MA, Tsang RW, Panzarella T, Brierley JD. Differentiated thyroid cancer with extrathyroidal extension: prognosis and the role of external beam radiotherapy. J Thyroid Res. 2010;2010:183461. Epub 2010/11/05
5. Tam S, Amit M, Boonsripitayanon M, Cabanillas ME, Busaidy NL, Gunn GB, et al. Adjuvant External Beam Radiotherapy in Locally Advanced Differentiated Thyroid Cancer. JAMA otolaryngology-- head & neck surgery. 2017;143(12):1244–51. Epub 2017/11/04
6. Romesser PB, Sherman EJ, Shaha AR, Lian M, Wong RJ, Sabra M, et al. External beam radiotherapy with or without concurrent chemotherapy in advanced or recurrent non-anaplastic non-medullary thyroid cancer. Journal of surgical oncology. 2014;110(4):375–82. Epub 2014/06/26
7. Servagi Vernat S, Khalifa J, Sun XS, Kammerer E, Blais E, Faivre JC, et al. 10-Year Locoregional Control with Postoperative External Beam Radiotherapy in Patients with Locally Advanced High-Risk Non-Anaplastic Thyroid Carcinoma De Novo or at Relapse, a Propensity Score Analysis. Cancers. 2019;11:6. Epub 2019/06/30
8. Fussey JM, Crunkhorn R, Tedla M, Weickert MO, Mehanna H. External beam radiotherapy in differentiated thyroid carcinoma: A systematic review. Head Neck. 2016;38(Suppl 1):E2297–305. Epub 2015/09/04
9. Cooper DS, Doherty GM, Haugen BR, Kloos RT, Lee SL, Mandel SJ, et al. Revised American Thyroid Association management guidelines for patients with thyroid nodules and differentiated thyroid cancer. Thyroid: official journal of the American Thyroid Association. 2009;19(11):1167–214. Epub 2009/10/29
10. Mitchell AL, Gandhi A, Scott-Coombes D, Perros P. Management of thyroid cancer: United Kingdom National Multidisciplinary Guidelines. The Journal of laryngology and otology. 2016;130(S2):S150–S60. Epub 2016/11/15
11. Kiess AP, Agrawal N, Brierley JD, Duvvuri U, Ferris RL, Genden E, et al. External-beam radiotherapy for differentiated thyroid cancer locoregional control: A statement of the American Head and Neck Society. Head Neck. 2016;38(4):493–8. Epub 2015/12/31

Chapter 23
A Patient with Papillary Carcinoma of the Thyroid with Elevated Serum Thyroglobulin but Negative Imaging Studies

Leonard Wartofsky

Case

A 39-year-old woman presented to our office for a first visit having recently moved to the area. She had presented in 2008 with a neck mass which on FNA biopsy was suspicious for papillary thyroid carcinoma (Bethesda class V), leading to a total thyroidectomy in early 2009. The surgical pathology revealed a 3.5 cm classic papillary cancer, with 2/6 central compartment nodes and 5/11 right lateral lymph nodes positive for metastasis, with report of tumor to the surgical margin and minimal extrathyroidal extension (pT3, N1b, Mx—stage I according to AJCC/UICC TNM staging system, eighth edition). She received 90 mCi of radioiodine in April 2009. Her course until the present time had been one of repeated measurable serum thyroglobulin (Tg) ranging from 8 to 20 ng/mL on TSH suppression without any success in localizing the source of the Tg by imaging studies. Anti-Tg antibodies were negative. Since 2009, she had undergone annual ultrasonography of the neck, neck and chest CT scans on two occasions, MRI of the neck on two occasions, and recombinant human TSH (rhTSH; Thyrogen®)-stimulated iodine-131 scans on two occasions, all without identification of tumor. On two occasions, mildly suspicious lymph nodes in both the right and left neck underwent ultrasound-guided FNA for cytology and Tg measurement of the aspirate, but both were negative. She is well educated, well read on her disease, concerned about the continuing measurable levels of Tg, and asked if there are any other diagnostic or therapeutic options.

L. Wartofsky (✉)
MedStar Health Research Institute, MedStar Washington Hospital Center, Washington, DC, USA

Georgetown University School of Medicine, Washington, DC, USA
e-mail: leonard.wartofsky@medstar.net

G. Grani et al. (eds.), *Thyroid Cancer*,
https://doi.org/10.1007/978-3-030-61919-0_23

Assessment

The case illustrates a patient with a biochemically incomplete response to treatment (i.e., persistent measurable Tg levels) but no evidence of structural disease. Ruling out the possibility of stable iodine contamination negating radioiodine uptake, we can explain the fact that her residual tumor is not seen on ultrasound, CT, MRI, or iodine-131 scans either because the tumor deposits are small and below the detection sensitivity of the various imaging modalities or because the tumor has dedifferentiated and is no longer taking up iodine. She is anti-Tg antibody negative, and there should be no reason for an artifactually or falsely elevated serum Tg.

Relevant Literature

The current guidelines of the American Thyroid Association (ATA) [1] suggest that imaging with ^{18}F-fluorodeoxyglucose (FDG) positron emission tomography (PET) coupled with a CT scan should be considered in patients in whom the serum Tg is elevated to >10 ng/ml and the usual iodine-131 diagnostic scan is negative. Studies have confirmed the efficacy of FDG-PET scanning when radioiodine uptake is absent [2, 3]. Leboulleux et al. [4] performed a meta-analysis of a total of 789 patients in 25 separate studies who were without radioiodine uptake for whom the sensitivity of FDG-PET/CT was found to be 83% and the specificity was 84%. FDG-PET/CT imaging may be enhanced with TSH stimulation [5] and is most likely to be helpful with larger tumors that have dedifferentiated, i.e., lost ability to trap radioiodine. Similarly, FDG-PET-positive tumors tend to have a significantly worse prognosis due in large part to the absence of RAI uptake that precludes therapy with radioiodine [6].

Given the situation of measurable Tg but negative imaging, obtaining an FDG-PET/CT scan would be advisable and consistent with the recommendations in the guidelines. Should the latter imaging disclose a locoregional metastasis or any localizable lesion, the therapeutic options to be considered include surgical excision, local ablative therapy such as radiofrequency or thermal ablation under CT guidance [7], or empiric radioiodine therapy (in spite of the prior history of little uptake). RAI has been given in this clinical scenario [8] to patients with ostensibly no RAI uptake on preliminary diagnostic scans with a demonstrable salutary effect in perhaps a third of patients who demonstrate positive uptake on a post-therapy scan and a subsequent fall in serum Tg, but such empiric therapy has not been shown to be successful in the majority of studies [9–12]. The sensitivity of FDG-PET/CT scanning may be improved by TSH stimulation (by either rhTSH or thyroid hormone withdrawal) [5], and sensitivity of FDG-PET/CT is greatest when Tg levels are elevated to >10 ng/ml, either with or without TSH stimulation [1]. Because iodine-124 emits a positron and can be imaged by PET scanning and shares the same radio-pharmacokinetics as iodine-131, studies have suggested that iodine-124

PET may be more useful for the identification of metastatic lesions than FDG-PET. Moreover, when positive, the presence of radioiodine avidity suggests an opportunity for RAI therapy with iodine-131 [13, 14]. When the iodine-124 is given in low doses (~2 mCi), stunning of the tumor tissue, thereby decreasing the efficacy of subsequent iodine-131 treatment, has not been considered a problem [15]. It should be emphasized that just because tumor deposits take up RAI does not mean that the tumor is radiosensitive and will be destroyed by therapy [16], especially in those tumors that are FDG avid. Finally, should the iodine-124 scan show no uptake, as was seen with iodine-123 in the case presented, or should the tumor be noted to progress after therapy, then a repeat therapeutic dose of iodine-131 would not be recommended [1]. New radioisotope-labeled molecules are being evaluated for PET imaging that may have applicability to a patient like ours. One pilot study employed fibroblast activation protein inhibitor labeled with 68-Gallium with marginal success [17].

Back to the Case

When next seen, the patient had a serum Tg of 7.5 on levothyroxine suppression and underwent rhTSH stimulation with a poststimulation Tg of 94 ng/ml and a negative iodine-123 scan (1.2 mCi; 444 MBq). She then underwent PET/CT scanning with the non-FDA-approved agent iodine-124 (1.7 mCi;63 MBq) and iodine-131 dosimetry (2 mCi; 74 MBq) [18–20] (see Figs. 23.1 and 23.2). The iodine-131 scan (Fig. 23.1a) was largely negative, whereas the iodine-124 PET revealed a focus of uptake posteriorly (Fig. 23.1b) that was identified by CT (Fig. 23.2a) as being in the left pelvic bone (arrow). Figure 23.2b indicates fusion of the transverse CT image of the pelvis with the corresponding transverse iodine-124 PET image, which demonstrates the utility of fusing the iodine-124 PET image with the CT image. The fused images demonstrated that the abnormal iodine-124 uptake corresponded precisely to the abnormality on the CT scan. In addition to the identification of this abnormality, the iodine-124 images demonstrated a second focus of abnormal iodine-124 uptake that correlated with another abnormality in the sacrum on the CT image suggesting an additional metastasis. The dosimetry estimated that she could receive a 440 mCi dose of iodine-131 safely with less than 72 mCi retained at 48 h. Although the patient was advised of the small likelihood of cure or significant improvement with another dose of radioiodine in the face of negative diagnostic radioiodine scans [9–12], she nevertheless was desirous of one more therapy. She was treated with 392 mCi, and the findings on the post-therapy iodine-131 scan were consistent with those seen on the iodine-124 PET scan, i.e., positive uptake in the identified metastases. At 4 months post-therapy, her blood neutrophil and platelet counts were normal, and her serum Tg has fallen to 1.9 ng/ml on suppression therapy. The follow-up plan is to continue twice yearly monitoring with serum Tg measurements, and a repeat iodine-124 PET/CT scan will be considered in

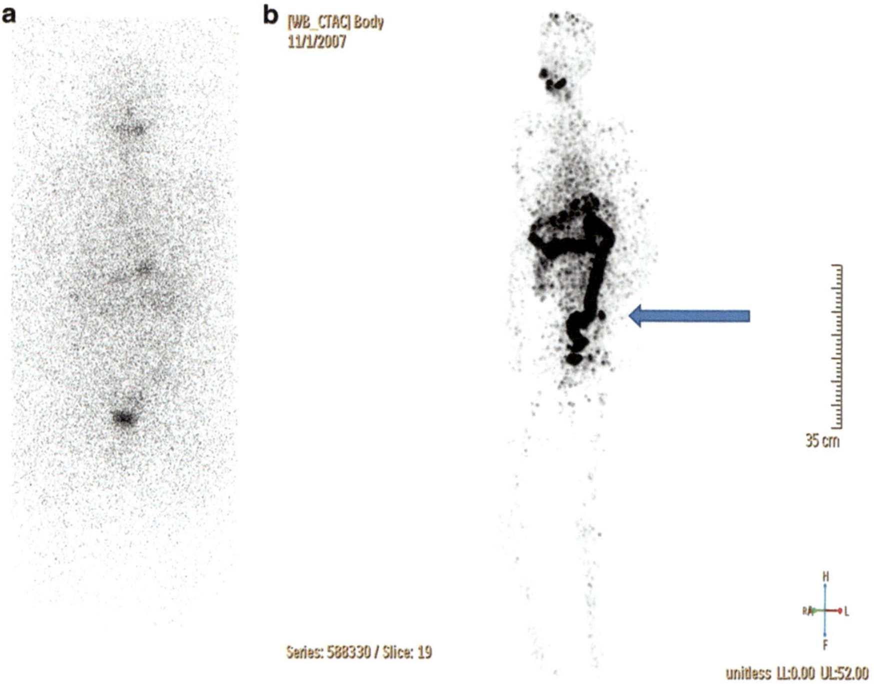

Fig. 23.1 (**a**) Iodine-123 scan (1.2 mCi; 444 MBq) indicating little detectable uptake. (**b**) Iodine-124 PET/CT (1.7 mCi;63 MBq) revealing a focus of uptake posteriorly

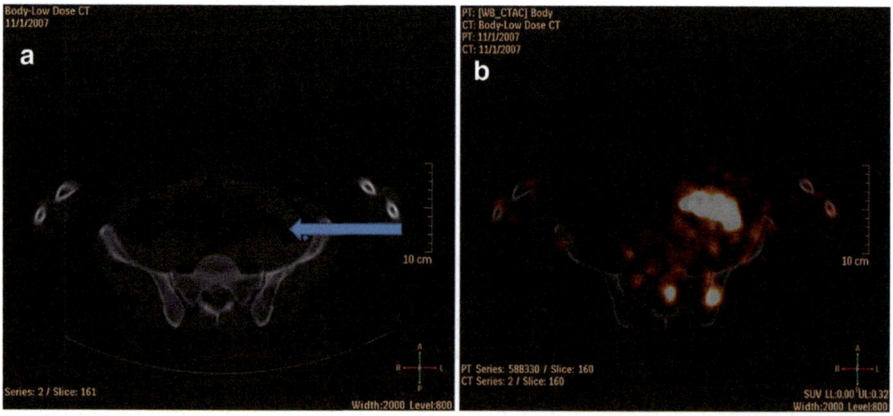

Fig. 23.2 (**a**) Computerized tomographic scan of pelvis indicating that the focus positive on PET scan was located in the left pelvic bone (arrow). (**b**) Fusion of the transverse CT image of the pelvis with the corresponding transverse iodine-124 PET image demonstrating localization of the lesion. The fused images demonstrated that the abnormal iodine-124 uptake corresponded precisely to the abnormality on the CT scan. In addition to localizing this abnormality, the ^{124}I images demonstrated a second focus of abnormal iodine-124 uptake that correlated with another abnormality in the sacrum on the CT image suggesting an additional metastasis

12–18 months unless her serum Tg becomes undetectable with time. She would be declared refractory to radioiodine and not considered for additional therapy should there be evidence of progressive disease as indicated by a rising Tg level and/or increased structural disease. In the latter circumstance, we will consider external radiation therapy or other attempts at local ablation. Multikinase inhibitors such as sorafenib or lenvatinib have also been considered for thyroglobulin-positive/scan-negative patients [21].

Clinical Pearls/Pitfalls

1. It is useful to tailor therapeutic interventions by risk stratification of patients according to the 2015 ATA guidelines on outcome status after initial treatment, which in this case indicated a biochemically incomplete response that was subsequently shown after iodine-124 PET scanning to be structurally incomplete.
2. Iodine-124 is associated with improved imaging over iodine-123 and lower radiation dose than iodine-131, thereby avoiding stunning. Although iodine-124 availability is currently confined to larger academic centers (because it is not an FDA-approved radioisotope and an IND is required), iodine-124 PET/CT scan should be considered in patients in whom the serum Tg is elevated to >10 ng/ml and the traditional iodine-131 scan is negative.
3. Another difference between iodine-124 and iodine-123 or iodine-131 is that iodine-124 emits a positron and can be imaged with a positron emission tomography (PET) scanner. The positron-emitting iodine-124 in combination with PET/CT makes it possible to measure the spatial distribution of radioiodine in tumors and normal organs at high resolution and sensitivity. Thus, iodine-124 PET/CT may provide improved delineation of the extent of metastases in well-differentiated thyroid cancer.
4. Radioiodine refractory tumors or those that fail to take up radioiodine should not be given additional doses of iodine-131.

References

1. Haugen BR, Alexander EK, Bible KC, Doherty GM, Mandel SJ, Nikiforov Y, et al. American Thyroid Association Management Guidelines for patients with thyroid nodules and differentiated thyroid cancer. Thyroid. 2016;26:1–133.
2. Marcus C, Whitworth PW, Surasi DS, Pai SI, Subramaniam RM. PET/CT in the management of thyroid cancers. Am J Roentgenol. 2014;202(6):1316–29.
3. Riemann B, Uhrhan K, Dietlein M, Schmidt D, Kuwert T, Dorn R, et al. Diagnostic value and therapeutic impact of (18)F-FDG-PET/CT in differentiated thyroid cancer. Results of a German multicentre study. Nucl Med. 2013;52:1):1–6.
4. Leboulleux S, Schroeder PR, Schlumberger M, Ladenson PW. The role of PET in follow-up of patients treated for differentiated epithelial thyroid cancers. Nat Clin Pract Endocrinol Metab. 2007;3:112–21.

5. Leboulleux S, Schroeder PR, Busaidy NL, Auperin A, Corone C, Jacene HA, Ewertz ME, Bournaud C, Wahl RL, Sherman SI, Ladenson PW, Schlumberger M. Assessment of the incremental value of recombinant thyrotropin stimulation before 2-[18F]-Fluoro-2-deoxy-D-glucose positron emission tomography/computed tomography imaging to localize residual differentiated thyroid cancer. J Clin Endocrinol Metab. 2009;94:1310–6.
6. Robbins RJ, Wan Q, Grewal RK, Reibke R, Gonen M, Strauss HW, Tuttle RM, Drucker W, Larson SM. Real-time prognosis for metastatic thyroid carcinoma based on 2-[18F]fluoro-2-deoxy-D-glucose-positron emission tomography scanning. J Clin Endocrinol Metab. 2006;91:498–505.
7. Wartofsky L. Adjunctive local approaches to metastatic thyroid cancer. In: Thyroid cancer: a comprehensive guide to clinical management. 2nd ed. New York: Humana/Springer; 2006. p. 509–13.
8. Mazzaferri EL. Empirically treating high serum thyroglobulin levels. J Nucl Med. 2005;46:1079–88.
9. Kim WG, Ryu JS, Kim EY, Lee JH, Baek JH, Yoon JH, et al. Empiric high-dose 131-iodine therapy lacks efficacy for treated papillary thyroid cancer patients with detectable serum thyroglobulin but negative cervical sonography and 18F-fluorodeoxy-glucose positron emission tomography scan. J Clin Endocrinol Metab. 2010;95:1169–73.
10. Leboulleux S, El Bez I, Borget I, Elleuch M, Deandreis D, Al Ghuzlan A, et al. Postradioiodine treatment whole-body scan in the era of 18-florodeoxyglucose positron emission tomography for differentiated thyroid carcinoma with elevated serum thyroglublin levels. Thyroid. 2012;22:832–8.
11. Rosario PW, Mourao GF, dos Santos JB, Calsolari MR. Is empirical radioactive iodine therapy still a valid approach to patients with thyroid cancer and elevated thyroglobulin? Thyroid. 2014;24:533–6.
12. Sabra MM, Grewal RK, Tala H, Larson SM, Tuttle RM. Clinical outcomes following empiric radioiodine therapy in patients with structurally identified metastatic follicular cell-derived thyroid carcinoma with negative diagnostic but positive post-therapy 131-I whole-body scans. Thyroid. 2012;22:877–83.
13. Phan HT, Jager PL, Paans AM, Plukker JT, Sturkenboom MG, Sluiter WJ, Wolffenbuttel BH, Dierckx RA, Links TP. The diagnostic value of 124I-PET in patients with differentiated thyroid cancer. Eur J Nucl Med Mol Imaging. 2008;35:958–65.
14. Freudenberg LS, Jentzen W, Stahl A, Bockisch A, Rosenbaum-Krumme SJ. Clinical applications of 124I-PET/CT in patients with differentiated thyroid cancer. Eur J Nucl Med Mol Imaging. 2011;38(Suppl 1):S48–56.
15. Van Nostrand D, Moreau S, Bandaru VV, Atkins F, Chennupati S, Mete M, Burman K, Wartofsky L. (124)I positron emission tomography versus (131)I planar imaging in the identification of residual thyroid tissue and/or metastasis in patients who have well-differentiated thyroid cancer. Thyroid. 2010;20:879–83.
16. Deandreis D, Al GA, Leboulleux S, Lacroix L, Garsi JP, Talbot M, Lumbroso J, Baudin E, Caillou B, Bidart JM, Schlumberger M. Do histological, immunohistochemical, and metabolic (radioiodine and fluorodeoxyglucose uptakes) patterns of metastatic thyroid cancer correlate with patient outcome? Endocr Relat Cancer. 2011;18:159–69.
17. Kratochwil C, Flechsig P, Lindner T, Abderrahim L, Altmann A, Mier W, et al. 68-Ga-FAPI PET/CT: tracer uptake in 28 different kinds of cancer. J Nucl Med. 2019;60:801–5.
18. Eschmann SM, Reischl G, Bilger K, Kuperferschlager J, Thelen MH, Dohmen BM, Bares R. Evaluation of dosimetry of radioiodine therapy in benign and malignant thyroid disorders by means of iodine-124 and PET. Eur J Nucl Med Mol Imaging. 2002;29:760–7.

19. Barth A, Robbins RJ, Larson SM. Patient-specific dosimetry for 131-I thyroid cancer therapy using 124-I PET and 3-dimensional-internal dosimetry (3D-ID) software. J Nucl Med. 2004;45:1366–72.
20. Freudenberg LS, Jentzen W, Gorges R, Petrich T, Marlowe RJ, Knust J, Bockrish A. 124-I PET dosimetry in advanced differentiated thyroid cancer: therapeutic impact. Nuclearmedizin. 2007;46:121–8.
21. Shinohara S, Kikuchi M, Suehiro A, Kishimoto I, Harada H, Hino M, Ishihara T. Characteristics and prognosis of patients with thyroglobulin-positive and radioactive iodine whole-body scan-negative differentiated thyroid carcinoma. Japan J Clin Oncol. 2015;45:427–32.

Chapter 24
A Child with Papillary Thyroid Cancer and Metastatic Pulmonary Disease: Role of Radioactive Iodine Therapy

Monica L. Arango and Steven G. Waguespack

Introduction

Papillary thyroid carcinoma is rare in the pediatric population and is optimally treated with surgery by a high-volume thyroid surgeon, followed by possible radioactive iodine (RAI) therapy, which is given in the context of postoperative staging (a diagnostic thyroid scan and a stimulated thyroglobulin [Tg] level) [1, 2], especially in cases of known or suspected distant metastases. Children with PTC and metastatic pulmonary disease typically respond satisfactorily to ^{131}I therapy and demonstrate a continuous improvement of Tg levels, even years after treatment [3–6]. However, some patients may need more than one course of ^{131}I, and the optimal approach to the evaluation and treatment of children with pulmonary metastases remains unresolved [7]. Given the excellent prognosis of children with PTC and pulmonary metastases, as well as the possible risk for second malignancies [4, 8, 9] and increased overall mortality among pediatric PTC survivors [10], the risks of multiple RAI doses must be weighed against the potential benefits.

M. L. Arango (✉)
Division of Pediatric Endocrinology, McGovern Medical School, UTHealth, Houston, TX, USA
e-mail: monica.L.Arango@uth.tmc.edu

S. G. Waguespack
Department of Endocrine Neoplasia & Hormonal Disorders, University of Texas MD Anderson Cancer Center, Houston, TX, USA
e-mail: swagues@mdanderson.org

G. Grani et al. (eds.), *Thyroid Cancer*,
https://doi.org/10.1007/978-3-030-61919-0_24

Case Presentation

A 9-year-old Hispanic male with a history of multiple upper respiratory infections but no risk factors for thyroid cancer presented to an otolaryngologist with an enlarged cervical lymph node, which had been present for at least a year. He underwent an excisional lymph node biopsy, which revealed metastatic PTC. Initial comprehensive staging included a normal TSH and a Tg of 354 ng/ml (normal <55 for an intact thyroid) with negative Tg antibodies; a neck ultrasound and contrast-enhanced computed tomography (CT) scan of the neck that revealed a diffusely infiltrating primary tumor with clinical N1b disease; and a chest X-ray (CXR) negative for pulmonary metastases. The patient had a total thyroidectomy and bilateral central and lateral neck dissections with final pathologic staging revealing a multifocal, bilateral T3bN1bMx (AJCC 8th edition) PTC, conventional type; the tumor was negative for the *BRAF* V600E mutation. Postoperative staging 2 months after surgery (after ensuring a normal 24-h urine iodine level) included a withdrawal ^{123}I thyroid scan and a stimulated Tg level (concomitant TSH 191 mU/L). There was no uptake identified on the diagnostic scan, but the stimulated Tg was 145 ng/ml (<0.9 post-thyroidectomy), suggesting residual metastatic disease. Given the high Tg level and risk for distant metastases, he was treated empirically with 45 mCi (1.7 GBq) of ^{131}I (weight-adjusted dose equivalent to a 150 mCi (5.6 GBq) dose in a 70 kg adult; ^{131}I dose = 150 mCi (5.6 GBq) × weight of patient (kg)/70). Posttreatment scan showed minimal diffuse bilateral pulmonary uptake as well as uptake bilaterally in the nodes of Rouviere (retropharyngeal lymph nodes), best seen with single-photon emission computed tomography (SPECT)-CT imaging (Fig. 24.1).

Assessment and Literature Review

Thyroid cancer is rare in the pediatric population. Adolescents are the most commonly affected pediatric age group (34 cases/million/year), and thyroid cancer is the most common cancer, representing 14% of all malignancies diagnosed at the ages of 15–19 years [11]. PTC is the most common type and accounts for about 90% of childhood thyroid malignancies. Initial clinical presentation is commonly a thyroid nodule or cervical lymphadenopathy, which is sometimes misinterpreted as reactive lymph node enlargement. Pediatric PTC is frequently multifocal and bilateral; regional lymph node metastases occur in up to 80% of cases [12, 13]. Children with a significant cervical disease burden are at the highest risk of hematogenous metastases to the lungs, which occur in up to 25% of cases [7, 12, 14–19]. Despite the apparent aggressive clinical presentation of PTC when diagnosed during childhood, and a higher rate of pulmonary metastases compared with adults, who have approximately a 4% rate of distant metastases [11], disease-specific mortality in pediatric PTC is extremely low (~2% or less decades after diagnosis) [5–7, 9, 10,

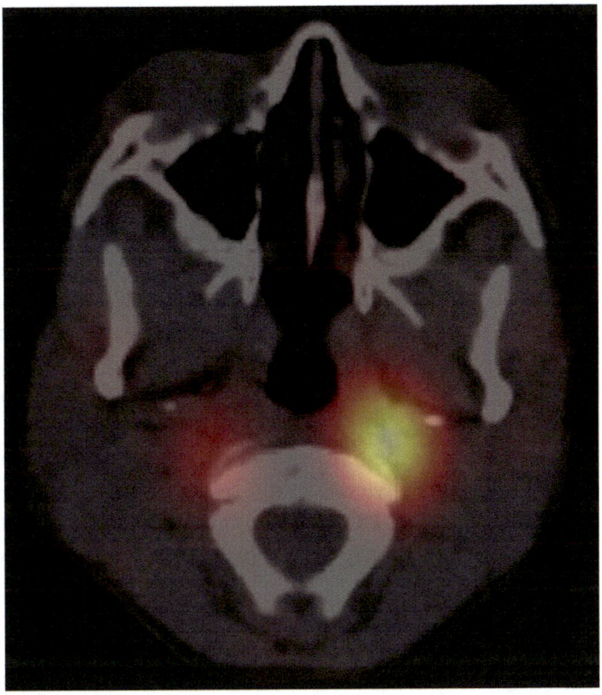

Fig. 24.1 Posttreatment ^{131}I SPECT-CT reveals intense uptake in a left retropharyngeal LN (node of Rouviere) and to a lesser extent in a right retropharyngeal LN

17, 18, 20–23]. This excellent long-term prognosis, coupled with unique concerns regarding the potential late sequelae related to overzealous treatment at a young age (e.g., second malignancies and pulmonary fibrosis) [4, 8–10, 24, 25], makes the management of pediatric PTC with lung metastases challenging. Furthermore, there have been no prospective clinical trials to guide decision-making; indeed, our understanding of pediatric PTC primarily comes from adult PTC, in addition to clinical reviews, pediatric PTC case series, and expert opinion. Only recently have formal society guidelines for the management of pediatric PTC been developed [1, 26].

Over the last few decades, the molecular pathogenesis of PTC has been better elucidated. Point mutations and gene fusions that activate the mitogen-activated protein kinase pathway play a major role in PTC development and propagation [27]. In pediatric PTC, a chromosomal rearrangement is the most likely molecular event [28–35]. Fusions involving the *RE*arranged during *T*ransfection (*RET*) proto-oncogene and the neurotropic tyrosine receptor kinase (*NTRK*) genes (*NTRK1/3*) are the most common, although some series have also reported rearrangements involving the v-raf murine sarcoma viral oncogene homolog B (*BRAF*) and anaplastic lymphoma kinase (*ALK*) genes [33, 36, 37]. The $BRAF^{V600E}$ point mutation is also prevalent in childhood PTC [28–31, 33–36, 38–40], although not as common as in adults. Knowledge regarding tumor genotype may inform the expected clinical course and response to RAI, although more research needs to be done in this area as relates to pediatric PTC.

In most cases, it is recommended that the initial evaluation of children with PTC includes a preoperative CXR to assess for macroscopic lung metastases; the finding of which may alter plans for subsequent RAI therapy [2]. However, a CXR is not sensitive enough to identify small-volume micronodular pulmonary metastases [6, 16], and for that reason, some centers also consider chest CT at diagnosis, especially in children with bulky cervical disease who are at the highest risk for distant metastases [2, 14]. Current pediatric guidelines do not advocate routine chest CT in all patients [1, 26], with the additional understanding that postoperative staging with RAI, if indicated, will effectively identify most children with pulmonary metastases, even those with negative baseline radiographic imaging [5, 6, 16]. In the end, knowledge regarding the presence or absence of pulmonary metastases does not alter the plan for initial therapy, which is the appropriate oncologic surgery (total thyroidectomy ± compartment-oriented neck dissection) by a high-volume thyroid surgeon.

The inaugural pediatric American Thyroid Association (ATA) guidelines introduced a postoperative risk categorization (ATA pediatric low, intermediate, and high risk) based upon AJCC TNM staging that helps to identify patients at risk of distant metastases and thereby determine which children should undergo routine postoperative staging with RAI [1]. Using this novel classification, children with significant central or lateral neck lymph node involvement are considered ATA pediatric intermediate or high risk, depending on the extent and volume of disease. In most intermediate-risk (clinical N1a or microscopic N1b disease) and in all high-risk (clinical N1b disease) patients, including patients already known to have distant metastases, postoperative staging with a diagnostic RAI scan and a TSH-stimulated Tg is recommended [1, 2].

In some children, as seen in the current case, the diagnostic whole-body scan (WBS) may be negative for lung uptake (Fig. 24.2a), but the Tg may be significantly elevated, thereby suggesting the presence of distant metastases. The absolute value of hyper-thyroglobulinemia that predicts lung metastases in children remains largely unknown. Recent studies suggest the value of a pre-ablation Tg and Tg/TSH ratio in predicting more accurately patients with pulmonary metastasis [41–43]. Until further studies elucidate the optimal Tg threshold, empiric RAI therapy is typically administered to a child who is at high risk for distant metastases and whose stimulated Tg is >10 ng/ml [1, 2]. Although the empiric use of ^{131}I is not associated with clear benefit in adults with negative diagnostic RAI scans and known structural disease [44], this issue remains unstudied in children, who may be more prone to benefit from RAI in this setting due to the inherent differences in tumor biology and iodine responsiveness. In all cases, after ^{131}I therapy, a post-therapy scan is recommended 4–7 days in order to identify iodine-avid disease that may not have been readily visible on the diagnostic WBS and also to help determine iodine avidity in known or suspected metastatic disease previously seen on radiographic imaging (Fig. 24.2b).

The goal of ^{131}I therapy in children with pulmonary metastases is to decrease the risk of thyroid cancer progression and in turn, to improve mortality by eliminating

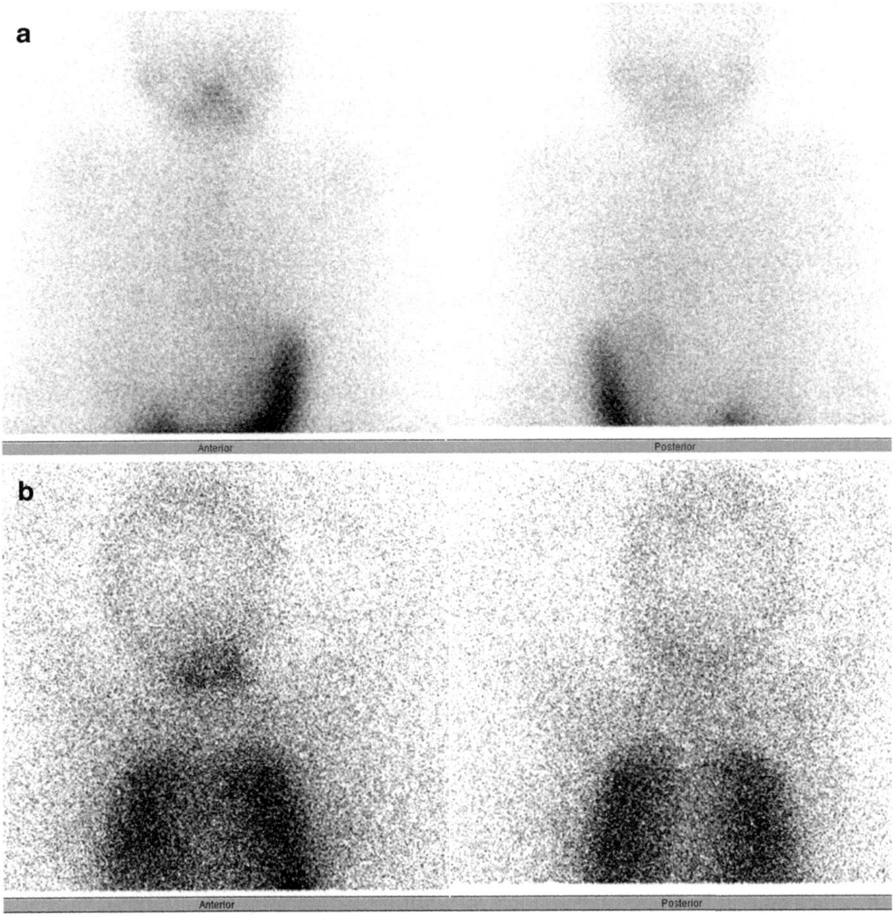

Fig. 24.2 Diagnostic (**a**) and posttreatment (**b**) ^{131}I scans in a 12-year-old boy with stage II PTC. The diagnostic study revealed no evidence of iodine-avid pulmonary metastases, but he was treated empirically with ^{131}I due to a stimulated Tg of 767 ng/ml and known pulmonary metastases that previously demonstrated iodine avidity. The posttreatment scan 7 days after ^{131}I clearly demonstrates diffuse pulmonary metastases

iodine-avid disease while minimizing the risk of late complications. The intent of therapy is no longer to treat every patient until they have an undetectable thyroglobulin level, since that is achievable in only about 50% or less of pediatric patients with pulmonary metastases [1, 6, 7]. Although some series report a higher rate of response [22], others have described more persistent disease despite multiple courses of RAI [5, 6, 45]. Factors affecting long-term outcome in children with pulmonary metastases include tumor doubling time and size of the pulmonary metastases [22, 45]; there have been no pediatric specific studies that have looked at thyroglobulin doubling time as a prognostic indicator.

Those children identified to have iodine-avid distant disease will likely benefit from ^{131}I therapy. Therefore, ^{131}I is typically administered at an activity that is proportionately equivalent to a 150–200 mCi (5.6–7.4 GBq) dose in an adult (sometimes less, if significant diffuse pulmonary uptake is present). For example, in a 30 kg child, an administered activity of 64 mCi ^{131}I would be considered (150 mCi × [30 kg/70 kg]). Dosimetry is considered in children with diffuse pulmonary metastases but is not readily available in all centers. When dosimetry is employed, the goal is to ensure that the whole-body retention 48 h after ^{131}I administration does not exceed 80 mCi (3 GBq) in the presence of iodine-avid diffuse lung metastases [46], which should minimize the concern about pulmonary fibrosis in this population.

Children with small-volume, iodine-avid micronodular (<1 cm) lung disease are the most likely to respond to treatment [22, 45], and they may ultimately become disease-free, whereas others, especially those with a more extensive metastatic disease burden, may never become cancer-free as assessed by Tg levels [3, 4, 7, 22, 45]. The nadir response to RAI can take 1–2 years or more [3, 5, 6]. Because of this, current recommendations are to wait until the disease either progresses or unequivocally remains persistent before proceeding to subsequent evaluation and possible retreatment with ^{131}I [1]. The thought is that such a cautious approach to repeated ^{131}I therapy may help to mitigate the long-term sequelae of RAI while also ensuring durable control of disease.

Further studies are required regarding the optimal dosing and timing of ^{131}I for children with PTC and iodine-avid pulmonary metastases. In all cases, the decision to treat a child with RAI should be individualized [1, 2, 26], preferably by clinicians experienced in the management of advanced pediatric PTC. After initial ^{131}I therapy, children with PTC and lung metastases should be monitored while continuing TSH suppression (goal TSH <0.1 mU/L). Monitoring the TSH-suppressed Tg is the optimal approach in most children with distant metastases. Periodic imaging with CXR or CT chest can be done to assess for structural disease progression, but CT should not be more frequent than every 1–2 years (or even less, depending on the case), in light of the added risk of repeated diagnostic radiation exposure and the fact that significant radiographic progression warranting additional therapy is unexpected in the vast majority of pediatric PTC cases. Once the nadir radiographic and biochemical Tg response is reached, repeat evaluation with a diagnostic WBS is considered in those with documented iodine-avid disease, but retreatment with RAI should be limited to those children who still have evidence of disease and who also benefited from prior ^{131}I therapy [1].

In children who develop iodine non-avid or non-responsive PTC, continued observation and TSH suppression are indicated. The development of progressive PTC that warrants further systemic treatment is rare, and in the event a child with metastatic PTC needs such an approach, consultation with providers who are experienced in the use of systemic therapy in children is recommended. A review of the currently available, molecularly targeted agents for the treatment of pediatric PTC is beyond the purview of this chapter, but there are both FDA-approved medications and other novel therapeutics in clinical trials that can be considered [47–51].

Back to the Case

Following initial ^{131}I therapy, expectant monitoring and TSH suppressive therapy commenced, and the patient's suppressed Tg over the following 2 years never reached a nadir; instead, it slowly rose from 13.5 to 29.5 ng/ml. Cross-sectional imaging revealed no overt evidence for cervical disease (outside of prominent nodes of Rouviere) and multiple tiny pulmonary nodules measuring up to 3 mm (noting that this was an initial diagnostic CT chest and that the pulmonary nodules were not as clearly seen on SPECT-CT previously obtained after initial RAI therapy). At the age of 12, he had a hypothyroid ^{131}I thyroid scan and a stimulated Tg that revealed no evidence of pathologic RAI uptake (Fig. 24.2a) and a value of 767 ng/ml, respectively. A second empiric ^{131}I dose of 58 mCi (2.1 GBq; weight-adjusted dose equivalent to a 156 mCi (5.8 GBq) dose in a 70 kg adult) was administered, and the posttreatment scan obtained 7 days after high-dose RAI revealed diffuse bilateral lung uptake (Fig. 24.2b). A year later, CT neck/chest and cervical US revealed no evidence of progression, and a non-suppressed Tg (TSH 2.4 mU/L) was 60 ng/ml. Due to persistent metastatic disease, molecular testing of his tumor was undertaken and revealed an *NCOA4-RET* fusion. Currently 18 years of age, the patient has persistent yet overall stable micronodular pulmonary metastases and continues to be monitored expectantly with TSH suppression.

Clinical Pearls

- Young children with PTC often present with extensive locoregional and pulmonary metastatic disease.
- The risk for pulmonary metastases is highest in children with extensive cervical disease.
- Despite the presence of pulmonary metastases, disease-specific mortality is low with survival over decades anticipated.
- RAI is indicated for children with known or suspected pulmonary metastases. A diagnostic whole-body scan may fail to reveal iodine-avid pulmonary metastases, and so a delayed posttreatment scan obtained 4–7 days after RAI is critical for identifying iodine-avid disease.
- Use of dosimetry (if available) in children with diffuse pulmonary metastases can ensure that the administered activity of ^{131}I is below that which would place the child at risk for pulmonary fibrosis.
- The clinical response of pulmonary metastases to ^{131}I may take years to fully appreciate. Given the long-term risks of RAI in children, the current approach is to retreat with ^{131}I only if there is evidence of disease beyond 1 year, or if there is disease progression in a patient who was previously felt to respond/benefit to therapeutic RAI; RAI therapy every 6–12 months until the patient becomes Tg and/or diagnostic scan negative is no longer the approach to treatment.

- It is unclear how best to define iodine non-avid/nonresponsive disease in children, although there will be a subset of children who do not respond to ^{131}I as anticipated.
- TSH suppression is indicated as an adjunct to RAI, and the goal of TSH is <0.1 mU/L in a child with pulmonary metastatic disease.
- Gene fusions are common oncogenic drivers in pediatric PTC, and knowledge regarding tumor genotype should help to improve risk stratification and provide a more individualized treatment approach, especially for those rare cases of disease progression despite RAI.

References

1. Francis GL, Waguespack SG, Bauer AJ, Angelos P, Benvenga S, Cerutti JM, et al. Management guidelines for children with thyroid nodules and differentiated thyroid cancer. Thyroid. 2015;25(7):716–59.
2. Waguespack SG, Wasserman JD. Pediatric differentiated thyroid carcinoma. In: Mallick U, Harmer C, Mazzaferri EL, Kendall-Taylor P, editors. Practical management of thyroid cancer: a multidisciplinary approach. 2nd ed. Cham: Springer International Publishing; 2018. p. 273–94.
3. Biko J, Reiners C, Kreissl MC, Verburg FA, Demidchik Y, Drozd V. Favourable course of disease after incomplete remission on (131)I therapy in children with pulmonary metastases of papillary thyroid carcinoma: 10 years follow-up. Eur J Nucl Med Mol Imaging. 2011;38(4):651–5.
4. Dottorini ME, Vignati A, Mazzucchelli L, Lomuscio G, Colombo L. Differentiated thyroid carcinoma in children and adolescents: a 37-year experience in 85 patients. J Nucl Med. 1997;38(5):669–75.
5. Alzahrani AS, Alswailem M, Moria Y, Almutairi R, Alotaibi M, Murugan AK, et al. Lung metastasis in pediatric thyroid cancer: radiological pattern, molecular genetics, response to therapy, and outcome. J Clin Endocrinol Metab. 2019;104(1):103–10.
6. Samuel AM, Rajashekharrao B, Shah DH. Pulmonary metastases in children and adolescents with well-differentiated thyroid cancer. J Nucl Med. 1998;39(9):1531–6.
7. Pawelczak M, David R, Franklin B, Kessler M, Lam L, Shah B. Outcomes of children and adolescents with well-differentiated thyroid carcinoma and pulmonary metastases following (1)(3)(1)I treatment: a systematic review. Thyroid. 2010;20(10):1095–101.
8. Iyer NG, Morris LG, Tuttle RM, Shaha AR, Ganly I. Rising incidence of second cancers in patients with low-risk (T1N0) thyroid cancer who receive radioactive iodine therapy. Cancer. 2011;117(19):4439–46.
9. Vassilopoulou-Sellin R, Goepfert H, Raney B, Schultz PN. Differentiated thyroid cancer in children and adolescents: clinical outcome and mortality after long-term follow-up. Head Neck. 1998;20(6):549–55.
10. Hay ID, Gonzalez-Losada T, Reinalda MS, Honetschlager JA, Richards ML, Thompson GB. Long-term outcome in 215 children and adolescents with papillary thyroid cancer treated during 1940 through 2008. World J Surg. 2010;34(6):1192–202.
11. Howlader N, Noone AM, Krapcho M, Miller D, Brest A, Yu M, et al. SEER cancer statistics review, 1975–2016, based on November 2018 SEER data submission, posted to the SEER web site, April 2019. Bethesda, MD: National Cancer Institute; [cited 2020 March 31]. Available from: https://seer.cancer.gov/csr/1975_2016/.

12. Zimmerman D, Hay ID, Gough IR, Goellner JR, Ryan JJ, Grant CS, et al. Papillary thyroid carcinoma in children and adults: long-term follow-up of 1039 patients conservatively treated at one institution during three decades. Surgery. 1988;104(6):1157–66.
13. Frankenthaler RA, Sellin RV, Cangir A, Goepfert H. Lymph node metastasis from papillary-follicular thyroid carcinoma in young patients. Am J Surg. 1990;160(4):341–3.
14. Wada N, Sugino K, Mimura T, Nagahama M, Kitagawa W, Shibuya H, et al. Treatment strategy of papillary thyroid carcinoma in children and adolescents: clinical significance of the initial nodal manifestation. Ann Surg Oncol. 2009;16(12):3442–9.
15. Vassilopoulou-Sellin R, Klein MJ, Smith TH, Samaan NA, Frankenthaler RA, Goepfert H, et al. Pulmonary metastases in children and young adults with differentiated thyroid cancer. Cancer. 1993;71(4):1348–52.
16. Bal CS, Kumar A, Chandra P, Dwivedi SN, Mukhopadhyaya S. Is chest x-ray or high-resolution computed tomography scan of the chest sufficient investigation to detect pulmonary metastasis in pediatric differentiated thyroid cancer? Thyroid. 2004;14(3):217–25.
17. Golpanian S, Perez EA, Tashiro J, Lew JI, Sola JE, Hogan AR. Pediatric papillary thyroid carcinoma: outcomes and survival predictors in 2504 surgical patients. Pediatr Surg Int. 2016;32(3):201–8.
18. Klein Hesselink MS, Nies M, Bocca G, Brouwers AH, Burgerhof JG, van Dam EW, et al. Pediatric differentiated thyroid carcinoma in the Netherlands: a nationwide follow-up study. J Clin Endocrinol Metab. 2016;101(5):2031–9.
19. Jeon MJ, Kim YN, Sung TY, Hong SJ, Cho YY, Kim TY, et al. Practical initial risk stratification based on lymph node metastases in pediatric and adolescent differentiated thyroid cancer. Thyroid. 2018;28(2):193–200.
20. Hogan AR, Zhuge Y, Perez EA, Koniaris LG, Lew JI, Sola JE. Pediatric thyroid carcinoma: incidence and outcomes in 1753 patients. J Surg Res. 2009;156(1):167–72.
21. Demidchik YE, Demidchik EP, Reiners C, Biko J, Mine M, Saenko VA, et al. Comprehensive clinical assessment of 740 cases of surgically treated thyroid cancer in children of Belarus. Ann Surg. 2006;243(4):525–32.
22. Bal CS, Garg A, Chopra S, Ballal S, Soundararajan R. Prognostic factors in pediatric differentiated thyroid cancer patients with pulmonary metastases. J Pediatr Endocrinol Metab. 2015;28:745–51.
23. Hay ID, Johnson TR, Kaggal S, Reinalda MS, Iniguez-Ariza NM, Grant CS, et al. Papillary thyroid carcinoma (PTC) in children and adults: comparison of initial presentation and long-term postoperative outcome in 4432 patients consecutively treated at the mayo clinic during eight decades (1936–2015). World J Surg. 2018;42(2):329–42.
24. Hebestreit H, Biko J, Drozd V, Demidchik Y, Burkhardt A, Trusen A, et al. Pulmonary fibrosis in youth treated with radioiodine for juvenile thyroid cancer and lung metastases after Chernobyl. Eur J Nucl Med Mol Imaging. 2011;38(9):1683–90.
25. Albano D, Bertagna F, Panarotto MB, Giubbini R. Early and late adverse effects of radioiodine for pediatric differentiated thyroid cancer. Pediatr Blood Cancer. 2017;64:e26595.
26. Niedziela M, Handkiewicz-Junak D, Malecka-Tendera E, Czarniecka A, Dedecjus M, Lange D, et al. Diagnostics and treatment of differentiated thyroid carcinoma in children - Guidelines of Polish National Societies. Endokrynol Pol. 2016;67(6):628–42.
27. Cancer Genome Atlas Research Network. Integrated genomic characterization of papillary thyroid carcinoma. Cell. 2014;159(3):676–90.
28. Bauer AJ. Molecular genetics of thyroid cancer in children and adolescents. Endocrinol Metab Clin North Am. 2017;46(2):389–403.
29. Prasad ML, Vyas M, Horne MJ, Virk RK, Morotti R, Liu Z, et al. NTRK fusion oncogenes in pediatric papillary thyroid carcinoma in Northeast United States. Cancer. 2016;122(7):1097–107.
30. Picarsic JL, Buryk MA, Ozolek J, Ranganathan S, Monaco SE, Simons JP, et al. Molecular characterization of sporadic pediatric thyroid carcinoma with the DNA/RNA ThyroSeq v2 next-generation sequencing assay. Pediatr Dev Pathol. 2016;19(2):115–22.

31. Nikita ME, Jiang W, Cheng SM, Hantash FM, McPhaul MJ, Newbury RO, et al. Mutational analysis in pediatric thyroid cancer and correlations with age, ethnicity, and clinical presentation. Thyroid. 2016;26(2):227–34.
32. Cordioli MI, Moraes L, Bastos AU, Besson P, Alves MT, Delcelo R, et al. Fusion oncogenes are the Main genetic events found in sporadic papillary thyroid carcinomas from children. Thyroid. 2017;27(2):182–8.
33. Vanden Borre P, Schrock AB, Anderson PM, Morris JC 3rd, Heilmann AM, Holmes O, et al. Pediatric, adolescent, and young adult thyroid carcinoma harbors frequent and diverse targetable genomic alterations, including kinase fusions. Oncologist. 2017;22(3):255–63.
34. Pekova B, Dvorakova S, Sykorova V, Vacinova G, Vaclavikova E, Moravcova J, et al. Somatic genetic alterations in a large cohort of pediatric thyroid nodules. Endocr Connect. 2019;8:796–805.
35. Mostoufi-Moab S, Labourier E, Sullivan L, LiVolsi V, Li Y, Xiao R, et al. Molecular testing for oncogenic gene alterations in pediatric thyroid lesions. Thyroid. 2018;28(1):60–7.
36. Sisdelli L, Cordioli M, Vaisman F, Moraes L, Colozza-Gama GA, Alves PAG Jr, et al. AGK-BRAF is associated with distant metastasis and younger age in pediatric papillary thyroid carcinoma. Pediatr Blood Cancer. 2019;66(7):e27707.
37. Park G, Kim TH, Lee HO, Lim JA, Won JK, Min HS, et al. Standard immunohistochemistry efficiently screens for anaplastic lymphoma kinase rearrangements in differentiated thyroid cancer. Endocr Relat Cancer. 2015;22(1):55–63.
38. Cordioli MI, Moraes L, Cury AN, Cerutti JM. Are we really at the dawn of understanding sporadic pediatric thyroid carcinoma? Endocr Relat Cancer. 2015;22(6):R311–24.
39. Ballester LY, Sarabia SF, Sayeed H, Patel N, Baalwa J, Athanassaki I, et al. Integrating molecular testing in the diagnosis and management of children with thyroid lesions. Pediatr Dev Pathol. 2016;19(2):94–100.
40. Alzahrani AS, Murugan AK, Qasem E, Alswailem M, Al-Hindi H, Shi Y. Single point mutations in pediatric differentiated thyroid cancer. Thyroid. 2017;27(2):189–96.
41. Vali R, Rachmiel M, Hamilton J, El Zein M, Wasserman J, Costantini DL, et al. The role of ultrasound in the follow-up of children with differentiated thyroid cancer. Pediatr Radiol. 2015;45(7):1039–45.
42. Livhits MJ, Pasternak JD, Xiong M, Li N, Gosnell JE, Yeh MW, et al. Pre-ablation thyroglobulin and thyroglobulin to thyroid-stimulating hormone ratio may be associated with pulmonary metastases in children with differentiated thyroid cancer. Endocr Pract. 2016;22(11):1259–66.
43. Liu L, Huang F, Liu B, Huang R. Detection of distant metastasis at the time of ablation in children with differentiated thyroid cancer: the value of pre-ablation stimulated thyroglobulin. J Pediatr Endocrinol Metab. 2018;31(7):751–6.
44. Sabra MM, Grewal RK, Tala H, Larson SM, Tuttle RM. Clinical outcomes following empiric radioiodine therapy in patients with structurally identifiable metastatic follicular cell-derived thyroid carcinoma with negative diagnostic but positive post-therapy 131I whole-body scans. Thyroid. 2012;22(9):877–83.
45. Zhang XY, Song HJ, Qiu ZL, Shen CT, Chen XY, Sun ZK, et al. Pulmonary metastases in children and adolescents with papillary thyroid cancer in China: prognostic factors and outcomes from treatment with (131)I. Endocrine. 2018;62(1):149–58.
46. Verburg FA, Reiners C, Hanscheid H. Approach to the patient: role of dosimetric RAI Rx in children with DTC. J Clin Endocrinol Metab. 2013;98(10):3912–9.
47. Waguespack SG, Sherman SI, Williams MD, Clayman GL, Herzog CE. The successful use of sorafenib to treat pediatric papillary thyroid carcinoma. Thyroid. 2009;19(4):407–12.
48. Iyer P, Mayer JL, Ewig JM. Response to sorafenib in a pediatric patient with papillary thyroid carcinoma with diffuse nodular pulmonary disease requiring mechanical ventilation. Thyroid. 2014;24(1):169–74.

49. Mahajan P, Dawrant J, Kheradpour A, Quintanilla NM, Lopez ME, Orth RC, et al. Response to lenvatinib in children with papillary thyroid carcinoma. Thyroid. 2018;28(11):1450–4.
50. Laetsch TW, DuBois SG, Mascarenhas L, Turpin B, Federman N, Albert CM, et al. Larotrectinib for paediatric solid tumours harbouring NTRK gene fusions: phase 1 results from a multicentre, open-label, phase 1/2 study. Lancet Oncol. 2018;19:705–14.
51. Subbiah V, Cote GJ. Advances in targeting RET-dependent cancers. Cancer Discov. 2020;10:498–505.

Chapter 25
A Patient with Bone Metastases from Follicular Carcinoma of the Thyroid

Leonard Wartofsky

Case

The patient is a 55-year-old man referred to us from his endocrinologist in Morgantown, West Virginia. He had originally presented in West Virginia during August 2013 complaining of numbness in his right leg extending up to his abdomen. He was found to have tumor involving the thoracic spine on CT scan. Emergency surgery in late August 2013 included a corpectomy of the T8 vertebral body with decompression of T8-T11 with a laminectomy and debulking of the tumor. The surgical pathology of the spine tumor suggested thyroid cancer, and at that evaluation, he was noted to complain of hoarseness and have a neck mass. He underwent thyroidectomy in early September 2013, and the surgical pathology revealed his tumor to be a widely invasive follicular thyroid cancer. The right recurrent laryngeal nerve was sacrificed due to its being encased in tumor, and he remained hoarse postoperatively. A follow-up MRI of the thoracic spine in November 2013 disclosed probable metastasis to the first rib on the left, as well as tumor involving the right pedicle of T12 with additional metastases to L1, L3, L4, and L5. He underwent external radiation therapy for ten treatments (dosage unknown) in late November 2013. A CT scan of the head (without contrast) done in late November 2013 described a lytic lesion in the left anteroparietal calvarium. In addition, CT scan of the chest and abdomen with contrast in December 2013 described a lesion in the right lung, some hypodensities in the liver, and a 1.7 × 1.5 cm nodule in the adrenal gland. In the other facility, he was treated with 120 mCi radioactive iodine. His tumor was apparently producing sufficient thyroid hormone that his serum TSH level failed to elevate post thyroidectomy, and he was prepared for scanning and

L. Wartofsky (✉)
MedStar Health Research Institute,
MedStar Washington Hospital Center, Washington, DC, USA

Georgetown University School of Medicine, Washington, DC, USA
e-mail: leonard.wartofsky@medstar.net

G. Grani et al. (eds.), *Thyroid Cancer*,
https://doi.org/10.1007/978-3-030-61919-0_25

Table 25.1 Laboratory values

Date	TSH (mIU/L)	Tg (ng/ml)	*TgAb* (IU/ml)	Course
10/04/13	4.18	16,340	<2	Thyroidectomy 9/7/13
10/26/13	1.09	12,503	<2	IMRT to lumbar spine 11/13
12/22/13	0.36	9517	<2	120 mCi 131-I (12/23/13)
01/13/14	2.99	3303	<2	
02/23/14	3.72	1662	<20 (different assay)	
03/12/14	54	2840	<2	360 mCi 131-I (3/17/14)
06/02/14	1.92	142	<2	
08/22/14	0.09	64	<2	

TSH thyrotropin, *Tg* thyroglobulin, *TgAb* antithyroglobulin antibodies

radioiodine therapy with recombinant human TSH. The posttreatment scan disclosed foci of uptake in the head, neck, chest, shoulders, abdomen, and pelvis. Plain films of the lumbar spine in January 2014 again described metastasis at L4 and L5 and in his left rib. His physical examination was totally unremarkable except for the thyroidectomy scar and subjective numbness in the right lower extremity (Table 25.1).

Assessment

This 55-year-old man presented with widespread metastases to multiple bones, which were subsequently confirmed to be from a follicular carcinoma of the thyroid. According to his medical record notes, his serum thyroglobulin levels were quite high and fell after surgery and radioiodine ablation (Table 25.1) but remained markedly elevated. His post-therapy scan indicates fairly good radioiodine uptake suggesting potential benefit from additional radioactive iodine treatment. Our approach will be to do additional imaging to assess the current extent and location of residual disease in order to determine possible therapeutic approaches.

Relevant Literature

Features of follicular thyroid carcinoma distinct from papillary thyroid carcinoma have been reviewed recently [1, 2]. In general, distant metastases from differentiated thyroid cancer can be seen in 4–6% of patients at initial presentation [3, 4]. Distant metastatic disease can subsequently develop in 10–30% of patients [5, 6], depending on the histology (about 10% in papillary cancer and 20–30% in follicular and Hurthle cell cancers), most commonly to the lungs and bones. Distant metastases of follicular carcinoma are most commonly found in bone and lung but metastases to brain and liver may also occur. Bone metastases are more common with follicular than papillary thyroid carcinoma and are associated with poor prognosis [7]. The presence of distant metastases may be heralded by an extremely elevated serum thyroglobulin, with the findings confirmed by plain radiography, 131-I whole body scan, CT, MRI, PET/CT, or bone scan. Radioiodine uptake in a bone lesion will indicate that it is derived from thyroid cancer, but absent that, a bone biopsy is advisable to confirm the diagnosis. Other imaging modalities for bone lesions may include thallium-201, technetium-99 m, or iodine-124 PET [8]. Newer radiolabeled peptides such as ^{68}Ga-FAPI-04 and PSMA ligands have been proposed for diagnostic imaging in patients with lesions that are negative on both radioiodine scanning and ^{18}F-fluorodeoxyglucose (FDG)-PET imaging [9]. The more common bony sites for metastases are the spine, pelvis, ribs, femur, and skull. Clinically, patients will present with bone pain or fracture, swelling at the site, or spinal metastases with symptoms of cord compression. Bone metastases connote a significantly poorer prognosis than that noted in the majority of thyroid cancer patients. In a retrospective analysis by Shoup et al. [10] of 242 patients, 40% had metastases on presentation, and they had a 10-year survival of 26% with a median survival of 4.1 years. The importance of age is apparent as seen with a 10-year survival in those patients <45 years old of 58% compared to only 13% in those >45 years old. Survival with metastatic disease will also depend upon the site of the metastases, and whether or not the lesions are radioiodine avid. Radioiodine avidity does not necessarily imply radioiodine sensitivity, and bulky metastases are rarely cured by radioiodine [11]. Other factors influencing prognosis and which are statistically significant by univariate analysis include gender, extent of surgery, and histologic type [3, 5].

The treatment of bone metastases typically involves radioiodine, assuming that the lesions are RAI avid, and it is the younger patients who are more likely to have RAI uptake, a fact that likely is linked to their better survival statistics. This may account for why some studies show clear benefit of RAI therapy [12, 13], while others do not [14, 15]. Preparation for radioiodine therapy requires an elevated serum TSH level, which may be achieved by either thyroid hormone withdrawal or off-label administration of recombinant human TSH [16, 17]. Those lesions that are FDG/PET avid tend to be less differentiated and more resistant to RAI treatment [18, 19]. RAI may be administered either as a standard or "empiric" dose or activity based upon consensus guidelines and physician experience or as a "dosimetric" activity based on how the patient's body handles (retains and excretes) a given activity of radioiodine. When there is RAI uptake, arguments have been made for administering the highest dose feasible that is within safe limits as can be determined by dosimetry [20], and dosimetric approaches have been shown to be potentially more efficacious than empiric dosage [21]. However, relatively lower doses appear to be appropriate in older patients [22]. In the absence of RAI uptake, other therapeutic modalities may be tried but will be associated with less salutary effect. There is hope that redifferentiating agents such as selumetinib might prove useful for these patients in the future by resensitizing tumors to radioiodine [23, 24]. When feasible, particularly for isolated and/or symptomatic bone metastasis, other approaches to management could include surgical resection with or without cementoplasty, radiofrequency ablation, external radiation, arterial embolization, or targeted chemotherapy [25], along with adjunctive use of bisphosphonates [26]. Pak et al. [27] reviewed a 32-year experience with surgical metastasectomy with 51 metastases excised in 29 patients who had a variety of types of thyroid cancer. Many of the patients received adjunctive therapy with XRT and RAI as well with a resultant 78% survival at 5 years that dropped to 50% at 10 years, with age > 45, a poor prognostic factor. Wu et al. [28] in 77 patients followed long-term noted improved median survival with adjunctive external radiation and denosumab therapy.

External beam radiation is employed for pain relief and for lesions in critical or weight-bearing areas, as well as for those lesions not amenable to surgery or RAI treatment. It is typically given in doses of 50 Gy in 25 fractions for solitary bone lesions and 40 Gy in 20 fractions for vertebral lesions. Arterial embolization has been employed by Eustatia-Rutten and colleagues [29] with 41 embolizations in 16 patients resulting in clinical improvement in 60% of subjects. The procedure requires visualization of the artery feeding the metastasis by selective catheterization, and then particles of isobutyl, Gelfoam, or polyvinyl alcohol are injected with relief of pain and improvement in neurologic symptoms. The best results are seen in those patients who also have had RAI, XRT, or surgical treatment. Radiofrequency ablation (RFA) [30, 31] uses probes inserted under CT guidance to generate thermal energy to achieve local tissue temperatures >50 °C inducing cell death. RFA has rarely been applied to bone lesions and has found greater application to lesions in the liver or kidney. While planar radioiodine scanning with iodine-131 is the primary imaging procedure for differentiated thyroid cancer, scanning with iodine-124 PET offers advantages of detecting both positron emission, as well as the spatial distribution of radioiodine uptake, and allows improved detection of the extent of residual disease [32–36].

Subsequent Management

The degree of thyroglobulin elevation indicated persistent residual disease. Given that his earlier post-therapy radioiodine scan showed significant uptake and the actual activity administered (120 mCi) was relatively low, the patient was deemed a good candidate for higher-dose radioiodine therapy to be determined by dosimetry [20]. He was withdrawn from his levothyroxine therapy, and after 3 weeks, his serum TSH level had risen to 42 mU/L. He then underwent routine total body scanning with iodine-131 (Fig. 25.1), as well as iodine-124 PET scanning, which again clearly delineated good isotope uptake, with particularly better visualization of the extent of bone metastases by the iodine-124 PET images (Fig. 25.2). Regional lesional dosimetry afforded by iodine-124 indicated that sufficient uptake of activity in specific lesions could be achieved for therapeutic benefit based on earlier data on locoregional dosimetry [34, 37]. The dosimetry calculations predicted that he could receive as much as 410 mCi of iodine-131 safely and have less than 100 mCi retained in total body at 48 h. He was treated with 360 mCi iodine-131 in late March 2014 at a time that his TSH measured 54 mU/L; the post-therapy scan was

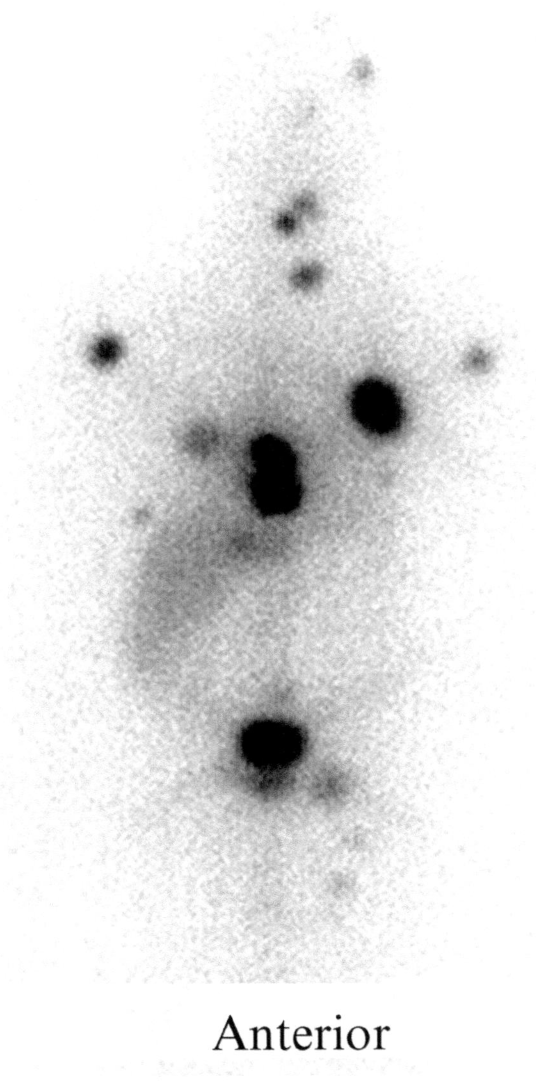

Fig. 25.1 Post-thyroid hormone withdrawal total body scan after 4 mCi iodine-131

essentially identical to the pretreatment diagnostic scan demonstrating good uptake in multiple sites estimated to approximate 72 Gy or 7200 rads. Follow-up studies by his physicians in West Virginia on June 2, 2014, included a serum thyroglobulin of 142 ng/ml and a TSH of 1.92 mU/L. His dose of levothyroxine was increased, and the last studies recorded to date on August 22, 2014, included a thyroglobulin of 64 ng/ml and a TSH of 0.09 mU/L. His total white blood cell, absolute neutrophil, and platelet counts have remained within normal limits. Recommendations to his physicians included continuing suppressive dosage of levothyroxine, adjunctive therapy with bisphosphonates or denosumab, monitoring serum thyroglobulin every

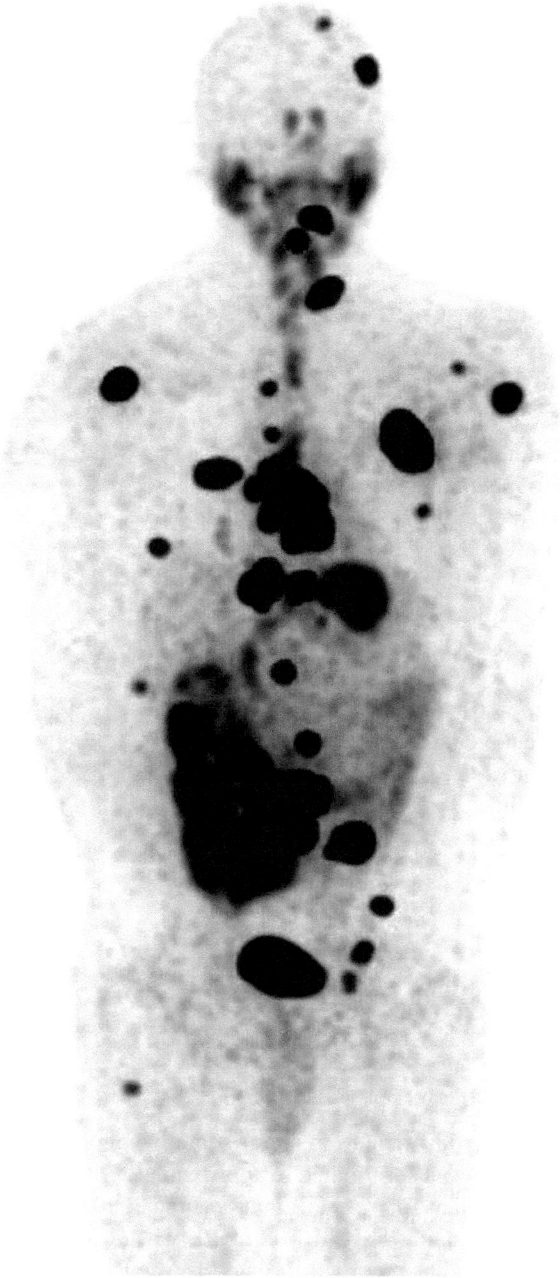

Fig. 25.2 Total body iodine-124 PET/CT scan with 1.7 mCi iodine-124

6 months, considering local intervention on selective lesions by XRT or RFA as warranted, and a potential additional dosimetric radioiodine dose based upon demonstrated progressive disease, persistent iodine uptake, and relatively normal blood counts.

Clinical Pearls/Pitfalls

1. Lesions positive on FDG/PET scanning are likely to represent poorly differentiated thyroid cancer, not demonstrate radioiodine uptake, and have a poor prognosis.
2. Follicular thyroid carcinoma metastatic to bone heralds a poor prognosis for cure, especially in older patients with extensive disease that does not take up radioiodine.
3. While several therapeutic approaches to bone metastases exist, the best opportunity for palliative stabilization of progression or remission rests with a combination of surgical resection when feasible, radioactive iodine and external radiation therapy. Radioiodine uptake by lesions does not necessarily indicate radiosensitivity.
4. Although the current ATA Guidelines [38] indicate that no recommendation can be made about the superiority of dosimetric RAI administration over empiric dosage, they do acknowledge that there are theoretical advantages to dosimetric approaches to the treatment of both locoregional and metastatic diseases.
5. While currently available only in major academic centers, iodine-124 PET/CT scans are superior to either traditional iodine-131 scans or FDG/PET scans for more definitive imaging of metastases from thyroid cancer.
6. High-dosage radioiodine therapy by dosimetry can be administered safely and has proven effective in at least one study.

Acknowledgments Grant support from the Catherine Heron and Al Schneider Thyroid Cancer Fellowship Fund.

References

1. Daniels GH. Follicular thyroid carcinoma: a perspective. Thyroid. 2018;28:1229–42.
2. Grani G, Lamartina L, Durante C, Filetti S, Cooper DS. Follicular thyroid cancer and Hurthle cell carcinoma: challenges in diagnosis, treatment, and clinical management. Lancet Diabetes Endocrinol. 2018;6:500–14.
3. Verburg FA, Mader U, Tanase K, Thies E-D, Diessl S, Buck AK, Luster M, Reiners C. Life expectancy is reduced in differentiated thyroid cancer patients>45 years old with extensive local tumor invasion, lateral lymph node, or distant metastases at diagnosis and normal in all other DTC patients. J Clin Endocrinol Metab. 2013;98:172–80.
4. Klubo-Gwiezdzinska J, Morowitz D, Van Nostrand D, Burman KD, Vasko V, Soberman M, Wartofsky L. Metastases of well-differentiated thyroid cancer to the gastrointestinal system. Thyroid. 2010;20:381–7.

5. Schlumberger MJ. Papillary and follicular thyroid carcinoma. N Engl J Med. 1998;338:297–306.
6. Shaha AR, Ferlito A, Rinaldo A. Distant metastases from thyroid and parathyroid cancer. ORL J Otorhinolaryngol Relat Spec. 2001;63:243–9.
7. Choksi P, Papaleontiou M, Guo C, Worden F, Banerjee M, Haymart M. Skeletal complications and mortality in thyroid cancer: a population-based study. J Clin Endocrinol Metab. 2017;102:1254–60.
8. Jentzen W, Verschure F, van Zon A, van de Kolk R, Wierts R, Schmitz J, Bockisch A, Binse I. 124-I PET assessment of response of bone metastases to initial radioiodine treatment of differentiated thyroid cancer. J Nucl Med. 2016;57:1499–504.
9. Kratochwill C, Flechsig P, Lindner T, Abderrahim L, Altmann A, Mier W, et al. ^{68}Ga-FAPI PET/CT tracer uptake in 28 different kinds of cancer. J Nucl Med. 2019;60:801–5.
10. Shoup M, Stojadinovic A, Nissan A, Ghossein RA, Freedman S, Brennan MF, et al. Prognostic indicators of outcomes in patients with distant metastases from differentiated thyroid carcinoma. J Am Coll Surg. 2003;197(2):191–7.
11. Sabra MM, Dominguez JM, Grewal RK, Larson SM, Ghossein RA, Tuttle RM, Fagin JA. Clinical outcomes and molecular profile of differentiated thyroid cancers with radioiodine-avid distant metastases. J Clin Endocrinol Metab. 2013;98:E829–36.
12. Hindie E, Melliere D, Lange F, Hallaj I, de Labriolle-Vaylet C, Jeanguillaume C, et al. Functioning pulmonary metastases of thyroid cancer: does radioiodine influence the prognosis? Eur J Nucl Med Mol Imaging. 2003;30(7):974–81.
13. Bernier MO, Leenhardt L, Hoang C, Aurengo A, Mary JY, Menegaux F, et al. Survival and therapeutic modalities in patients with bone metastases of differentiated thyroid carcinomas. J Clin Endocrinol Metab. 2001;86(4):1568–73.
14. Dinneen SF, Valimaki MJ, Bergstralh EJ, Goellner JR, Gorman CA, Hay ID. Distant metastases in papillary thyroid carcinoma: 100 cases observed at one institution during 5 decades. J Clin Endocrinol Metab. 1995;80(7):2041–5.
15. Pittas AG, Adler M, Fazzari M, Tickoo S, Rosai J, Larson SM, Robbins RJ. Bone metastases from thyroid carcinoma: clinical characteristics and prognostic variables in one hundred forty-six patients. Thyroid. 2000;10(3):261–8.
16. Van Nostrand D, Khorjekar G, O'Neil J, Moreau S, Atkins F, Kharazi P, Mete M, Chennupati S, Burman KD, Wartofsky L. Recombinant human thyroid stimulating hormone versus thyroid hormone withdrawal in the identification of metastasis in differentiated thyroid cancer with 131I planar whole body and 124I PET. J Nucl Med. 2012;53:359–62.
17. Klubo-Gwiezdzinska J, Burman KD, Van Nostrand D, Mete M, Jonklaas J, Wartofsky L. Radioiodine treatment of metastatic thyroid cancer: relative efficacy and side effect profile after preparation by thyroid hormone withdrawal vs. recombinant human TSH. Thyroid. 2012;22:310–7.
18. Wang W, Larson SM, Tuttle RM, Kalaigian H, Kolbert K, Sonenberg M, Robbins RJ. Resistance of [18f]-fluorodeoxyglucose-avid metastatic thyroid cancer lesions to treatment with high-dose radioactive iodine. Thyroid. 2001;11(12):1169–75.
19. Robbins RJ, Wan Q, Grewal RK, Reibke R, Gonen M, Strauss HW, Tuttle RM, Drucker W, Larson SM. Real-time prognosis for metastatic thyroid carcinoma based on 2-[18F]fluoro-2-deoxy-D-glucose-positron emission tomography scanning. J Clin Endocrinol Metab. 2006;91:498–505.
20. Van Nostrand D, Atkins F, Yeganeh F, Acio E, Bursaw R, Wartofsky L. Dosimetrically-determined doses of radioiodine for the treatment of metastatic thyroid carcinoma. Thyroid. 2002;12(2):121–34.
21. Klubo-Gwiezdzinska J, Van Nostrand D, Atkins FB, Burman KD, Jonklaas J, Mete M, Wartofsky L. Efficacy of dosimetric versus empirically determined prescribed activity of 131-I for therapy of differentiated thyroid Cancer. J Clin Endocrinol Metab. 2011;96:3217–25.
22. Kulkarni K, Van Nostrand D, Atkins F, Aiken M, Burman K, Wartofsky L. The relative frequency in which empiric dosages of radioiodine would potentially "over-" or "under-" treat patients who have metastatic well-differentiated thyroid cancer. Thyroid. 2006;16:1019–51.

23. Ho AL, Grewal RK, Leboeuf R, Sherman EJ, Pfister DG, Deandreis D, et al. Selumetinib-enhanced radioiodine uptake in advanced thyroid cancer. N Engl J Med. 2013;368(7):623–32.
24. Jaber T, Waguespeack SG, Cabanillas ME, Elbanan M, Vu T, Dadu R, et al. Targeted therapy in advanced thyroid cancer to resensitize tumors to radioactive iodine. J Clin Endocrinol Metab. 2018;103:3698–705.
25. Chen H, Luthra R, Routbort MJ, Patel KP, Cabanillas ME, Broaddus RR, Williams MD. Molecular profile of advanced thyroidcarcinomas by next-generation sequencing: characterizing tumors beyond diagnosis for targeted therapy. Mol Cancer Ther. 2018;17:1575–84.
26. Vitale G, Fonderico F, Martignetti A, Caraglia M, Ciccarelli A, Nuzzo V, et al. Pamidronate improves the quality of life and induces clinical remission of bone metastases in patients with thyroid cancer. Br J Cancer. 2001;84(12):1586–90.
27. Pak H, Gourgiotis L, Chang WI, Guthrie LC, Skarulis MC, et al. Role of metastasectomy in the management of thyroid carcinoma: the NIH experience. J Surg Oncol. 2003;82(1):10–8.
28. Wu D, Lima CJG, Moreau SL, Kulkarni K, Zeymo A, Burman KD, et al. Improved survival after multimodal approach with 131-I treatment in patients with bone metastases secondary to differentiated thyroid cancer. Thyroid. 2019;29:971–8.
29. Eustatia-Rutten CF, Romijn JA, Guijt MJ, Vielvoye GJ, van den Berg R, Corssmit EP, et al. Outcome of palliative embolization of bone metastases in differentiated thyroid carcinoma. J Clin Endocrinol Metab. 2003;88(7):3184–9.
30. Dupuy DE, Monchik JM, Decrea C, Pisharodi L. Radiofrequency ablation of regional recurrence from well-differentiated thyroid malignancy. Surgery. 2001;130:971–7.
31. Wartofsky L. Adjunctive local approaches to metastatic thyroid cancer. In: Wartofsky L, Van Nostrand D, editors. Thyroid cancer: a comprehensive guide to clinical management. 3rd Edition, Springer, 2016, pp. 745–50.
32. Eschmann SM, Reischl G, Bilger K, Kuperferschlager J, Thelen MH, Dohmen BM, Bares R. Evaluation of dosimetry of radioiodine therapy in benign and malignant thyroid disorders by means of iodine-124 and PET. Eur J Nucl Med Mol Imaging. 2002;29:760–7.
33. Van Nostrand D, Moreau S, Bandaru VV, Atkins F, Chennupati S, et al. (124)I positron emission tomography versus (131)I planar imaging in the identification of residual thyroid tissue and/or metastasis in patients who have well-differentiated thyroid cancer. Thyroid. 2010;20:879–83.
34. Sgouros G, Kolbert KS, Sheikh A, Pentlow KS, Mun EF, Barth A, et al. Patient-specific dosimetry for 131-I thyroid cancer therapy using 124-I PET and 3-dimensional-internal dosimetry (3D-ID) software. J Nucl Med. 2004;45:1366–72.
35. Phan HT, Jager PL, Paans AM, Plukker JT, Sturkenboom MG, Sluiter WJ, Wolffenbuttel BH, Dierckx RA, Links TP. The diagnostic value of 124I-PET in patients with differentiated thyroid cancer. Eur J Nucl Med Mol Imaging. 2008;35:958–65.
36. Maxon HR, Thomas SR, Samaratunga RC. Dosimetric considerations in the radioiodine treatment of macrometastases and micrometastases from differentiated thyroid cancer. Thyroid. 1997;7(2):183–7.
37. Hobbs RF, Wahl RL, Lodge MA, Javadi MS, Cho SY, Chien DT, et al. 124-I PET-based 3D-RD dosimetry for a pediatric thyroid cancer patient: real=time treatment planning and methodologic comparison. J Nucl Med. 2009;50:1844–7.
38. Haugen BR, Alexander EK, Bible KC, Doherty GM, Mandel SJ, Nikiforov Y, et al. American Thyroid Association Management guidelines for patients with thyroid nodules and differentiated thyroid cancer. Thyroid. 2016;26:1–133.

Chapter 26
Radioiodine Therapy in Lactating Women with Higher-Risk Differentiated Thyroid Cancer

Swaytha Yalamanchi and David S. Cooper

Case Presentation

A 30-year-old woman presents 1 month status post total thyroidectomy with left and central neck dissection for management of papillary thyroid carcinoma (PTC). Pathology demonstrated multifocal and BRAF-positive PTC with the largest tumor focus being 6 cm in diameter. A total of 6 of the 14 central lymph nodes and 7 of 33 lateral lymph nodes were positive for disease. The patient gave birth approximately 5 months earlier and stopped breastfeeding 2 weeks prior to presenting to endocrinology clinic.

Assessment and Literature Review

Both lactating and non-lactating women may have breast uptake on scintigraphy. In the former group, uptake may persist up to 32 weeks following cessation of lactation. Dopamine agonists may shorten the time interval between cessation of breastfeeding and initiation of radioiodine therapy in patients with differentiated thyroid cancer. Regardless of the use of dopamine agonist therapy, it is imperative to perform a pre-treatment I-123 scan in women with recent lactation or galactorrhea to confirm that breast uptake is absent prior to proceeding with I-131 radioiodine therapy.

S. Yalamanchi
Division of Endocrinology, Diabetes, and Metabolism, Palo Alto Medical Foundation, Palo Alto, CA, USA

D. S. Cooper (✉)
Division of Endocrinology, Diabetes, and Metabolism, The Johns Hopkins University School of Medicine, Baltimore, MD, USA
e-mail: dscooper@jhmi.edu

G. Grani et al. (eds.), *Thyroid Cancer*,
https://doi.org/10.1007/978-3-030-61919-0_26

Definitions/Background

The incidence of thyroid cancer has increased more rapidly than other malignancies in recent years, independent of age and ethnicity. From 1974 to 2013, the incidence of thyroid cancer increased by 3% annually. This growth is likely partly due to a rise in subclinical disease detected on imaging studies performed for alternate reasons, though the incidence of large tumors, including those >4 cm, has also increased; the incidence rate and mortality of advanced stage papillary thyroid cancer have additionally increased [1–3]. While uncommon in pregnancy or the postpartum period, thyroid cancer is the second most common cancer among pregnant women after breast cancer, with an incidence of approximately 25 per 100,000 pregnant or postpartum women [4]. Surgery is the primary therapy for papillary thyroid cancer, with the approach dictated by the extent of disease, age, and comorbidities.

Radioiodine Ablation

Postoperative radioactive iodine (RAI) ablation therapy is used in specific cases to achieve the following interrelated goals: remnant ablation to facilitate initial staging and subsequent detection of recurrent disease via serum thyroglobulin and I-131 scan, adjuvant therapy to decrease the risk of recurrence and mortality by eliminating suspected disease, and documentation and treatment of known persistent disease [5]. Guidelines from the American Thyroid Association (ATA) recommend RAI therapy in all patients with known distant metastases, gross extrathyroidal extension, or primary tumor size greater than 4 cm. RAI is also recommended for selected patients with a thyroid cancer focus 1–4 cm in size without extrathyroidal extension if lymph node metastases and/or other high-risk features (e.g., age greater than 55, certain histological subtypes, intrathyroidal vascular invasion, multifocal disease) exist that would place individuals into the category of intermediate to high risk of recurrence or death [5].

Relative and Absolute Contraindications to RAI Therapy

Both relative and absolute contraindications to radioiodine therapy exist. Radioiodine is concentrated in thyroid follicular cells via the membrane sodium-iodide symporter (NIS) [6]. Pregnancy is an absolute contraindication to therapeutic I-131 administration due to risk of fetal exposure. Thyroid fetal tissue, which begins to form at 10–12 weeks, may be destroyed, potentially resulting in cretinism [7]. Potential adverse effects associated with radioiodine vary depending on gestational age and administered activity, but may include risk of miscarriage, growth retardation, fetal hypothyroidism, fetal malformation, and effects on fetal IQ as noted above [8]. In a series of 237 women, 55 of whom ultimately underwent a therapeutic abortion, six infants developed hypothyroidism, with four having intellectual disabilities. Three of these six women received radioiodine in the second trimester. The rates of fetal and neonatal complications were otherwise similar to that of uncomplicated pregnancies [9].

Women either who are actively breastfeeding or who have recently stopped breastfeeding should not receive radioiodine therapy because of risks of exposure to I-131 to the child, and risk of breast tissue exposure to radiation secondary to high levels of NIS expression in breast tissue during lactation [7].

Women may have breast uptake on pretreatment scintigraphy for a multitude of other reasons besides lactation, including hyperprolactinemia from any cause [10, 11], breast cancer/tumor (including but not limited to breast cysts and current/previously excised fibroadenoma) [12–15], and mastitis [16] (Fig. 26.1). False-positive breast uptake may also occur due to contamination or uptake in the ribs, lung, liver, and soft tissue.

Prevalence

A retrospective study performed from 2000 to 2006 to examine the utility of radioiodine scans prior to RAI therapy in patients with DTC showed that 6% of non-lactating women had evidence of breast uptake on pretreatment scans [17]. Similarly, Hammami et al. demonstrated that approximately 6% of all nonpregnant and non-lactating women (23 had not breastfed for an average of 11.4 months; 4 were nulliparous; 3 were postmenopausal) with iatrogenic hypothyroidism following thyroid hormone withdrawal also had breast uptake on radioiodine scans. The authors noted four different patterns of radioiodine breast uptake: "full," "focal," "crescentic," and "irregular." No association, however, could be made between scintigraphy patterns and etiology of breast uptake. The majority of women did not have expressible galactorrhea (52%) and were normoprolactinemic (76%; the remainder had prolactin levels <2.5 times the upper limit of normal, likely due to iatrogenic hypothyroidism) [18].

Pathophysiology

Iodide is an essential component of thyroid hormones tri-iodothyronine (T3) and thyroxine (T4). Intracellular iodide stores are maintained by NIS, located on the basolateral plasma membrane of thyroid follicular cells. NIS expression facilitates the use of radioiodine for both diagnostic and therapeutic purposes in the management of thyroid cancer. Active iodide transport also occurs in extrathyroidal tissues,

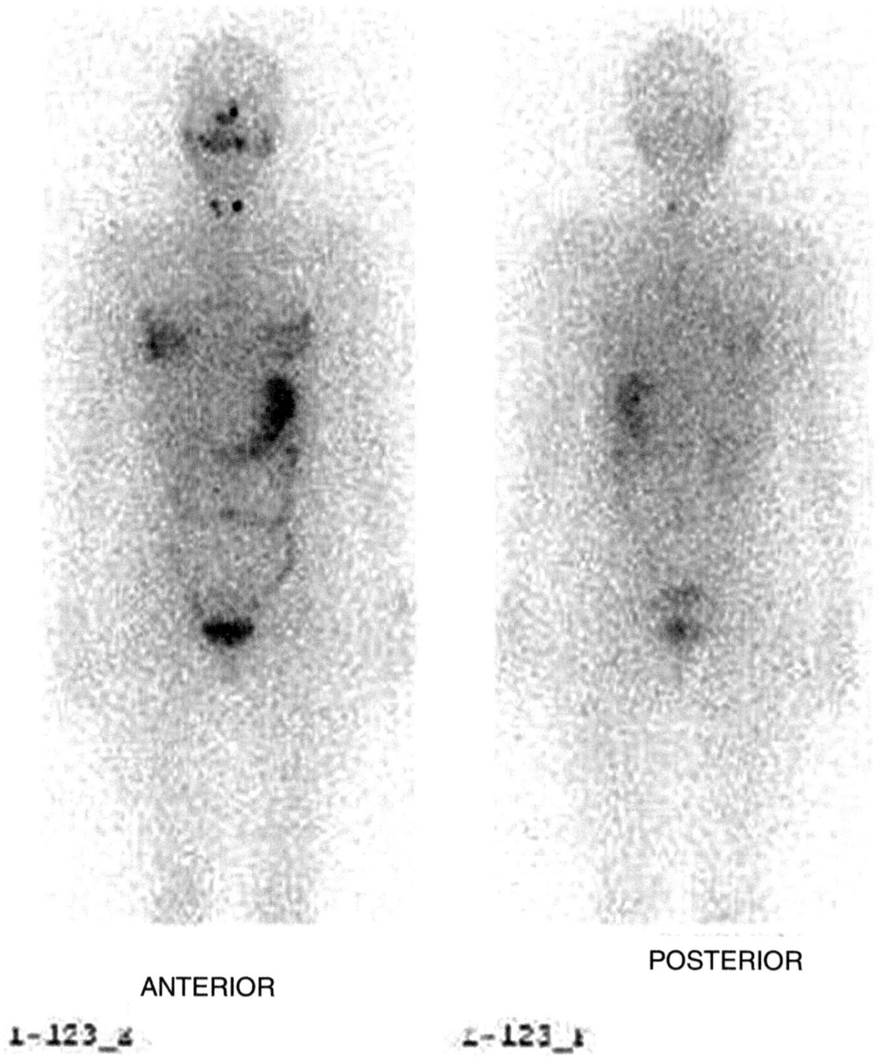

Fig. 26.1 Pretreatment I-123 scan in a patient with low-risk papillary thyroid cancer, idiopathic hyperprolactinemia, and mild galactorrhea demonstrating bilateral breast uptake. The decision was made not to treat this patient with radioiodine based on the scan

including the lactating breasts, salivary glands, small intestine, and stomach [6]. In lactating breast tissue, expression of NIS allows iodide to be concentrated and secreted into breast milk for neonatal nutrition. NIS is generally present in breast tissue only during gestation and lactation. This is likely due in part to a threshold level of estrogen necessary for both direct effects on mammary gland NIS transcription, as well as effects via oxytocin and prolactin [19]. Expression of NIS has also been found to be high in fibroadenomas and, to a lesser extent, malignant breast tissue [12]. NIS expression in breast and ovarian cancers, which would allow for radioiodine for diagnostic and therapeutic purposes, is being explored [20–23].

Role of Prolactin

Hyperprolactinemia, even in the postmenopausal woman with baseline atrophic breast tissue, may also result in increased breast uptake on scintigraphy that is reversible with normalization of prolactin levels [10, 24]. Both animal models and cultured human breast cancer cells respond to prolactin stimulation with increased expression of NIS and thus radioiodine uptake [10].

Medical Therapy

False-positive breast uptake should first be ruled out by taking a focused history with consideration of lateral radiographic views and SPECT imaging. Subsequently, if the decision is made to proceed with radioiodine therapy, breastfeeding should be discontinued, and/or offending agents resulting in hyperprolactinemia should be stopped if medically feasible. Current guidelines recommend discontinuation of drugs causing hyperprolactinemia at least 6 weeks and, ideally, 3 months prior to administration of radioiodine, to allow for NIS transporter activity to return to baseline; a pretreatment 123-I scan is recommended if more urgent treatment is needed or if there is concern regarding residual breast uptake [7].

Little data exist regarding therapeutic options. Hsiao et al. published a case report of a single postpartum woman treated with bromocriptine with subsequent minimal breast uptake on scintigraphy 8 weeks after cessation of breastfeeding [25]. Brzozowska et al. reported an observational case series of eight postpartum women who were followed by I-123 scintigraphy; five women received dopamine agonist therapy (cabergoline or bromocriptine), and three women received no therapy. The duration of ongoing breast uptake on scintigraphy was quite variable, but lasted up to 32 weeks in women who did not receive dopamine agonist therapy. In contrast, women who received dopamine agonist therapy had negative uptake studies sooner (3–10 weeks in four of the five women in the treatment group) [26]. Although data are limited in this clinical setting, cabergoline is generally regarded to be more efficacious in normalizing prolactin levels compared to bromocriptine [27]. Thus, patients may be initiated on cabergoline 0.25 mg twice/week (titrated up to 1 mg twice/week) or bromocriptine 7.5 mg twice/day based on existing data. Although dopamine agonists may shorten the time interval between cessation of breastfeeding and radioiodine therapy, it is unlikely that a delay in the administration of I-131 will change the thyroid cancer-related outcome of the patient. Diagnostic scintigraphy with an I-123 scan should be performed prior to administration of therapeutic I-131 to confirm absence of breast uptake [17, 26].

Management of the Case

Our patient qualifies for RAI therapy on the basis of her bulky primary tumor focus and metastatic disease. As she had stopped breastfeeding only 2 weeks prior to her visit, she was initiated on cabergoline 0.5 mg twice/week. Six weeks later, she underwent a pretreatment scan with I-123 that showed no evidence of breast uptake. The patient was treated with 75 mCi of radioiodine and had a posttreatment scan showing only two foci of uptake in the thyroid bed. She has done well subsequently without clinical, sonographic, or biochemical evidence of recurrent disease, including a negative total body scan and an undetectable serum thyroglobulin after recombinant TSH 9 months later.

Clinical Pearls/Pitfalls

- Breast uptake on I-123 scintigraphy is possible in the setting of recent cessation of breastfeeding or in non-lactating women with hyperprolactinemia, breast cancer/tumor, or mastitis.
- Breast uptake of radioiodine is likely mediated by hormonal control of mammary gland NIS with interplay between estrogen, oxytocin, and prolactin.
- The 2015 ATA guidelines recommend deferring RAI for at least 6–8 weeks after women have stopped breastfeeding [3]. The ATA guidelines on Radiation Safety after RAI recommend waiting 3 months after cessation of lactation before administration of therapeutic RAI, with a 123-I pretreatment scan if treatment is urgent or if there is concern regarding residual breast uptake [5]. However, breast uptake has been reported to persist for up to 8 months after cessation of lactation. In contrast with both of the aforementioned guidelines, we thus recommend a pretreatment scan prior to radioiodine administration in all women with a history of recent lactation (within 6 months), galactorrhea, breast cancer/tumor, and mastitis.
- Dopamine agonist therapy may shorten the time interval between cessation of breastfeeding and the ability to safely administer radioiodine therapy.

References

1. SEER Cancer Statistics Review, 1975–2011. National Cancer Institute. Bethesda, MD. Based on November 2013 SEER data submission, released, April 2014. http://Seer.cancer.gov/csr/1975_2011/
2. Pellegriti G, Frasca F, Regalbuto C, Squatrito S, Vigneri R. Worldwide increasing incidence of thyroid cancer: update on epidemiology and risk factors. J Cancer Epidemiol. 2013;965212
3. Lim H, Devesa SS, Sosa JA, Check D, Kitahara CM. Trends in thyroid cancer incidence and mortality in the United States, 1974–2013. JAMA. 2017;317(13):1338–48.

4. Cottreau CM, Dashevsky I, Andrade SE, Li DK, Nekhlyudov L, Raebel MA, Ritzwoller DP, Partridge AH, Pawloski PA, Toh S. Pregnancy-Associated Cancer: a U.S. population-based study. J Womens Health (Larchmt). 2019;28(2):250–7.
5. Haugen BR, Alexander EK, Bible KC, Doherty GM, Mandel SJ, Nikiforov YE, Pacini F, Randolph GW, Sawka AM, Schlumberger M, Schuff KG, Sherman SI, Sosa JA, Steward DL, Tuttle RM, Wartofsky L. 2015 American Thyroid Association management guidelines for adult patients with thyroid nodules and differentiated thyroid cancer. Thyroid. 2016;26(1):1–133.
6. Portulano C, Paroder-Belenitsky M, Carrasco N. The Na+/I- symporter (NIS): mechanism and medical impact. Endocr Rev. 2014;35(1):106–49.
7. American Thyroid Association Taskforce on Radioiodine Safety, Sisson JC, Freitas J, et al. Radiation safety in the treatment of patients with thyroid diseases by radioiodine 131-I: practice recommendations of the American Thyroid Association. Thyroid. 2011;21(4):335–46.
8. Hyer S, Pratt B, Newbold K, Hamer K. Outcome of pregnancy after exposure to radioiodine in utero. Endocr Pract. 2011;17:1–10.
9. Stoffer SS, Hamburger JI. Inadvertent 131I therapy for hyperthyroidism in the first trimester of pregnancy. J Nucl Med. 1976;17(02):146–9.
10. Ronga G, Bruno R, Puxeddu E, et al. Radioiodine uptake in non-lactating mammary glands: evidence for a causative role of hyperprolactinemia. Thyroid. 2007;17(4):363–6.
11. Hu LH, Wang SJ, Liu RS. Hyperprolactinemia-related 131-I uptake in nonlactating breasts. Clin Nucl Med. 2012;37(3):e57–8.
12. Ryan J, Curran CE, Hennessy E, et al. The sodium iodide symporter (NIS) and potential regulators in normal, benign and malignant human breast tissue. PLoS One. 2011;6(1):e16023.
13. Serafini A, Sfakianakis G, Georgiou M, Morris J. Breast cyst simulating metastases on iodine-131 imaging in thyroid carcinoma. J Nucl Med. 1998;39(11):1910–2.
14. Ranade R, Pawar S, Mahajan A, Basu S. Unusual false positive radioiodine uptake on (131) I whole body scintigraphy in three unrelated organs with different pathologies in patients of differential thyroid carcinoma: a case series. World J Nucl Med. 2016;15(2):137–41.
15. Kim MH, Kim HS, Park SA. Extrathyroidal accumulation in a fibroadenoma of the breast. Clin Nucl Med. 2017;42(2):e123–5.
16. Bakheet SM, Hammami MM. Patterns of radioiodine uptake by the lactating breast. Eur J Nucl Med. 1994;21(7):604–8.
17. Van Nostrand D, Aiken M, Atkins F, et al. The utility of radioiodine scans prior to iodine 131 ablation in patients with well-differentiated thyroid cancer. Thyroid. 2009;19(8):849–55.
18. Hammami MM, Bakheet S. Radioiodine breast uptake in nonbreastfeeding women: clinical and scintigraphic characteristics. J Nucl Med. 1996;37(1):26–31.
19. Tazebay UH, Wapnir IL, Levy O, et al. The mammary gland iodide transporter is expressed during lactation and in breast cancer. Nat Med. 2000;6(8):871–8.
20. Angelousi A, Nonni A, Kassi E, Kontzoglou K. Expression of sodium iodide symporter in human breast tissues. J BUON. 2016;21(1):53–60.
21. Yao C, Pan Y, Li Y, Xu X, Lin Y, Wang W, Wang S. Effect of sodium/iodide symporter (NIS)-mediated radioiodine therapy on estrogen-receptor negative breast cancer. Oncol Rep. 2015;34(1):59–66.
22. Riesco-Eizaguirre G, Leoni SG, Mendiola M, Estevez-Cebrero MA, Gallego MI, Redondo A, Hardisson D, Santisteban P, De la Vieja A. NIS mediates iodide uptake in the female reproductive tract and is a poor prognostic factor in ovarian cancer. J Clin Endocrinol Metab. 2014;99(7):E1199–208.
23. Micali S, Bulotta S, Puppin C, Territo A, Navarra M, Bianchi G, Damante G, Filetti S, Russo D. Sodium iodine symporter (NIS) in extrathyroidal malignancies: focus on breast and urological cancer. BMC Cancer. 2014;30(14):303.
24. Sinha A, Bradley KM, Steatham J, Weaver A. Asymmetric breast uptake of radioiodine in a patient with thyroid malignancy: metastases or not? J R Soc Med. 2008;101(6):319–20.

25. Hsiao E, Huynh T, Mansberg R, Bautovich G, Roach P. Diagnostic I-123 scintigraphy to assess potential breast uptake of I-131 before radioiodine therapy in a postpartum woman with thyroid cancer. Clin Nucl Med. 2004;29(8):498–501.
26. Brzozowska M, Roach PJ. Timing and potential role of diagnostic I-123 scintigraphy in assessing radioiodine breast uptake before ablation in postpartum women with thyroid cancer: a case series. Clin Nucl Med. 2006;31(11):683–7.
27. Wang AT, Mullan RJ, Lane MA, et al. Treatment of hyperprolactinemia: a systematic review and meta-analysis. Syst Rev. 2012;1:33.

Part V
Differentiated Thyroid Cancer: Beyond Radioactive Iodine Therapy

Chapter 27
A Case of a Patient with RAI-Refractory Differentiated Thyroid Cancer with Progressive Neck Disease and Stable Lung Metastases

Dana M. Hartl, Joanne Guerlain, and Ingrid Breuskin

Case Presentation

A 69-year-old male patient was referred to our department for management of neck recurrence from papillary thyroid carcinoma.

Comorbidities included type II diabetes, hypertension, asymptomatic stenosis of one femoral artery, tobacco consumption (50 pack-years), and stable low-grade idiopathic sideroblastic anemia.

Ten years earlier, the patient had undergone total thyroidectomy and therapeutic central and right lateral neck dissection, at an outside institution, followed by two therapeutic doses of RAI after thyroid hormone withdrawal for a 3 cm, pT3N1b papillary thyroid carcinoma. No ectopic uptake was noted on the whole-body scans performed post-iodine. Three years later, an increase in serum thyroglobulin (Tg) led to the discovery on chest CT of two small (<10 mm) lung metastases. A third therapeutic dose of RAI was delivered, but no uptake was seen in the metastases, which remained stable over serial CTs. Three years after this treatment, neck ultrasound revealed a metastatic node in neck level III on the right. A reoperative right lateral neck dissection was performed, revealing 13 metastatic nodes out of 20 resected. A fourth administration of RAI followed surgery, with no uptake on single-photon emission computed tomography (SPECT) whole body scan. Tg after thyroid hormone withdrawal remained elevated at 37 ng/ml, however. Over the next 4 years, thyroxine-suppressed Tg increased from 2 to 18 ng/ml. Ultrasound with fine-needle aspiration cytology (FNAC) revealed three previously non-identified lymph node metastases in neck levels II and VIB on the right side, measuring 15–20 mm each.

D. M. Hartl (✉) · J. Guerlain · I. Breuskin
Department of Head and Neck Oncology, Thyroid Surgery Unit, Gustave Roussy and Paris-Sud University, Villejuif, France
e-mail: dana.hartl@gustaveroussy.fr

G. Grani et al. (eds.), *Thyroid Cancer*,
https://doi.org/10.1007/978-3-030-61919-0_27

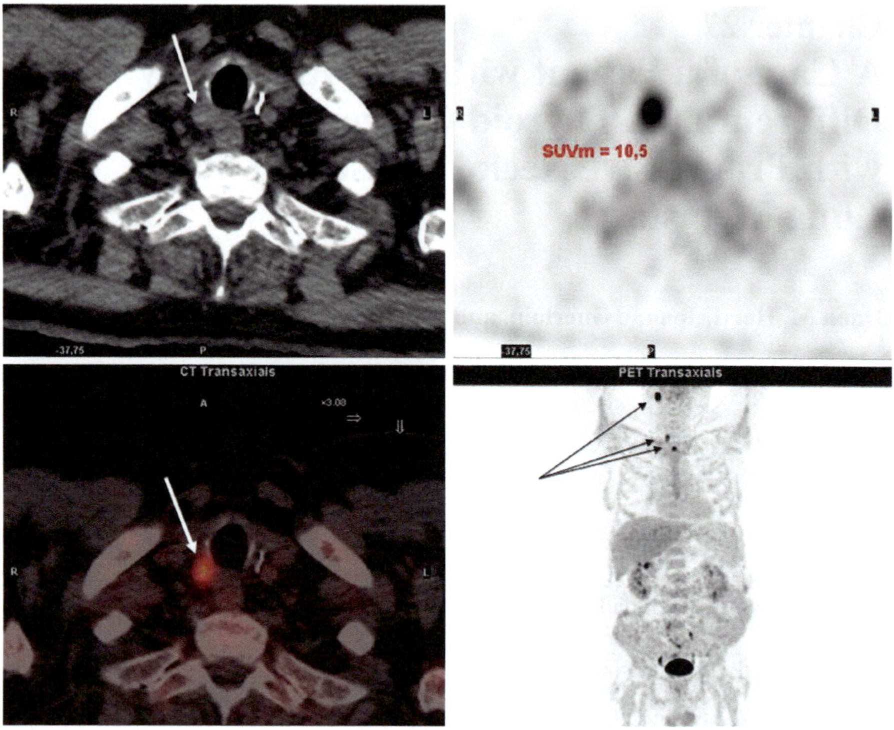

Fig. 27.1 Upper left: non-contrast-enhanced CT showing right paratracheal mass (white arrow). Lower left: 18FDG-PET-CT showing right paratracheal recurrent tumor (white arrow). Upper right: 18FDG uptake with a standard uptake value of 10.5. Lower right: 18FDG-PET showing uptake in three lesions on the right side of the neck—from top to bottom—level II, paratracheal and pretracheal, shown by black arrows

All three lymph nodes were ^{18}FDG-PET positive (Fig. 27.1). The lung micrometastases were ^{18}FDG-PET-negative and still stable. The patient was addressed to our center for management.

Due to the size and progressive nature of the tumor, and the location near the great vessels and the esophagus, reoperative surgery in the neck and upper mediastinum was proposed by the multidisciplinary tumor board. Surgery was performed using intermittent recurrent nerve neuromonitoring. Intraoperative findings revealed that the level II metastasis invaded the posterior aspect of the internal jugular vein which was sacrificed. The paratracheal node completely surrounded the inferior laryngeal (recurrent) nerve and superficially invaded the esophageal muscle, which was resected with a shaving technique, with no perforation of the esophageal mucosa. The nerve was resected en-bloc with the tumor mass. The pretracheal node was also resected en bloc with the paratracheal mass. Final pathology revealed three lymph node metastases of a tall cell variant of papillary thyroid carcinoma with extranodal extension. The postoperative course was uneventful, with a satisfactory vocal outcome.

Follow-up ^{18}FDG-PET-CT performed at 10 months revealed retrosternal uptake in the middle mediastinum, with a 1 cm lesion visualized on contrast-enhanced CT. Postoperative levothyroxine-suppressed Tg was 4 ng/ml. This new recurrence will be monitored for progression and possibly resected via a sternotomy, if no new lesions are discovered and the lung metastases remain stable.

Workup/Diagnosis

- *How do we know that this patient has RAI-refractory disease?*

At the fourth administration of a therapeutic dose of RAI, no uptake was seen on SPECT, but the micrometastases were still visible on CT and Tg was still elevated, proof of persistent disease despite RAI [1]. The definition of RAI-refractory disease encompasses patients with metastases that never showed any uptake of RAI, even on the first therapeutic whole body scan, patients with lesions that initially were RAI avid and then lost the ability to concentrate RAI, patients harboring both RAI avid and RAI not-avid lesions, and, finally, disease that progresses despite a high cumulative dose of RAI [1].

- *Was FNAC necessary if ^{18}FDG-PET-CT showed significant uptake?*

The reported specificity of ^{18}FDG-PET-CT for recurrence in the neck is 67% [2], whereas the specificity of ultrasound is 89%. Ultrasound-guided FNAC with Tg measured in the needle aspirate fluid has a reported specificity of 95% [3]. Thus, FNAC with measurement of Tg in the needle washout fluid, when possible, improves diagnostic accuracy and avoids the pitfall of false-positive readings of ^{18}FDG-PET-CT. FNAC also rules out other tumors, such as lung or head and neck cancer, in this older patient with a history of smoking.

- *What does the previous course of the disease tell us about prognosis?*

The extrathyroidal extension of the disease (pT3), the initial stage of the neck disease (N1b), the age of the patient at first diagnosis (59 years old), and his gender are risk factors for lower disease-free survival [4, 5]. The aggressive histopathological variant of differentiated thyroid carcinoma (tall cell) has also been shown to be a risk factor for recurrent/persistent disease and worse survival [6, 7]. In rare cases, tall cell carcinoma ($\geq$ 50% tall cells) and carcinoma with tall cell features (30–49% tall cells) have also been found to show anaplastic transformation in the recurrent tumor [6].

The lymph node ratio—13/20 or 0.65 in this patient after the first reoperation—has also been shown to portend a lower rate of disease-free survival. A rate of 0.3 or above was associated with a 3.4 times higher rate of persistent or recurrent disease in the study by Vas Nunes et al. [8]. A cutoff of 0.7 was associated with worse prognosis for Schneider et al. [9]. Extranodal spread of disease—a further risk factor—was not noted on the pathological report from the first reoperation in the neck in our patient, although it was evident after the operation at our institution.

- *What other imaging or explorations could or should be performed to determine resectability of the neck disease?*

In a reoperative situation with macroscopic surgical targets in proximity to the carotid artery, trachea, and esophagus, morphological imaging such as contrast-enhanced CT or MRI may improve prediction of local invasion and aid surgical planning [10]. With recurrent disease close to the esophagus, endoscopic ultrasound may also be helpful in determining the depth of any invasion of the esophageal muscle wall [11]. Finally, laryngoscopy is highly recommended in cases with recurrent disease before reoperation to detect recurrent nerve paralysis from a previous operation or from locally invasive cancer [12, 13]. Preoperative laryngeal mobility was normal for our patient.

Management

- *What are the treatment options?*

For resectable lesions, surgery is generally recommended, unless undue morbidity is to be expected, due to the slowly progressive nature of the disease and the relatively good prognosis over the short to medium term [14, 15]. External beam radiation therapy to the neck is an option for progressive but unresectable disease [15–17]. Other local therapies such as alcohol injection, radiofrequency ablation, or cryotherapy have not been widely studied in the treatment of large (>1 cm) neck recurrences. Systemic therapy with small molecule multikinase inhibitors with approved drugs or within the framework of a clinical trial are generally reserved for progressive distant metastases of significant volume, due to the long-term nature of this treatment and its toxicities. Confirmed invasion of the visceral axis may contraindicate this type of systemic therapy with anti-angiogenic activity, however, due to the risk of perforation, fistula, or hemorrage [18, 19].

- *What extent of surgery is recommended?*

For our patient, several factors were in favor of surgery to remove the neck metastases: the good general health of the patient despite his comorbidities and age, the size of the metastases >1 cm, RAI-refractory disease, the progression of Tg, resectability ascertained on contrast-enhanced CT, the small volume of the lung metastases and their stability over 7 years, and the absence of other detectable lesions. The aim of surgery was to reduce tumor burden and to reduce the risk of symptoms in the neck from vascular and visceral invasion over time.

- *Why was the recurrent nerve resected if it was functional?*

Dissection of the tumor off of the nerve sheath is technically feasible, but generally leaves small disease on the nerve, with resection classified as R1 or R2 [20]. In our patient, however, the distal end of the nerve was entirely encased by the tumor, and nerve preservation would have required leaving macroscopic residual tumor near the larynx, trachea, and esophagus (R2 resection). Our aim was to optimize loco-regional control in the neck and minimize the risk of invasion of the trachea and/or esophagus. With RAI-refractory tumors, this goal can be attained only with a macroscopically complete surgical resection.

Swallowing may be affected postoperatively, with aspiration of liquids, and patients should be monitored and receive swallowing rehabilitation if necessary. Voice outcomes are variable after resection of the recurrent nerve due to several factors: compensation from the contralateral side, bilateral innervation of the interarytenoid muscle, variable muscle atrophy, and some degree of reinnervation from nerve anastomoses and from the regional autonomous nerve system. Voice can be surgically improved with several methods based on volume augmentation of the paralyzed vocal fold or medialization of the vocal fold or the arytenoid cartilage, generally with excellent results [21]. Our patient did not have any postoperative dysphagia and considered his voice satisfactory; he declined any type of intervention to improve voice.

- *What outcome can be expected?*

A survival rate of 10% at 10 years and 6% at 15 years has been reported for patients harboring RAI-refractory metastatic disease [22]. In the same study, however, an intermediate group of patients aged >40 with RAI-refractory disease but low tumor burden and micronodular lung metastases had a survival rate of 67% at 10 years. Our patient falls into this intermediate group with a relatively good prognosis (better than many other solid tumors). This prognosis justifies loco-regional treatments when possible to maintain a low tumor burden and avoid symptoms from progressive disease. For patients with multiple recurrences in the neck, Kim et al. [23] showed a 10-year disease-specific survival rate of 83% as compared to patients with no recurrence or only one recurrence whose 10-year disease-specific survival rate was 100%.

Reoperative surgery in the neck must be preceded by a meticulous preoperative imaging workup, in order to foresee possible complications or sequelae and inform the patient preoperatively, but also to find and completely map all of the neck metastases in order to resect all of them, and not "leave behind" persistent disease [24, 25]. Morbidity for reoperation is higher than for primary neck dissection, with a higher risk of unintended nerve injury (recurrent, spinal accessory, and phrenic nerves in particular), tracheal or esophageal injury, and chyle leak (due to damage to the lymphatic system, usually the thoracic duct) [25–27]. Patients should be informed of possible complications preoperatively, but also reassured that the surgical team has knowledge and experience in effectively managing these complications. Intentional resection of the recurrent nerve, more frequent in the reoperative setting [24], should be discussed with the patient preoperatively, with information regarding the effectiveness of a vocal rehabilitation procedure secondarily if needed.

Recurrence after reoperative surgery has been reported to occur in 40–66% of cases [25, 26, 28–30]. The main cause of recurrence is inherent disease aggressiveness, but insufficient workup, "missing" metastatic nodes at the first reoperation, can also cause recurrent/persistent disease [25]. A persistently elevated stimulated Tg level after reoperation is a risk factor for further recurrence [28].

Several techniques have been developed to aid in finding and resecting recurrences, often difficult to locate due to scarring from previous operation(s). Intraoperative ultrasound may be performed but requires training in ultrasonography or bringing the radiologist into the operating room. Radio-guided surgery with RAI (when uptake is present) may aid, particularly for metastatic nodes in the mediastinum or retropharyngeal nodes, not seen on ultrasound [31]. ^{18}FDG-PET-guided surgery has been described but is not yet widely employed due to technical constraints [32, 33]. Harpoon-guided (hooked-needle) surgery has been described but may be delicate for small metastases close to major vascular structures such as the carotid artery and internal jugular vein [34]. Ultrasound tattoo-guided surgery, using colloidal charcoal or methylene blue, is relatively simple to implement, with high rates of localization, but is only applicable to lesions that can be visualized on ultrasound and that are accessible with a needle [35–37]. Due to the size of the recurrences, which were well visualized on CT and their anatomic locations, we did not use localizing techniques in this patient, however.

Conclusions

Patients with a low tumor burden and stable disease generally have a relatively long survival, and aggressive surgery may be advantageous for resectable, progressive lesions in the neck, taking into account other treatment options and quality of life. Recurrent lesions near the visceral axis should be explored with morphological imaging techniques and laryngoscopy to determine resectability. In recurrent disease, a complete diagnostic workup is necessary, to avoid the pitfall of falsely positive lesions, but also to detect concurrent lesions. Patients should be informed of the surgical risks and be aware of the possibility of further recurrences despite macroscopically complete reoperative surgery.

References

1. Schlumberger M, Brose M, Elisei R, Leboulleux S, Luster M, Pitoia F, et al. Definition and management of radioactive iodine-refractory differentiated thyroid cancer. Lancet Diabetes Endocrinol. 2014;2(5):356–8.
2. Seo YL, Yoon DY, Baek S, Ku YJ, Rho YS, Chung EJ, et al. Detection of neck recurrence in patients with differentiated thyroid cancer: comparison of ultrasound, contrast-enhanced CT and (18)F-FDG PET/CT using surgical pathology as a reference standard: (ultrasound vs. CT vs. (18)F-FDG PET/CT in recurrent thyroid cancer). Eur Radiol. 2012;22(10):2246–54.
3. Kim MJ, Kim EK, Kim BM, Kwak JY, Lee EJ, Park CS, et al. Thyroglobulin measurement in fine-needle aspirate washouts: the criteria for neck node dissection for patients with thyroid cancer. Clin Endocrinol. 2009;70(1):145–51.

4. Mazzaferri EL. Long-term outcome of patients with differentiated thyroid carcinoma: effect of therapy. Endocrine Pract. 2000;6(6):469–76.
5. Tuttle RM, Tala H, Shah J, Leboeuf R, Ghossein R, Gonen M, et al. Estimating risk of recurrence in differentiated thyroid cancer after total thyroidectomy and radioactive iodine remnant ablation: using response to therapy variables to modify the initial risk estimates predicted by the new American Thyroid Association staging system. Thyroid. 2010;20(12):1341–9.
6. Ganly I, Ibrahimpasic T, Rivera M, Nixon I, Palmer F, Patel SG, et al. Prognostic implications of papillary thyroid carcinoma with tall-cell features. Thyroid. 2014;24(4):662–70.
7. Kazaure HS, Roman SA, Sosa JA. Aggressive variants of papillary thyroid cancer: incidence, characteristics and predictors of survival among 43,738 patients. Ann Surg Oncol. 2012;19(6):1874–80.
8. Vas Nunes JH, Clark JR, Gao K, Chua E, Campbell P, Niles N, et al. Prognostic implications of lymph node yield and lymph node ratio in papillary thyroid carcinoma. Thyroid. 2013;23(7):811–6.
9. Schneider DF, Mazeh H, Chen H, Sippel RS. Lymph node ratio predicts recurrence in papillary thyroid cancer. Oncologist. 2013;18(2):157–62.
10. Urken ML. Prognosis and management of invasive well-differentiated thyroid cancer. Otolaryngol Clin N Am. 2010;43(2):301–28, viii
11. Koike E, Yamashita H, Noguchi S, Ohshima A, Yamashita H, Watanabe S, et al. Endoscopic ultrasonography in patients with thyroid cancer: its usefulness and limitations for evaluating esophagopharyngeal invasion. Endoscopy. 2002;34(6):457–60.
12. Randolph GW, Kamani D. The importance of preoperative laryngoscopy in patients undergoing thyroidectomy: voice, vocal cord function, and the preoperative detection of invasive thyroid malignancy. Surgery. 2006;139(3):357–62.
13. Chandrasekhar SS, Randolph GW, Seidman MD, Rosenfeld RM, Angelos P, Barkmeier-Kraemer J, et al. Clinical practice guideline: improving voice outcomes after thyroid surgery. Otolaryngol Head Neck Surg. 2013;148(6 Suppl):S1–37.
14. Nixon IJ, Whitcher MM, Palmer FL, Tuttle RM, Shaha AR, Shah JP, et al. The impact of distant metastases at presentation on prognosis in patients with differentiated carcinoma of the thyroid gland. Thyroid. 2012;22(9):884–9.
15. Haugen BR, Alexander EK, Bible KC, Doherty GM, Mandel SJ, Nikiforov YE, et al. 2015 American Thyroid Association management guidelines for adult patients with thyroid nodules and differentiated thyroid cancer: the American Thyroid Association guidelines task force on thyroid nodules and differentiated thyroid cancer. Thyroid. 2016;26(1):1–133.
16. Kim JH, Kim MS, Yoo SY, Lim SM, Lee GH, Yi KH. Stereotactic body radiotherapy for refractory cervical lymph node recurrence of nonanaplastic thyroid cancer. Otolaryngol Head Neck Surg. 2010;142(3):338–43.
17. Romesser PB, Sherman EJ, Shaha AR, Lian M, Wong RJ, Sabra M, et al. External beam radiotherapy with or without concurrent chemotherapy in advanced or recurrent non-anaplastic non-medullary thyroid cancer. J Surg Oncol. 2014;110(4):375–82.
18. Leboulleux S, Bastholt L, Krause T, de la Fouchardiere C, Tennvall J, Awada A, et al. Vandetanib in locally advanced or metastatic differentiated thyroid cancer: a randomised, double-blind, phase 2 trial. Lancet Oncol. 2012;13(9):897–905.
19. Hartl DM, Guerlain J, Bresuskin I, Baudin E, Lamartina L, Hadoux J, et al. Surgery in the context of kinase inhibitor therapy for locally invasive thyroid cancer. Eur J Surg Oncol. 2020;46:650.
20. Brierley J, Gospodarowicz MK, Wittekind C. TNM classification of malignant tumours. 8th ed. Chichester, West Sussex; Hoboken: Wiley; 2017. xviii, 253 pages p.
21. Hartl DM, Travagli JP, Leboulleux S, Baudin E, Brasnu DF, Schlumberger M. Clinical review: current concepts in the management of unilateral recurrent laryngeal nerve paralysis after thyroid surgery. J Clin Endocrinol Metab. 2005;90(5):3084–8.

22. Durante C, Haddy N, Baudin E, Leboulleux S, Hartl D, Travagli JP, et al. Long-term outcome of 444 patients with distant metastases from papillary and follicular thyroid carcinoma: benefits and limits of radioiodine therapy. J Clin Endocrinol Metab. 2006;91(8):2892–9.
23. Kim KM, Park JB, Bae KS, Kang SJ. Analysis of prognostic factors in patients with multiple recurrences of papillary thyroid carcinoma. Surg Oncol. 2012;21(3):185–90.
24. Farrag TY, Agrawal N, Sheth S, Bettegowda C, Ewertz M, Kim M, et al. Algorithm for safe and effective reoperative thyroid bed surgery for recurrent/persistent papillary thyroid carcinoma. Head Neck. 2007;29(12):1069–74.
25. Onkendi EO, McKenzie TJ, Richards ML, Farley DR, Thompson GB, Kasperbauer JL, et al. Reoperative experience with papillary thyroid cancer. World J Surg. 2014;38(3):645–52.
26. Lang BH, Lee GC, Ng CP, Wong KP, Wan KY, Lo CY. Evaluating the morbidity and efficacy of reoperative surgery in the central compartment for persistent/recurrent papillary thyroid carcinoma. World J Surg. 2013;37(12):2853–9.
27. Ruggiero FP, Fedok FG. Outcomes in reoperative thyroid cancer. Otolaryngol Clin N Am. 2008;41(6):1261–8, xii
28. Yim JH, Kim WB, Kim EY, Kim WG, Kim TY, Ryu JS, et al. The outcomes of first reoperation for locoregionally recurrent/persistent papillary thyroid carcinoma in patients who initially underwent total thyroidectomy and remnant ablation. J Clin Endocrinol Metab. 2011;96:2049.
29. Clayman GL, Shellenberger TD, Ginsberg LE, Edeiken BS, El-Naggar AK, Sellin RV, et al. Approach and safety of comprehensive central compartment dissection in patients with recurrent papillary thyroid carcinoma. Head Neck. 2009;31(9):1152–63.
30. Al-Saif O, Farrar WB, Bloomston M, Porter K, Ringel MD, Kloos RT. Long-term efficacy of lymph node reoperation for persistent papillary thyroid cancer. J Clin Endocrinol Metab. 2010;95(5):2187–94.
31. Travagli JP, Cailleux AF, Ricard M, Baudin E, Caillou B, Parmentier C, et al. Combination of radioiodine (131I) and probe-guided surgery for persistent or recurrent thyroid carcinoma. J Clin Endocrinol Metab. 1998;83(8):2675–80.
32. Kim WW, Kim JS, Hur SM, Kim SH, Lee SK, Choi JH, et al. Radioguided surgery using an intraoperative PET probe for tumor localization and verification of complete resection in differentiated thyroid cancer: a pilot study. Surgery. 2011;149(3):416–24.
33. Gulec SA. PET probe-guided surgery. J Surg Oncol. 2007;96(4):353–7.
34. Triponez F, Poder L, Zarnegar R, Goldstein R, Roayaie K, Feldstein V, et al. Hook needle-guided excision of recurrent differentiated thyroid cancer in previously operated neck compartments: a safe technique for small, nonpalpable recurrent disease. J Clin Endocrinol Metab. 2006;91(12):4943–7.
35. Hartl DM, Chami L, Al Ghuzlan A, Leboulleux S, Baudin E, Schlumberger M, et al. Charcoal suspension tattoo localization for differentiated thyroid cancer recurrence. Ann Surg Oncol. 2009;16(9):2602–8.
36. Kang TW, Shin JH, Han BK, Ko EY, Kang SS, Hahn SY, et al. Preoperative ultrasound-guided tattooing localization of recurrences after thyroidectomy: safety and effectiveness. Ann Surg Oncol. 2009;16(6):1655–9.
37. Soprani F, Bondi F, Puccetti M, Armaroli V. Charcoal tattoo localization for differentiated thyroid cancer recurrence in the central compartment of the neck. Acta Otorhinolaryngol Ital. 2012;32(2):87–92.

Chapter 28
A Case of Fistula After Adjuvant External Beam Radiotherapy and Lenvatinib for High-Risk Follicular Thyroid Cancer

Carmen Kut, Angela Liang, and Ana P. Kiess

Initial Presentation

A 60-year-old man was initially diagnosed with thyroid cancer after presenting with a bulky left neck mass, dysphagia, and shortness of breath. He underwent total thyroidectomy with tracheal shave resection, which showed the presence of invasive follicular thyroid carcinoma with a poorly differentiated insular component. The tumor mass was over 10 cm, primarily in the left thyroid lobe, with lymphovascular invasion and substernal extension adherent to the trachea. He subsequently received radioactive iodine, but presented to the hospital 18 months later for acute respiratory distress and voice hoarseness. Direct laryngoscopy showed left vocal cord paralysis and a mass involving the anterior tracheal wall. Computed tomography (CT) imaging of the neck showed a tumor in the left thyroid operative bed with erosion through the left cricoid cartilage, first tracheal ring, and esophagus. Computed tomography (CT) imaging of the chest was concerning for numerous small pulmonary nodules. Neck ultrasound showed enlarged lymph nodes in the left level VI.

Surgical Resection and Pathologic Findings

The patient underwent fine needle aspiration (FNA) of a left level VI lymph node in the neck, which was consistent with recurrence of follicular thyroid carcinoma. Consequently, he proceeded with total laryngectomy, bilateral central neck

---

C. Kut · A. P. Kiess (✉)
Department of Radiation Oncology, Johns Hopkins School of Medicine, Baltimore, MD, USA
e-mail: akiess1@jhmi.edu

A. Liang
Johns Hopkins School of Medicine, Baltimore, MD, USA

G. Grani et al. (eds.), *Thyroid Cancer*,
https://doi.org/10.1007/978-3-030-61919-0_28

dissection, left selective neck dissection (levels IIA-V), cricopharyngeal myotomy, removal of the esophageal muscularis, and placement of a tracheoesophageal puncture voice prosthesis (TEP). Pathology showed a 3.5 cm invasive follicular carcinoma with predominantly poorly differentiated insular component, extending through the cricoid into the laryngeal submucosa; surgical margins were negative. There was positive lymphovascular invasion. Left neck dissection yielded metastatic carcinoma in 1 of 26 lymph nodes without extracapsular extension. The 4-month postoperative thyroglobulin level was elevated at 192 ng/mL. Genetic analysis of his surgical resection specimens (Foundation One) showed a telomerase reverse transcriptase (TERT) promoter mutation but no actionable findings for systemic therapy. BRAF mutation was not detected.

Consideration of Adjuvant Radiation Treatment in High-Risk Follicular Thyroid Cancer

Overall, this 60-year-old patient presented to the radiation oncology clinic with recurrent poorly differentiated follicular thyroid cancer (initially staged pT4aN0M0 by AJCC eighth edition). He had many high-risk features for locoregional recurrence including poorly differentiated histology with insular component, extrathyroidal extension with involvement of the cricoid, trachea and esophagus, and recurrence after prior radioactive iodine. While his imaging showed numerous small pulmonary nodules suspicious for distant metastases, these nodules were asymptomatic and in thyroid cancer may have relatively indolent growth. As a result, we recommended adjuvant radiation treatment for local control of his thyroid cancer.

External beam radiotherapy (EBRT) is optimally used in the subset of thyroid cancer patients at high risk for locoregional recurrence or progression. These risk factors can be described as follows: locally invasive disease, older age, unfavorable histology (poorly differentiated, insular, tall cell, columnar, Hurthle cell), and low RAI uptake [1–3]. Recent literature has indicated that gross extrathyroidal extension is strongly associated with risk of locoregional recurrence when compared with minimal extrathyroidal extension [1, 4–6]. Per AJCC eighth edition, stage T4a is defined as involvement of the recurrent laryngeal nerve, trachea, larynx, esophagus, and/or subcutaneous tissues. Surgical resection for patients with T4a disease is often challenging and may require shaving tumor off the recurrent laryngeal nerve, trachea, larynx or esophagus, with associated risk for gross or microscopic residual disease and high risk of locoregional recurrence.

For these high-risk patients, EBRT has been shown to significantly decrease the rate of locoregional recurrence. For example, Keum et al. evaluated 68 patients with papillary thyroid cancer invading the trachea who underwent shave excision of the tracheal cartilage and found that the locoregional recurrence rate with adjuvant EBRT (8%, 2 of 25 patients) was much lower than that with surgery only (51%, 22 of 43 patients) [6]. Similarly, Chow et al. evaluated 131 patients with resection of pT4a papillary thyroid cancer and found that adjuvant EBRT (compared to RAI alone) improved 10-year locoregional failure-free survival from 72% to 88% [7]. Thus, while current American Thyroid Association guidelines do not recommend routine indications for adjuvant EBRT for differentiated thyroid carcinomas, they do recommend consideration of EBRT for individual patients after serial neck reoperation for locoregionally recurrent disease [8]. Also, the American Head and Neck Society (AHNS) Endocrine Surgery Guidelines recommend consideration of adjuvant EBRT for differentiated thyroid carcinomas in select patients over 45 years old with high likelihood of microscopic residual disease and low likelihood of responding to RAI [9].

Considerations in Radiation Planning: Balancing Local Control and Toxicity

In radiation planning, it is important to strike a balance between therapeutic benefit and toxicity risks. While drug therapies tend to cause systemic side effects, the side effects associated with external beam radiation therapy are primarily in tissues that have been irradiated [10].

Early (or acute) side effects for thyroid cancer irradiation manifest within the first 3 months of radiation treatment and often include skin erythema, dry or moist desquamation of the skin, and inflammation of mucous membranes in the head and neck region. Early toxicities can also include dry mouth, hoarseness, and dysphagia. Late (or long-term) side effects, on the other hand, can manifest months to years following radiation treatment and are often caused by tissue hypoxia, activation of cytokine cascades, and macrophage accumulation leading to fibrosis and excessive extracellular matrix and collagen depositions [10, 11]. Over time, these late treatment-related side effects can lead to esophageal fibrosis/stenosis, dysphagia, lymphedema, hoarseness, and dry mouth. As a result, careful radiation planning is essential in optimizing local control while minimizing radiation-related toxicity to various tissues/organs and maintaining overall quality of life for the patient.

Intensity-modulated radiation therapy (IMRT) is the preferred modality for head and neck cancer irradiation as it facilitates the delivery of differential radiation doses to different areas at risk [12]. In other words, IMRT allows higher doses to small, high-risk areas to maximize locoregional control while distributing lower doses to low-risk areas to minimize side effects. To achieve this, we generally use IMRT to prescribe several distinct dose levels for differentiated thyroid cancer. For example, the AHNS Endocrine Surgery Guidelines recommend 70 Gy for gross disease, 66 Gy for areas with positive surgical margins or shave excision, 60 Gy for high-risk microscopic disease areas (including thyroid bed, tracheoesophageal groove, and level VI cervical nodes), and 54 Gy for low-risk microscopic disease areas [9]. These doses are similar to those reported in previous studies. Terezakis et al. (2009) and Rosenbluth et al. (2015) used 63–70 Gy for gross disease, 59.4–63 Gy for high-risk microscopic disease areas, and 54 Gy for low-risk microscopic disease areas, including nodal regions in the neck [3, 13]. Romesser et al. (2014) and Beckham et al. (2018) similarly used 70 Gy for gross disease, 66 Gy for close or microscopically positive margins, 60 Gy for high-risk areas, and 54 Gy for low-risk areas [1, 14].

Furthermore, it is important to consider radiation dose to at-risk organs including the parotid and submandibular glands (for xerostomia risk), the esophagus and cricopharyngeus (for dysphagia risk), and the larynx (for dysphonia and dysphagia risk) [15]. For thyroid cancer irradiation, sparing uninvolved cervical nodes superiorly can be safe in certain circumstances and can help to reduce xerostomia [15]. For example, this patient underwent bilateral neck dissection with only one involved lymph node in the left neck level VI. As a result, we spared the upper neck to limit xerostomia and taste change. As for the esophagus, even the best IMRT plan cannot completely spare this organ. The esophagus is often partially included in the clinical target volume (CTV), especially in cases of invasive disease in the tracheoesophageal groove. However, careful delineation of the CTV and the use of IMRT with differential doses for high and elective risk areas can reduce the volume of the esophagus receiving high-dose radiation.

For our patient with recurrent poorly differentiated follicular thyroid cancer and multiple high-risk features for additional locoregional recurrences in the future, we provided adjuvant image-guided, intensity-modulated radiotherapy (IGIMRT) to the thyroid bed and bilateral neck. This included 6000 cGy in 30 fractions to the local postoperative bed and 5400 cGy in 30 fractions to the bilateral central neck and left lateral neck with sparing of the upper neck to limit xerostomia (Figs. 28.1, 28.2, and 28.3). Overall, our goal was to provide adequate radiation dose for long-term disease control while limiting treatment-related side effects.

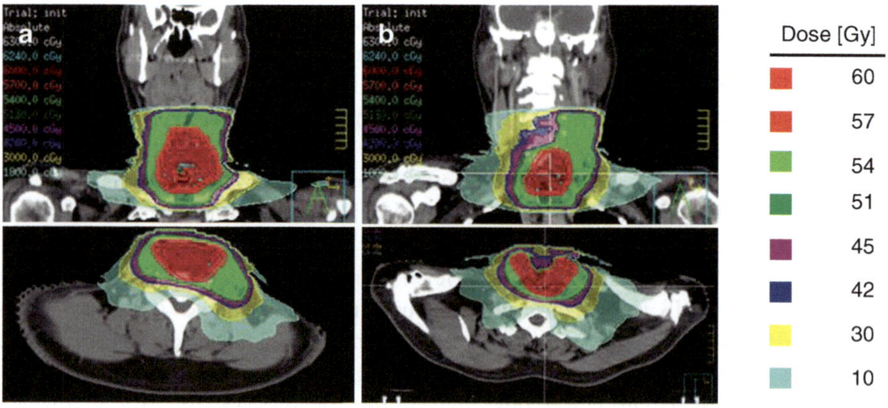

Fig. 28.1 Patient's radiation dose distribution at cross sections (**a**) and (**b**) in coronal (top) and axial (bottom) views

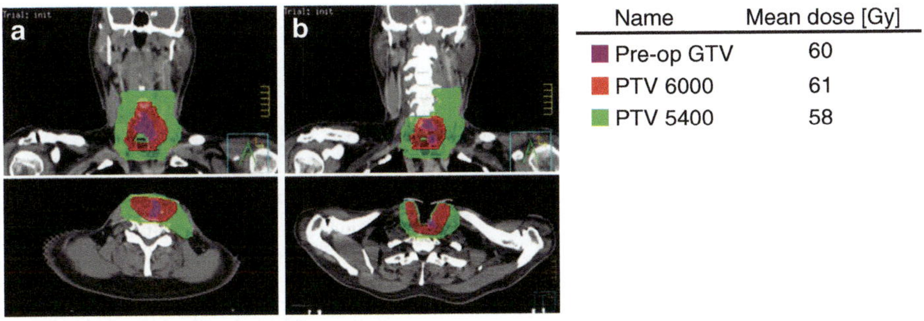

Fig. 28.2 Patient's planning treatment volumes (PTV) at cross sections (**a**) and (**b**) in coronal (top) and axial (bottom) views

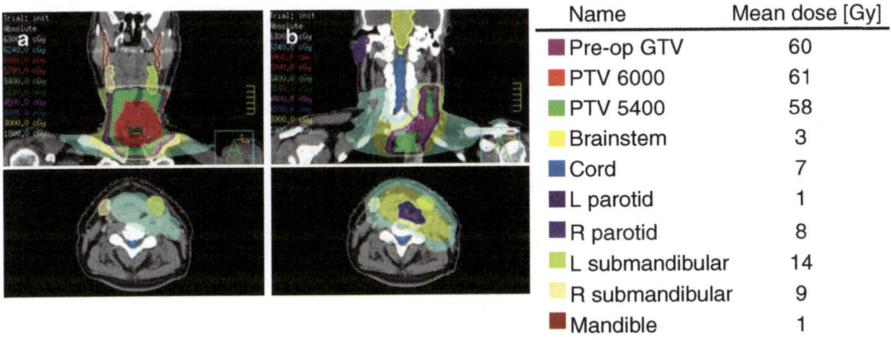

Fig. 28.3 Patient's contours and average radiation dose to normal tissues at cross sections (**a**) and (**b**) in coronal (top) and axial (bottom) views

Patient Outcome with Radiation Treatment: Side Effects and Locoregional Control

With careful radiation planning, our patient experienced relatively mild acute treatment-related side effects (Table 28.1) with grade 1 xerostomia, grade 1 dysphagia, and grade 2 mucositis. This is in comparison with recent literature that quotes relatively higher rates of acute treatment-related toxicities with grade 3 rates at 0–2% for xerostomia, 2–11% for dysphagia, and 14–23% for mucositis [1, 14].

However, this patient did develop significant late treatment-related side effects due to the combination of EBRT, the use of tracheoesophageal puncture (TEP), and subsequent treatment with tyrosine kinase inhibitors (TKIs) starting 5 months after EBRT (Table 28.1). This combination resulted in the development of a rare late complication of grade 3 tracheoesophageal fistula by 15-month follow-up.

Over time, his symptoms gradually improved with careful titration of his TKIs and multiple additional interventions including the removal of his tracheoesophageal puncture prosthesis, placement of a feeding tube, and surgical repair of the

Table 28.1 Acute and late treatment-related side effects

Time after RT start (mo)	Xerostomia (Grade)	Dysphagia (Grade)	Oral mucositis (Grade)	Weight change	Fatigue	Appetite	Feeding tube (Y/N)
Acute treatment-related side effects							
1	0	1	0	Baseline	Mild	Baseline	N
3	1	0	2	Baseline	Mild	Baseline	N
Late treatment-related side effects							
6	1	0	0	−7 lbs	Mild	Baseline	N
10	1	1	0	−20 lbs	Mild	Decreased	N
15	1	3	0	−50 lbs	Severe	Baseline	Y
25	1	3	0	N/A	Baseline	Baseline	Y
29	0	1	0	+60 lbs	Baseline	Baseline	Y
39	0	0	0	N/A	Baseline	Baseline	N
45	0	0	0	N/A	Baseline	Baseline	N

N/A Data not available at that time point

tracheoesophageal fistula. By 39 months of follow-up, his fistula was healed and he reported no evidence of dysphagia; his weight returned to baseline, and he was able to tolerate a regular oral diet.

In terms of disease control, the patient achieved long-term locoregional control with no evidence of recurrence in the neck at any point after EBRT. However, he developed an increase in number and size of pulmonary nodules, which prompted the initiation of systemic TKI therapy 5 months after the completion of EBRT.

Initiation of Systemic Therapy for Locally Advanced or Metastatic Thyroid Cancer

Following surgical resection and radiation treatment, the patient's 5-month postoperative thyroglobulin levels remained elevated at 192 ng/mL, consistent with residual thyroid cancer. His follow-up CT scans showed progression of small pulmonary nodules bilaterally, consistent with metastatic lung disease.

Generally, radioactive iodine (iodine-131) is the mainstay of systemic therapy for patients with advanced metastatic thyroid cancer. In approximately 30–40% of these patients (primarily young patients with small metastases and well-differentiated thyroid tumors), there is very high uptake of radioactive iodine and good long-term disease control with this treatment [16–18]. However, the remaining 60–70% of patients develop recurrence after radioactive iodine treatment with disease that is refractory to radioactive iodine [16, 18]. This is the case with our patient, who received radioactive iodine treatment after his initial thyroidectomy and unfortunately relapsed with significant tumor burden 18 months after initial presentation. As a result, following EBRT, he was started on an alternative systemic therapy, the tyrosine kinase inhibitor lenvatinib.

Lenvatinib is FDA-approved for use in patients with locally advanced or metastatic differentiated thyroid cancer that is refractory to radioactive iodine [16]. It is an oral multi-kinase inhibitor that targets a broad-spectrum kinases, including VEGF receptors 1–3, FGF receptors 1–4, and oncogenes RET, KIT, and PDGF receptor α [19]. Data from the SELECT trial, a phase 3 clinical study, demonstrate that lenvatinib significantly improves median progression-free survival to 18.3 months (compared with placebo at 3.6 months) [20]. While the SELECT trial data is very promising, it also links lenvatinib with multiple potential adverse events. The most common side effects include hypertension, fatigue, rash, diarrhea, nausea/vomiting, and weight loss. Since lenvatinib is an anti-VEGF tyrosine kinase inhibitor, it has a 3–15% incidence of cardiac dysfunction, with 1–10% developing symptomatic heart failure [16, 21, 22]. It can also increase the risk of acute coronary syndrome and arrhythmias [16]. In the kidneys, the anti-VEGF action of lenvatinib can lead to proteinuria and kidney failure [20]. While less common, lenvatinib can also cause arterial and venous thromboembolic events (5.4% incidence) and liver failure (0.4%) [20]. Furthermore, lenvatinib has been associated with rare but serious adverse events such as bleeding and increased risk of fistulas (both gastrointestinal and autodigestive; 1.5%). As a result, patients on TKIs such as lenvatinib must be closely monitored for adverse events. While the recommended initial dose of lenvatinib is 24 mg once a day in 28-day cycles [16], the SELECT trial showed that 78% of patients required dose reduction and 14% of patients required discontinuation of lenvatinib due to adverse events [20].

Considering the above data, our patient was initiated on lenvatinib at 24 mg daily (9-months postoperatively, 5 months s/p completion of radiation treatment) and closely monitored for possible side effects. He did very well initially. While he required a brief treatment break at 2 months after initiation of lenvatinib due to soft tissue sores at the tracheostomy site, his thyroglobulin levels reached <10 ng/ml and his CT chest showed interval decrease in the number and size of pulmonary nodules. However, after 6 months of lenvatinib, he started to experience significant side effects including neck pain and a 50-lb weight loss. As a result, his lenvatinib dose was reduced to 20 mg, then 14 mg, and ultimately discontinued 8 months later when he was diagnosed with a tracheoesophageal fistula (Fig. 28.4). He required an enteral feeding tube for nutritional support (first a nasogastric tube, later replaced by a jejunostomy tube).

Development of Tracheoesophageal Fistularization and Associated Risk Factors

Targeted therapy with tyrosine kinase inhibitors with antiangiogenic activity has now become standard of care in most types of metastatic, progressive, radioiodine-resistant thyroid cancer [23]. While these drugs were thought initially to be less toxic compared with traditional chemotherapy, they can induce rare and severe toxicities. These include aerodigestive fistula formation and associated bleeding, respiratory distress, and abscess formation [23]. While rare, thyroid cancer patients who

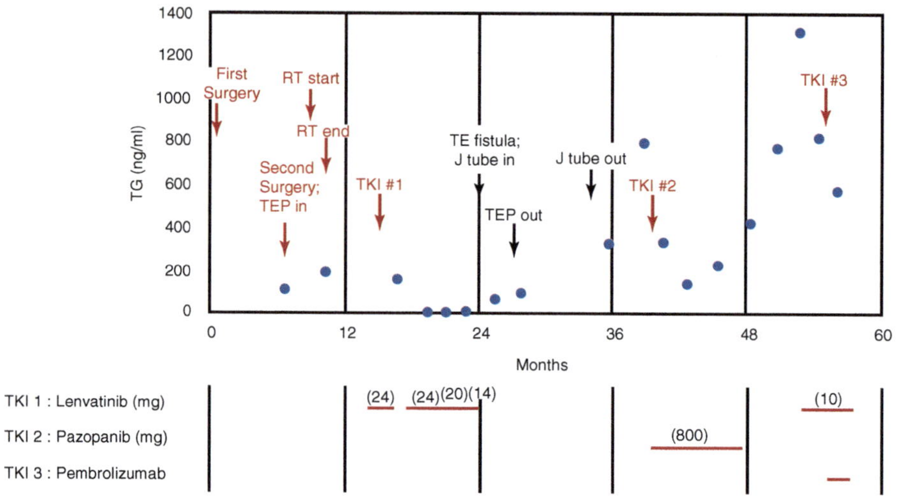

Fig. 28.4 Patient's thyroglobulin (TG) levels over time. Upper limit of normal is 35 ng/mL. Systemic therapy duration and doses are shown on the same timeline, as well as events related to tracheoesophageal (TE) fistula. Pembrolizumab was given at 200 mg IV every 3 weeks. (RT: radiation treatments, TKI: tyrosine kinase inhibitors, TE fistula: tracheoesophageal fistula, J tube: jejunostomy tube)

developed tracheoesophageal fistulas tend to share one or more of the following risk factors: (1) invasion of thyroid cancer into the esophagus or trachea (in this patient's case, requiring laryngectomy and partial esophageal resection); (2) history of external beam radiotherapy; (3) instrumentation of the trachea or esophagus (in this patient's case, the presence of tracheoesophageal puncture prosthesis) [23].

Tracheoesophageal puncture (TEP) is an elective procedure introduced in the 1980s [24]. In this simple procedure, a small puncture is created between the trachea and the esophagus, and a one-way air valve system diverts the tracheal air into the pharynx. The patient can then occlude the stoma and use one-way airflow to cause vibrations of the pharyngoesophageal sphincter to create speech. This option has become increasingly popular due to its high success rate of vocal rehabilitation and fast time frame to achieve intelligible speech [25]. However, use of a TEP relies on the contractile properties of the soft tissues surrounding the prosthesis to both retain the prosthesis and also to prevent salivary and food leakage around the prosthesis, which can predispose the patient to aspiration pneumonia [24]. This is especially a concern if the patient has predisposing risk factors (e.g., radiation therapy, impaired nutrition, diabetes, or liver disease) that may reduce the integrity of the TEP tract [24, 26]. Recent literature has found that there is considerable risk of fistula tract enlargement at the TEP site (ranging from 4% to 26%). As a result, for patients with advanced thyroid cancer, the consideration of placing a TEP must take into account the potential need for future neck radiotherapy and/or antiangiogenic medications such as TKIs.

Given multiple risk factors, this patient was closely monitored with imaging and clinical exams. Approximately 18 months postoperatively (13 months s/p completion of radiation treatment, 8 months after initiation of lenvatinib), he developed

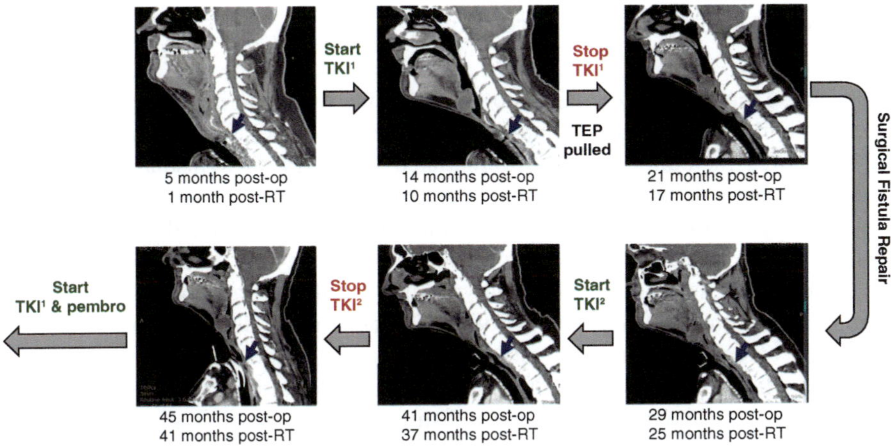

Fig. 28.5 Sagittal CT images showing development of tracheoesophageal fistula (blue arrow) requiring multiple interventions including cessation of tyrosine kinase inhibitors and surgical fistula repair (TKI¹: lenvatinib, TKI²: pazopanib, TEP: tracheoesophageal prosthesis)

profuse leakage of both liquids and solids around the TEP. As a result, lenvatinib was discontinued. He was restricted to NPO (nothing by mouth) and required feeding tube placement for enteral nutrition. The tracheoesophageal voice prosthesis was removed and closed. He underwent two reconstructive surgeries for repair of the persistent tracheoesophageal fistula with local flaps. Over time, the fistula healed and the patient was able to tolerate an oral diet (12 months s/p cessation of lenvatinib) (Figs. 28.4 and 28.5).

However, after lenvatinib was discontinued, the patient's thyroglobulin increased from <10 ng/mL to 803 ng/mL and his CT chest showed worsening metastatic disease with increased size and number of pulmonary nodules. As a result, he ultimately resumed TKI therapy with 800 mg pazopanib (16 months s/p cessation of lenvatinib) (Figs. 28.4 and 28.5). Pazopanib is a multi-kinase inhibitor which inhibits VEGF receptors, PDGF receptors, FGF receptors, cytokine receptors (cKIT), IL-2 receptor inducible T cell kinase, lymphocyte specific protein tyrosine kinase, and transmembrane glycoprotein tyrosine kinase. Pazopanib has lower reported fistularization risk (1%) compared to lenvatinib.

Our patient responded to pazopanib therapy with a reduction in his thyroglobulin level to 138 ng/mL and associated radiographic response. Eventually, pazopanib was also discontinued due to radiographic evidence of a recurrent, small tracheoesophageal fistula. His fistula healed, but thyroglobulin levels increased again to 1322 ng/mL (Figs. 28.4 and 28.5). Single-agent anti-PD1 agents such as pembrolizumab were considered but have only been associated with 10–20% partial response rates in thyroid cancer [27]. Therefore, he is currently being treated with salvage pembrolizumab (200 mg IV every 3 weeks) and low-dose TKI therapy (10 mg lenvatinib daily). A recent retrospective study with 12 patients has shown 42% partial response rate with the combination of pembrolizumab and TKI [27]. He is tolerating this therapy well to date with no evidence of recurrent fistula.

Conclusion and Future Directions

In this case report, we presented a 60-year-old man with recurrent poorly differentiated follicular thyroid cancer (initially staged pT4aN0M0). He had multiple high-risk features including poorly differentiated histology with insular component, extrathyroidal extension with involvement of the cricoid, trachea and esophagus, and recurrence after prior radioactive iodine treatment. As a result, he underwent extensive surgical resection including total laryngectomy, bilateral neck dissection, tracheal shave resection, and cricopharyngeal myotomy. A tracheoesophageal puncture was performed with placement of a voice prosthesis. He was also treated with adjuvant external beam neck radiotherapy and subsequent systemic therapies including the antiangiogenic multi-kinase inhibitors lenvatinib and pazopanib. Over time, he developed a tracheoesophageal fistula requiring multiple surgical interventions, enteral feeding, and therapy changes. At 6.5 years after his initial diagnosis, the patient is now doing well, eating an oral diet with no evidence of locoregional recurrence and continued control of lung metastases. However, in our practice, we are now very cautious about placing TEP prostheses in patients who may require adjuvant EBRT and/or antiangiogenic therapy. In addition to fistularization risks, multi-kinase inhibitors harbor activity against a broad range of targets and can lead to other significant toxicities (including cardiac dysfunction, kidney failure, thromboembolic events, and liver failure). As a result, when prescribing multi-kinase inhibitors, it is essential to closely monitor these patients for complications and provide early interventions when indicated.

Novel, selective kinase inhibitors are under development for advanced thyroid cancer that could provide similar therapeutic benefits with significantly less associated side effects. For example, for advanced thyroid cancers with RET mutation (e.g., medullary thyroid cancer or RET rearranged papillary thyroid carcinoma), the selective RET inhibitor selpercatinib has recently been FDA-approved based on results of the LIBRETTO-001 phase 1/2 trial, and multiple other trials with selpercatinib are underway [28, 29]. Since this drug does not have antiangiogenic targeting, it has significantly fewer associated risks and side effects. In addition, advances in external beam radiotherapy may reduce potential toxicities such as decreasing elective target volume in select patients and testing the use of proton therapy for thyroid cancers. These advances point toward a future with more personalized and targeted therapy options with less associated risks for patients with advanced thyroid cancer.

References

1. Romesser PB, et al. External beam radiotherapy with or without concurrent chemotherapy in advanced or recurrent non-anaplastic non-medullary thyroid cancer. J Surg Oncol. 2014;110:375–82. https://doi.org/10.1002/jso.23656.

2. Chow S-M, et al. Papillary thyroid carcinoma: prognostic factors and the role of radioiodine and external radiotherapy. Int J Radiat Oncol Biol Phys. 2002;52:784–95.
3. Terezakis SA, et al. Role of external beam radiotherapy in patients with advanced or recurrent nonanaplastic thyroid cancer: Memorial Sloan-Kettering Cancer Center experience. Int J Radiat Oncol Biol Phys. 2009;73:795–801.
4. Schwartz DL, et al. Postoperative external beam radiotherapy for differentiated thyroid cancer: outcomes and morbidity with conformal treatment. Int J Radiat Oncol Biol Phys. 2009;74:1083–91.
5. Azrif M, Slevin NJ, Sykes AJ, Swindell R, Yap BK. Patterns of relapse following radiotherapy for differentiated thyroid cancer: implication for target volume delineation. Radiother Oncol. 2008;89:105–13.
6. Keum KC, et al. The role of postoperative external-beam radiotherapy in the management of patients with papillary thyroid cancer invading the trachea. Int J Radiat Oncol Biol Phys. 2006;65:474–80.
7. Chow S-M, Yau S, Kwan C-K, Poon PCM, Law SCK. Local and regional control in patients with papillary thyroid carcinoma: specific indications of external radiotherapy and radioactive iodine according to T and N categories in AJCC 6th edition. Endocr Relat Cancer. 2006;13:1159. https://doi.org/10.1677/erc.1.01320.
8. Cooper DS, et al. Revised American Thyroid Association management guidelines for patients with thyroid nodules and differentiated thyroid cancer: the American Thyroid Association (ATA) guidelines taskforce on thyroid nodules and differentiated thyroid cancer. Thyroid. 2009;19:1167–214.
9. Kiess AP, et al. External-beam radiotherapy for differentiated thyroid cancer locoregional control: a statement of the American Head and Neck Society. Head Neck. 2016;38:493–8.
10. Bentzen SM. Preventing or reducing late side effects of radiation therapy: radiobiology meets molecular pathology. Nat Rev Cancer. 2006;6:702–13.
11. Fleckenstein K, et al. Temporal onset of hypoxia and oxidative stress after pulmonary irradiation. Int J Radiat Oncol Biol Phys. 2007;68:196–204.
12. Brierley JD, Giuliani ME. Practical management of thyroid cancer. Cham: Springer; 2018. p. 147–52.
13. Rosenbluth BD, et al. Intensity-modulated radiation therapy for the treatment of nonanaplastic thyroid cancer. Int J Radiat Oncol Biol Phys. 2005;63:1419–26.
14. Beckham TH, et al. Intensity-modulated radiation therapy with or without concurrent chemotherapy in nonanaplastic thyroid cancer with unresectable or gross residual disease. Thyroid. 2018;28:1180–9.
15. Brierley JD, Tsang RW. External beam radiation therapy for thyroid cancer. Endocrinol Metab Clin North Am. 2008;37:497–509, xi. https://doi.org/10.1016/j.ecl.2008.02.001.
16. Capdevila J, et al. Optimisation of treatment with lenvatinib in radioactive iodine-refractory differentiated thyroid cancer. Cancer Treat Rev. 2018;69:164–76.
17. Schmidt A, Iglesias L, Klain M, Pitoia F, Schlumberger MJ. Radioactive iodine-refractory differentiated thyroid cancer: an uncommon but challenging situation. Arch Endocrinol Metabol. 2017;61:81–9.
18. Schlumberger M, et al. Definition and management of radioactive iodine-refractory differentiated thyroid cancer. Lancet Diabet Endocrinol. 2014;2:356–8.
19. Kim SY, et al. Safety of tyrosine kinase inhibitors in patients with differentiated thyroid cancer: real-world use of lenvatinib and sorafenib in Korea. Front Endocrinol. 2019;10:384.
20. Schlumberger M, et al. A phase 3, multicenter, double-blind, placebo-controlled trial of lenvatinib (E7080) in patients with 131I-refractory differentiated thyroid cancer. 2014. https://ascopubs.org/doi/abs/10.1200/jco.2014.32.18_suppl.lba6008.
21. Qi WX, Shen Z, Tang LN, Yao Y. Congestive heart failure risk in cancer patients treated with vascular endothelial growth factor tyrosine kinase inhibitors: a systematic review and meta-analysis of 36 clinical trials. Br J Clin Pharmacol. 2014;78:748–62.

22. Steingart RM, et al. Management of cardiac toxicity in patients receiving vascular endothelial growth factor signaling pathway inhibitors. Am Heart J. 2012;163:156–63.
23. Blevins DP, et al. Aerodigestive fistula formation as a rare side effect of antiangiogenic tyrosine kinase inhibitor therapy for thyroid cancer. Thyroid. 2014;24:918–22. https://doi.org/10.1089/thy.2012.0598.
24. Dewey EH, et al. Reconstruction of expanding tracheoesophageal fistulae in post-radiation therapy patients who undergo total laryngectomy with a bipaddled radial forearm free flap: report of 8 cases. Head Neck. 2016;38:E172–8. https://doi.org/10.1002/hed.23966.
25. Pawar P, Sayed S, Kazi R, Jagade M. Current status and future prospects in prosthetic voice rehabilitation following laryngectomy. J Cancer Res Ther. 2008;4:186–91. https://doi.org/10.4103/0973-1482.44289.
26. Cavalot AL, et al. Pharyngocutaneous fistula as a complication of total laryngectomy: review of the literature and analysis of case records. Otolaryngol Head Neck Surg. 2000;123:587–92. https://doi.org/10.1067/mhn.2000.110617.
27. Iyer PC, et al. Salvage pembrolizumab added to kinase inhibitor therapy for the treatment of anaplastic thyroid carcinoma. J Immunother Cancer. 2018;6:68. https://doi.org/10.1186/s40425-018-0378-y.
28. https://ClinicalTrials.gov/show/NCT04211337.
29. https://ClinicalTrials.gov/show/NCT04194944.

Chapter 29
RAI Refractory Differentiated Thyroid Cancer with Multiple-Organ Progressive Disease

Steven I. Sherman

Case Presentation

A 44-year-old woman presented for treatment for progressive follicular variant of papillary thyroid carcinoma despite surgeries and radioiodine. She had undergone a total thyroidectomy and adjuvant radioiodine with 175 mCi 131-I at age 39 for a 5.5 cm tumor with extensive lymphovascular invasion. Given persistently abnormal serum thyroglobulin levels, she received an additional radioiodine treatment with 150 mCi, but posttreatment scan was negative. After referral to a comprehensive cancer center for further management, she underwent two additional surgeries for recurrent tumor in the right thyroid bed and upper mediastinum, including multiple soft tissue deposits. A chest computed tomography (CT) demonstrated numerous subcentimeter lung nodules bilaterally that subsequently demonstrated no uptake of either fluorodeoxyglucose on positron emission tomography or radioiodine on a 5 mCi diagnostic scan. Despite aggressive TSH-suppressive thyroid hormone therapy, she developed a chronic, nonproductive cough without hemoptysis, and recurrent tumor was palpable at the junction of the right cricoid and trachea. Her lung nodules had grown significantly over a 6 month interval, and right tracheoesophageal groove recurrence with involvement of the tracheal wall was confirmed on CT (Fig. 29.1). Tumor mutation profiling revealed an activating mutation in codon 61 in the *NRAS* gene, without *RET* or *NTRK* gene rearrangements. The patient's case was presented at Multidisciplinary Tumor Board for treatment planning.

S. I. Sherman (✉)
University of Texas M.D. Anderson Cancer Center, Houston, TX, USA
e-mail: sisherma@mdanderson.org

G. Grani et al. (eds.), *Thyroid Cancer*,
https://doi.org/10.1007/978-3-030-61919-0_29

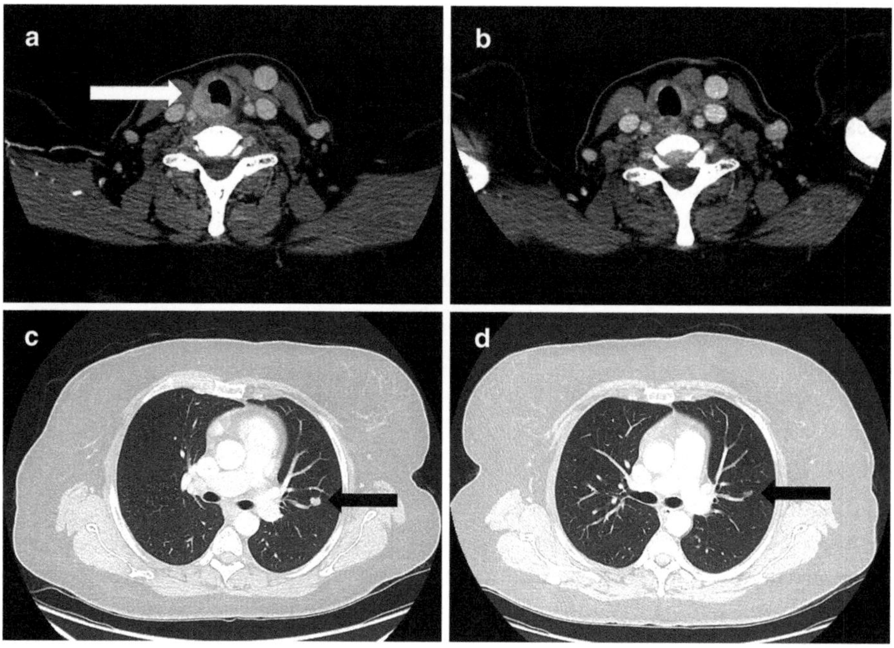

Fig. 29.1 Representative tumors and response to lenvatinib therapy in a 44-year-old woman with progressive radioiodine-refractory thyroid carcinoma. (**a**). Right tracheoesophageal groove recurrence with involvement of the tracheal wall prior to therapy. (**b**). Left lung metastasis prior to therapy. (**c**). Near resolution of the right tracheoesophageal groove recurrence after 2 months of lenvatinib therapy. (**d**). Near resolution of the left lung metastasis after 2 months of lenvatinib therapy

Literature Review

For patients with metastatic DTC who progress despite surgery, radioiodine, and TSH suppressive thyroid hormone, biologically targeted systemic therapies have emerged as effective treatments for progressive, radioiodine-refractory differentiated thyroid carcinoma (RR-DTC), although side effects can be considerable and overall survival has not yet been demonstrated to improve with treatment in most settings.

Given that these systemic therapies for patients with progressive RR-DTC are generally not curative and can have significant toxicities, careful attention must be paid to appropriate patient selection for these treatments. The first priority is to identify which patients actually have "radioiodine-refractory" and "progressive" disease, although debate still exists about clinically optimal definitions [1–3]. An evolving standard is to combine scintigraphic imaging findings with clinical outcomes, defining radioiodine-refractory disease as meeting *any* of the following four criteria: (1) tumors that are structurally evident on radiographic imaging that demonstrate no uptake on postthyroidectomy radioiodine imaging; (2) tumors that previously concentrated radioiodine but no longer demonstrate uptake on subsequent scanning; (3) mixed uptake, visualizing radioiodine concentration in some lesions but not others; and (4) disease that progresses radiographically despite uptake of therapeutic radioiodine. Careful review of previous radioiodine imaging and preparation regimens must be performed before declaring a patient as "radioiodine refractory," as proper dietary iodine restriction and TSH stimulation need to be assured to avoid false-negative imaging results [3]. Finally, patients may have metastatic disease that could benefit from further treatments with radioiodine, but in whom the potential toxicity of additional radioiodine on bone marrow, pulmonary or salivary function is considered excessive and therefore radioiodine is no longer a reasonable treatment option.

"Progression" of disease also requires careful definition. For purposes of identifying patients who should be considered candidates for therapy beyond radioiodine, a combination of the extent of metastatic disease, the rate of growth of that disease, and the potential for morbidity and mortality related to further tumor growth all need to be considered [2]. The extent of disease and rate of tumor growth can be assessed standardly by serial CT or magnetic resonance (MR) imaging. An emerging convention defines progressive disease warranting consideration of further therapy as metastatic lesions measuring at least 1–2 cm, with the sum of the diameters of the largest tumor deposits increasing by at least 20% over a 12–24 month period, or the appearance of significant new metastatic lesions, as these are the patients most likely at highest risk for near-term complications or death from their cancer [2]. The presence or absence of symptoms or complications from metastatic disease or appearance of more rapidly growing tumors may modify the assessment. For example, a patient with a critically located vertebral metastasis may not be optimally managed by active surveillance if a minimal degree of growth threatens vertebral collapse, pain, or neurologic compromise. Similarly, a patient with extensive micrometastatic pulmonary disease that is growing very rapidly should also be considered for systemic therapy before reaching the 1–2 cm threshold [2]. In addition, some patients who experience locally progressive disease in the neck may benefit from neoadjuvant therapy that could facilitate subsequent surgery even in the absence of progressive distant metastases [1].

In the setting of a limited number of progressing lesions, localized therapy can be considered. For example, palliative stereotactic radiotherapy can be administered to a patient with a painful skeletal metastasis or an enlarging pulmonary metastasis compressing a bronchus with excellent symptomatic benefit. Radiofrequency and cryoablation are also useful for a variety of metastatic lesions in both soft tissue and bone.

However, the patient with multiple measurable, progressive, radioiodine-refractory metastases in one or more organs is a candidate for systemic therapy, usually with an orally administered kinase inhibitor [1]. Various kinases have emerged as potentially valuable targets for such inhibition in the treatment of cancer. In particular, the pro-angiogenic vascular endothelial growth factor receptor

(VEGFR) has been demonstrated to be a prime target in the surrounding tumor microenvironment for treatment of several solid malignancies. In addition to being pro-angiogenic, VEGFR has also been identified on tumor cells themselves, thus providing a positive feedback loop by which the tumor secretes the stimulatory ligand, i.e., VEGF, which is capable of binding to the cognate receptor on the tumor cell whose kinase signals upstream of multiple pro-proliferative cascades. Other oncogenic kinases, such as BRAF, are commonly mutated in papillary thyroid carcinoma and offer a second opportunity to target the tumor cell's growth pathways. Less commonly found but highly promising targets are activated kinases that result from oncogenic gene rearrangements like *RET/PTC* and *NTRK*.

Several kinase inhibitors have regulatory approval for treatment of RR-DTC, including two multikinase inhibitors lenvatinib and sorafenib. Lenvatinib, in addition to targeting VEGFR and RET/PTC kinases, also inhibits several other angiogenic kinases and therefore is a highly potent antagonist of angiogenesis. In a randomized phase III trial in 392 patients with progressive RR-DTC, lenvatinib markedly improved median progression-free survival compared with placebo, 18.3 months versus 3.6 months (hazard ratio 0.21, 99% confidence interval [CI] 0.14–0.31; $p < 0.0001$) [4]. In addition, four patients experienced prolonged complete responses on lenvatinib, and the overall response rate (64.8% versus 1.5%) was significantly better in the lenvatinib group. Patients older than 65 years at the time of therapy initiation with lenvatinib had a significantly longer overall survival than those randomized to placebo (HR 0.53, 95% CI 0.31–0.91), but no survival benefit has been observed in ongoing follow-up of younger patients. The starting dose of lenvatinib was 24 mg by mouth, daily, although most patients required dose reductions and/or treatment interruptions. Common adverse events (in decreasing frequency) due to lenvatinib were hypertension, diarrhea, fatigue, decreased appetite, nausea or vomiting, decreased weight, and stomatitis. Although the immunotherapy drug pembrolizumab by itself appears to have minimal activity in RR-DTC, combining pembrolizumab, 200 mg intravenously every 3 weeks, with lenvatinib, 20 mg per day, yielded a 97% disease control rate and 12-month progression-free survival of 74% in a preliminary report from a small phase II trial.

Sorafenib targets multiple kinases including VEGFR, RET/PTC, RAF, and platelet-derived growth factor receptor β. In a randomized phase III trial in 417 patients with progressive RR-DTC, sorafenib significantly improved median progression-free survival compared with placebo, 10.8 months versus 5.8 months (hazard ratio 0.59, 95% CI 0.45–0.76; $p < 0.0001$) [5]. Although objective responses were uncommon, 6-month disease control rate was 54%. Preliminary analysis failed to suggest a significant impact of sorafenib on overall survival but follow-up continues. The starting dose of sorafenib was 400 mg by mouth, twice daily, and most patients required dose reductions and/or treatment interruptions. The most common adverse events (in decreasing frequency) due to sorafenib were hand-foot skin reaction, diarrhea, alopecia, rash or desquamation, fatigue, weight loss, and hypertension.

Beyond these two approved drugs, several other multikinase inhibitors have been reported in phase II trials to have promising activity in treating patients with progressive RR-DTC [1]. The antiangiogenic agents axitinib, cabozantinib, pazopanib, sunitinib, and vandetanib are all VEGFR inhibitors that yielded up to 50% partial response rates in limited phase II trials and offer additional treatment options for selected patients. For example, pazopanib appears to be particularly well tolerated in older patients. Cabozantinib is currently under study in a randomized trial for patients who have progressed on previous therapy with either lenvatinib or sorafenib.

In addition to the multitargeted kinase inhibitors that likely primarily affect the tumor microenvironment, more selective targeting of intracellular kinases critical to tumor proliferation is a developing approach to treatment of progressive RR-DTC. Rearrangements leading to *RET/PTC* oncogenes producing activated RET kinase are the third most common driver mutations in PTC. Selpercatinib and pralsetinib are both highly selective inhibitors of RET kinase. At this writing, selpercatinib has been FDA approved on the basis of an open-label, single arm trial in 27 patients with RR-DTC. The overall response rate was 100% in patients who had never been treated with a kinase inhibitor, and 79% in those who had previously progressed on a kinase inhibitor [6]. Median duration of response was 18 months, and among those patients previously treated, median progression-free survival was 20 months. The recommended starting dose is 160 mg orally twice daily. The most common side effects due to selpercatinib included dry mouth, diarrhea, constipation, nausea, abdominal pain, rash, hypertension, headache, fatigue, and edema. Pralsetinib remains under FDA review of results from its open label phase 1/2 trial that included 13 patients with *RET*-rearranged RR-DTC, who experienced a 91% partial response rate. Less commonly observed, rearrangements of *NTRK* genes can be similarly targeted with the highly selective kinase inhibitors larotrectinib and entrectinib, of which both have been FDA approved for RR-DTC, though the numbers of patients reported so far have been small.

Patients whose tumors contain activating mutations in *BRAF* have been treated with selective BRAF kinase inhibitors. In a single-arm phase II trial of vemurafenib, a highly selective antagonist of the V600E mutant BRAF kinase, a 38.5% response rate, and 18.8 month progression-free survival were reported in the primary cohort of 26 patients with BRAF-mutant RR-DTC who had not previously been treated with sorafenib [7]. Similar findings were also reported using a slightly less selective BRAF inhibitor, dabrafenib. By inhibiting signaling through a second, anti-apoptotic pathway, the mTOR inhibitor everolimus has also been shown to be active in RR-DTC, particularly in Hurthle cell tumors.

A very exciting and novel application of selective kinase inhibitors has been the attempt to "redifferentiate" RR-DTC. As first suggested in preclinical models, inhibition of signaling through the mitogen-activated protein kinase (MAPK) pathway may allow restoration of sensitivity to radioiodine therapy. This hypothesis has been supported by several recent trials and retrospective series, in which patients with RR-DTC were treated with either a MEK inhibitor, a BRAF inhibitor, or both. In one series of 41 patients with RR-DTC who were treated with a variety of MAPK pathway inhibitors, 78% acquired RAI uptake on diagnostic scans leading to subsequent therapy (median 131-I activity 154 mCi) [8]. Despite discontinuation of kinase inhibitor therapy after RAI treatment, durable partial response was reported in 40% of patients, and median time to progression following RAI administration without subsequent kinase inhibitor therapy was 14 months.

Cytotoxic chemotherapy has been used since the late 1960s in advanced DTC, but with little enthusiasm given early reports of limited efficacy and high toxicity [9]. Monotherapy with agents such as doxorubicin, cisplatin, or bleomycin yield very few responses that are of limited durability. A randomized trial compared the combination of doxorubicin and cisplatin with doxorubicin. Of the patients with metastatic DTC, complete or partial response was seen in 16% with combination therapy, whereas 31% had partial response with doxorubicin monotherapy. Notably, the two complete responses seen in the combination therapy arm lasted 33 and 40 months, respectively. The combination of epirubicin and carboplatin yielded similar outcomes, though it was suggested in one study that pre-chemotherapy administration of recombinant human TSH might increase the therapeutic efficacy of the regimen.

Bone metastases often lead to considerable morbidity and increased risk for death [10]. As first suggested with metastatic breast carcinoma, osteoclast inhibitors such as bisphosphonates may reduce the frequency of skeletal-related events (SRE) such as fracture and improve pain control from bone metastases. A retrospective study reported that monthly infusions of zoledronic acid, 4 mg, improved 3-year SRE-free rates by 50–86%, compared with no bisphosphonate treatment. Thyroid cancer bone metastases likely respond similarly to the anti-osteoclast monoclonal antibody denosumab, which is also approved for reduction of SREs from solid tumor bone metastases. In one retrospective series, survival was longer in patients treated with denosumab, often in addition to radioiodine.

Management of the Case

The patient had developed clear evidence of progressive, RR-DTC, having had a negative posttreatment radioiodine scan followed by a negative diagnostic scan despite growing, macronodular lung metastases and local neck recurrence. Her head and neck surgeon felt the palliative surgical option was a total laryngectomy and tracheostomy and recommended consideration of systemic therapy instead, given her progressing pulmonary metastases. After consensus treatment planning, she was started on lenvatinib, 24 mg by mouth daily. Within several weeks, she developed severe hypertension requiring lenvatinib dose reduction while antihypertensive therapy was titrated upward. After 4 weeks, she was able to reescalate her lenvatinib back to 24 mg daily, keeping her blood pressure controlled medically and tolerating grade 1 side effects of fatigue, decreased appetite, and pain on the soles of her feet while walking. After 2 months of therapy, restaging CT scans showed near-complete resolution of her lung metastases and tracheoesophageal groove recurrence (Fig. 29.1). Her serum thyroglobulin level declined from 220 ng/mL before lenvatinib to 5 ng/mL after 4 months of the kinase inhibitor. Due to worsening erythrodysesthesia of the feet, her lenvatinib dose was reduced over several steps to 14 mg daily for 3 weeks of every 4 week cycle. Other than development of a painful thoracic vertebral metastasis that required stereotactic beam radiosurgery for symptom palliation, she has maintained a stable response to lenvatinib therapy for 4 years.

Clinical Pearls

- Careful review of radioiodine imaging, clinical responses to radioiodine therapy, and serial tomographic imaging is necessary to identify patients with progressive, radioiodine-refractory DTC.
- Antiangiogenic multitargeted kinase inhibitors lenvatinib and sorafenib prolong progression-free survival, leading to frequent tumor shrinkage and partial responses, but evidence of improvement in overall survival remains lacking.
- Toxicities of multitargeted kinase inhibitors are considerable, but usually can be addressed by careful symptom management and dose modification.
- Highly selective kinase inhibitors targeting specific mutated oncogenic kinases are demonstrating high response rates and may lead to redifferentiation of RR-DTC.
- As a rapidly evolving area of therapy, further results from ongoing clinical trials will likely continue to change clinical practice paradigms in the near future.

References

1. Cabanillas ME, Ryder M, Jimenez C. Targeted therapy for advanced thyroid cancer: kinase inhibitors and beyond. Endocr Rev. 2019;40(6):1573–604.
2. Tuttle RM, Brose MS, Grande E, Kim SW, Tahara M, Sabra MM. Novel concepts for initiating multitargeted kinase inhibitors in radioactive iodine refractory differentiated thyroid cancer. Best Pract Res Clin Endocrinol Metab. 2017;31(3):295–305.
3. Van Nostrand D. Radioiodine refractory differentiated thyroid cancer: time to update the classifications. Thyroid. 2018;28(9):1083–93.
4. Schlumberger M, Tahara M, Wirth LJ, Robinson B, Brose MS, Elisei R, et al. Lenvatinib versus placebo in radioiodine-refractory thyroid cancer. N Engl J Med. 2015;372(7):621–30.
5. Brose MS, Nutting CM, Jarzab B, Elisei R, Siena S, Bastholt L, et al. Sorafenib in radioactive iodine-refractory, locally advanced or metastatic differentiated thyroid cancer: a randomised, double-blind, phase 3 trial. Lancet. 2014;384(9940):319–28.
6. Shah MH, Sherman EJ, Robinson B, Solomon BJ, Kang H, Lorch JH, et al. Selpercatinib (LOXO-292) in patients with RET-altered thyroid cancers. American Society of Clinical Oncology Virtual Online; May 29, 2020. p. 3594.
7. Brose MS, Cabanillas ME, Cohen EE, Wirth LJ, Riehl T, Yue H, et al. Vemurafenib in patients with BRAF(V600E)-positive metastatic or unresectable papillary thyroid cancer refractory to

radioactive iodine: a non-randomised, multicentre, open-label, phase 2 trial. Lancet Oncol. 2016;17(9):1272–82.

8. Falcone R, Waguespack S, Dadu R, Sherman S, Busaidy N, Hu M, et al. Redifferentiation radioiodine (RAI)-therapy in patients with metastatic papillary, follicular and poorly differentiated thyroid cancer (TC). Thyroid. 2019;29(S1):A180.
9. Sherman SI. Cytotoxic chemotherapy for differentiated thyroid carcinoma. Clin Oncol (R Coll Radiol). 2010;22:464–8.
10. Iniguez-Ariza NM, Bible KC, Clarke BL. Bone metastases in thyroid cancer. J Bone Oncol. 2020;21:100282.

Chapter 30
RAI-Refractory Differentiated Thyroid Cancer and Lung Lesions Causing Bleeding

Steven I. Sherman

Case Presentation

A 74-year-old woman presented for her routine follow-up noting recent development of a cough productive of blood-tinged sputum for the past 3 months, not associated with fever, shortness of breath, chest pain, or other systemic symptoms. By her report, she averaged about one to two teaspoons of bloody sputum each morning. Her past history is notable for a 3 cm, locally invasive, poorly differentiated carcinoma of the thyroid, treated with total thyroidectomy 6 years previously. Adjuvant radioiodine, 150 mCi, had been administered, with post-therapy scan uptake noted only in the thyroid bed. Two additional radioiodine treatments had been given during the next 2 years, 180 and 200 mCi, respectively, with concurrent stimulated thyroglobulin levels of about 20 ng/mL, but no pathologic uptake had been noted on post-therapy imaging. One month after her third radioiodine treatment, computed tomography (CT) scans had been performed, demonstrating extensive metastatic adenopathy in bilateral and central neck compartments and bilateral subcentimeter pulmonary nodules. Following a bilateral, central, and mediastinal neck dissection and postoperative adjuvant external beam radiotherapy, her TSH-suppressed serum thyroglobulin level had declined to 2 ng/mL. She had remained clinically and radiographically stable for the intervening 3 years until her current presentation with hemoptysis, although the serum thyroglobulin had risen to 88 ng/mL at her last evaluation 6 months ago. Examination of her upper airway including indirect laryngoscopy demonstrated no focal lesions or bleeding, there were no masses palpated in the neck, and her lungs were clear to percussion and auscultation. With an undetectable serum TSH, her thyroglobulin level was 2241 ng/mL. A CT scan demonstrated an enlarging 1.6 cm pulmonary

S. I. Sherman (✉)
University of Texas M.D. Anderson Cancer Center, Houston, TX, USA
e-mail: sisherma@mdanderson.org

G. Grani et al. (eds.), *Thyroid Cancer*,
https://doi.org/10.1007/978-3-030-61919-0_30

nodule in the left upper lobe and a 2.5 cm left lower paratracheal mass, along with numerous subcentimeter lung nodules that were unchanged compared with previous imaging studies.

Literature Review

Hemoptysis is commonly a distressing presenting symptom of neck and intrathoracic diseases, both benign and malignant [1]. Among patients without a known diagnosis of malignancy who present with mild hemoptysis (defined as blood-tinged or streaked sputum, blood clots, or <20 mL of blood expectorated within 24 hours), most will have nonmalignant etiologies of hemoptysis including bronchitis, pneumonia, bronchiectasis, or heart failure [2]. Rarer causes of hemoptysis which also require consideration include pulmonary embolism, vascular malformations, vasculitic disorders, coagulopathies, and immunologic diseases, although many of these conditions are more likely to cause larger amounts of acute bleeding or life-threatening massive hemoptysis [1]. However, in the setting of a preexisting diagnosis of non-hematologic malignancy, fewer than 10% will be found to have a benign cause of hemoptysis [3]. About half will have primary lung carcinoma, whereas the other half will have metastases from non-thoracic primary malignancies. When an endobronchial lesion is identified by bronchoscopy, carcinomas of the breast, colorectum, kidney, and larynx and melanoma are the most common primaries, whereas thyroid carcinoma accounts for only a few percent of reported cases [2–4]. Upper airway causes of bleeding also need to be considered, including intraluminal invasion of a malignancy of the head and neck (of which most will be differentiated thyroid carcinoma) and rarer complications of cancer therapy such as a tracheo-esophageal fistula after radiation or antiangiogenic therapy.

Given this differential diagnosis, a patient with DTC who develops hemoptysis requires a diagnostic evaluation before planning treatment [1]. The amount of bleeding should be assessed and the risk for hemodynamic compromise considered. Medications should be reviewed for use of anticoagulants, aspirin, nonsteroidal anti-inflammatories, and antiangiogenic drugs that increase bleeding risk. Given the amount of blood that can be lost either acutely or chronically, blood hematocrit and hemoglobin should be determined along with coagulation parameters. Computed tomography should be performed and compared with any available previous imaging studies to identify new or changing lesions, as chest X-ray has a very low sensitivity for identifying the etiology of hemoptysis. Combining chest CT with flexible bronchoscopy yields nearly 85% sensitivity to identify the source of hemorrhage [5]. Once a suspicious lesion is visualized by bronchoscopy, a biopsy can be obtained if it is necessary to determine the histology of the tumor; alternatively, transthoracic biopsy (either CT-guided needle biopsy or an excisional procedure) can also be performed if bronchoscopic biopsy is not feasible or unsuccessful. Bronchoscopic findings may also facilitate rapid prognostication. Among patients with solid tumors and hemoptysis, bronchoscopic detection of both active bleeding and an endobronchial lesion portends a worse prognosis with a median survival of 3.5 months, compared with 66 months for those with neither active bleeding nor endobronchial lesion visualized [3]; however, whether this analysis specifically applies to DTC is unknown.

Therapeutic options for hemoptysis from metastatic DTC include bronchoscopic modalities such as argon plasma coagulation (APC) or Nd-yttrium laser resection, surgery, radiotherapy, and occasionally systemic therapy. During bronchoscopic APC, brief jets of ionized argon gas are aimed at the targeted endobronchial lesion, creating sufficient heat to coagulate and destroy the tumor tissue [6]. APC causes immediate and durable cessation of bleeding and can significantly relieve symptoms due to obstruction from endobronchial lesions. Nd-yttrium laser therapy causes photocoagulation of tumor vessels, also provides rapid relief of symptoms, and facilitates precise cutting of endotracheal and endobronchial lesions. However, the Nd-yttrium laser is considerably more expensive than the equipment required for APC [7]. Neither APC nor laser resection is appropriate for patients whose bleeding lesions are primarily intramural or peribronchial, as the risks of luminal perforation are considerable and bronchoscopic visualization of the target lesion is obviously required.

Surgical metastasectomy can be considered in patients who are inappropriate for bronchoscopic therapy but who have good performance status, sufficient pulmonary function anticipated following partial lung resection, and at least 6 months expected survival assuming local control of the cause of the hemoptysis [8]. Operative resection is usually reserved for patients in whom a complete resection of the local disease can be anticipated, and the longest survival among solid tumor patients who undergo lung metastasectomy is associated with surgery for curative intent followed by at least a 3-year disease-free interval [8]. However, palliative metastasectomy has been reported to be of symptomatic value for many patients, including those with metastatic DTC. Even in the setting of residual metastatic disease following an initial surgical metastasectomy, the 5-year survival rate was more than 60%.

Stereotactic radiosurgery (SRS) and radiofrequency ablation may also be used to control intrathoracic lesions causing hemoptysis up to 4 cm in diameter [9]. By delivering a highly targeted intense dose of high energy radiation, SRS is capable of selectively destroying metastatic lesions that are thought to be causing hemoptysis. Synchronization of radiation delivery with the breath cycle is optimal to minimize radiation dose to surrounding uninvolved lung tissue, but this allows lesions to be safely treated in both the central and peripheral lung fields. Data regarding use for either of these modalities in DTC are lacking, however.

The systemic therapies available for use in symptomatic metastatic radioiodine-refractory DTC are primarily antiangiogenic, such as lenvatinib. Hemoptysis was observed in up to 9% of DTC patients treated with antiangiogenic kinase inhibitors in one recent report, particularly in those with poorly differentiated histologies or previous therapy with external beam radiotherapy [10]. Alternatively, selective kinase inhibitors that have not been implicated as increasing bleeding risk, such as RET, TRK, and BRAF inhibitors, may be of benefit for patients with intrathoracic metastases that demonstrate activating kinase mutations or rearrangements.

Rarely, metastatic cancer can lead to massive hemoptysis sufficient to cause respiratory failure, hypotension, and death [5]. Rapid assessment to identify the laterality of the intrathoracic bleeding source is critical, permitting turning the patient so that the hemorrhagic side is placed in decubitus position. Intubation and possible use of endobronchial blockers may isolate the bleeding site and prevent flooding of neighboring lung tissue. Subsequently, thermoablative procedures, bronchial artery embolization, and/or surgery can be used as therapy to control and stop the hemorrhage [5].

Management of the Case

Given the possibility that the patient's hemoptysis could be arising from either her new lower paratracheal adenopathy or her enlarging left upper lobe nodule, flexible bronchoscopy was performed. The tracheal mucosa was intact, without evidence of tumor invasion or bleeding. However, fresh blood was seen within a branch off the left mainstem bronchus arising from the upper lobe, suggesting a more distal source of the bleeding compatible with the enlarging mass. A median sternotomy was performed, allowing a wedge resection of the left upper lobe. In addition, metastatic adenopathy was identified encasing the recurrent laryngeal nerve but not invading the trachea, and this was successfully resected as well. Pathology confirmed metastatic poorly differentiated thyroid carcinoma in the metastasectomy specimens. Four months later, her TSH-suppressed serum thyroglobulin level was 5 ng/mL, and at her last follow-up 3 years after metastasectomy, she remained clinically and radiographically stable.

Clinical Pearls

- Hemoptysis is an uncommon symptom of intrathoracic metastases from radioiodine-refractory DTC.
- Careful clinical assessment is required to rule out other contributing causes of hemoptysis.
- CT scanning and flexible bronchoscopy are optimally combined to localize the cause of hemoptysis secondary to metastatic disease and to identify appropriate therapeutic options.
- Bronchoscopic treatment with argon plasma coagulation or Nd-yttrium laser is appropriate when the bleeding lesion is visualized through bronchoscopy.
- Surgical metastasectomy may be considered for palliative therapy when bronchoscopic treatment is not feasible.
- Massive hemoptysis is a life-threatening emergency that necessitates rapid localization of the bleeding source and critical care measures to stop the hemorrhage.

References

1. Larici AR, Franchi P, Occhipinti M, Contegiacomo A, del Ciello A, Calandriello L, et al. Diagnosis and management of hemoptysis. Diagn Interv Radiol. 2014;20:299–309.
2. Hirshberg B, Biran I, Glazer M, Kramer MR. Hemoptysis: etiology, evaluation, and outcome in a tertiary referral hospital. Chest. 1997;112:440–4.
3. Grosu HB, Casal RF, Morice RC, Nogueras-Gonzalez GM, Eapen GA, Ost D, et al. Bronchoscopic findings and bleeding control predict survival in patients with solid malignancies presenting with mild hemoptysis. Ann Am Thorac Soc. 2013;10:342–9.
4. Marchioni A, Lasagni A, Busca A, Cavazza A, Agostini L, Migaldi M, et al. Endobronchial metastasis: an epidemiologic and clinicopathologic study of 174 consecutive cases. Lung Cancer. 2014;84:222–8.
5. Davidson K, Shojaee S. Managing massive hemoptysis. Chest. 2020;157:77–88.
6. Morice RC, Ece T, Ece F, Keus L. Endobronchial argon plasma coagulation for treatment of hemoptysis and neoplastic airway obstruction. Chest. 2001;119:781–7.
7. Freitag L. Interventional endoscopic treatment. Lung Cancer. 2004;45(Suppl 2):S235–8.
8. Pfannschmidt J, Egerer G, Bischof M, Thomas M, Dienemann H. Surgical intervention for pulmonary metastases. Dtsch Arztebl Int. 2012;109:645–51.
9. Abbas G, Schuchert MJ, Pennathur A, Gilbert S, Luketich JD. Ablative treatments for lung tumors: radiofrequency ablation, stereotactic radiosurgery, and microwave ablation. Thorac Surg Clin. 2007;17:261–71.
10. Lamartina L, Ippolito S, Danis M, Bidault F, Borget I, Berdelou A, et al. Antiangiogenic tyrosine kinase inhibitors: occurrence and risk factors of hemoptysis in refractory thyroid cancer. J Clin Endocrinol Metab. 2016;101:2733–41.

Chapter 31
A Patient with Follicular Thyroid Cancer and a Painful Bone Metastases at Risk for Pathologic Fracture

Virginia Liberini, Monica Finessi, and Désirée Deandreis

Abbreviations

ATA	American Thyroid Association
BC	Blood clearance
CR	Complete response
CT	Computed tomography
DTC	Differentiated thyroid carcinoma
EANM	European Association of Nuclear Medicine
EBRT	External beam radiotherapy
ETA	European Thyroid Association
FDG	Fluorodeoxyglucose
GR	Gustave Roussy
HIFU	High-intensity focused ultrasound
MR	Magnetic resonance
NIS	Sodium-iodide symporter
OS	Overall survival
PET	Positron emission tomography
PFS	Progression-free survival
RAI	Radioactive iodine
RFA	Radiofrequency ablation
SEER-9	Surveillance, Epidemiology, and End Results-9
SNMMI	Society of Nuclear Medicine and Molecular Imaging
SPECT	Single-photon emission computed tomography
SRE	Skeletal-related event

V. Liberini · M. Finessi · D. Deandreis (✉)
Division of Nuclear Medicine, Department of Medical Sciences, University of Turin, AOU Città della Salute e della Scienza, Turin, Italy
e-mail: desiree.deandreis@unito.it

G. Grani et al. (eds.), *Thyroid Cancer*,
https://doi.org/10.1007/978-3-030-61919-0_31

SUV	Standardized uptake value
Tg	Thyroglobulin
TKi	Tyrosine kinase inhibitor
VRE	Vertebral-related events
WB	Whole body

Case Presentation

A 56-year-old man was referred to the Gustave Roussy (GR) Institute (courtesy of Dr. Livia Lamartina) for management of bone metastases from follicular thyroid cancer, which had been diagnosed before the primary thyroid tumor. Because of thoracic pain, a computed tomography (CT) scan had been performed and revealed a 4 cm lytic lesion of the third left rib. The CT scan showed also a 6 cm left thyroid mass and small lung nodules that were less than 1 cm in diameter. A biopsy of the rib lesion showed a metastasis from a well-differentiated follicular thyroid cancer. A ^{18}F-fluorodeoxyglucose positron emission tomography (^{18}F-FDG PET)/CT scan showed uptake in the thyroid tumor [maximum standardized uptake value (SUVmax) of 6] and in the rib lesion (SUVmax 3.4) and no significant uptake in multiple lung lesions (SUVmax 1.1) (Fig. 31.1).

Furthermore, a lytic lesion of the right ischium was visible on the CT scan coupled with PET, without ^{18}F-FDG uptake. Blood tests showed thyroglobulin (Tg) level at 7979 ng/ml with no detectable anti-Tg antibodies.

A total thyroidectomy and central neck dissection were performed. Final histology showed a polymorphic thyroid cancer measuring 10 cm with poorly differentiated areas, 6 mitoses Å ~ 2 mm ^{2}, Ki 67 15%, and several foci of necrosis. Due to massive extrathyroidal extension, the tumor was classified as pT4. No metastatic lymph nodes were found (N0). Two months after surgery, the patient received 100 mCi (3.7 GBq) of radioactive iodine (^{131}I) after thyroid hormone withdrawal for 4 weeks. Thyroglobulin level was 3726 ng/ml with a TSH level of 35 mIU/l.

Post-therapy whole-body (WB) scan showed high ^{131}I uptake in the thyroid remnants and diffuse uptake not only in the lung and in the rib lesion but also in T8 and right iliac bone lesions. Furthermore, ^{131}I single-photon emission computed tomography (SPECT)/CT scan detected three other bone lesions in the spine (C4 and L1) and in the pelvis (left iliac bone), respectively, not visible on WB scan (Fig. 31.2a, b). On the CT component, the rib and the ischial lesions both appeared as lytic lesions of 4 cm and 2.3 cm, respectively; in particular, the ischial lesion showed cortical lysis with risk of fracture (Fig. 31.2c–e). On the other hand, there was no evidence of bone lesions in the other bone segments evaluated at the ^{131}I scan, as in T8. Cryoablation for the rib lesion and cryoablation plus cementoplasty for the ischial lesion were performed. During local treatment, a biopsy of the ischial lesion was performed and was consistent with well-differentiated thyroid cancer.

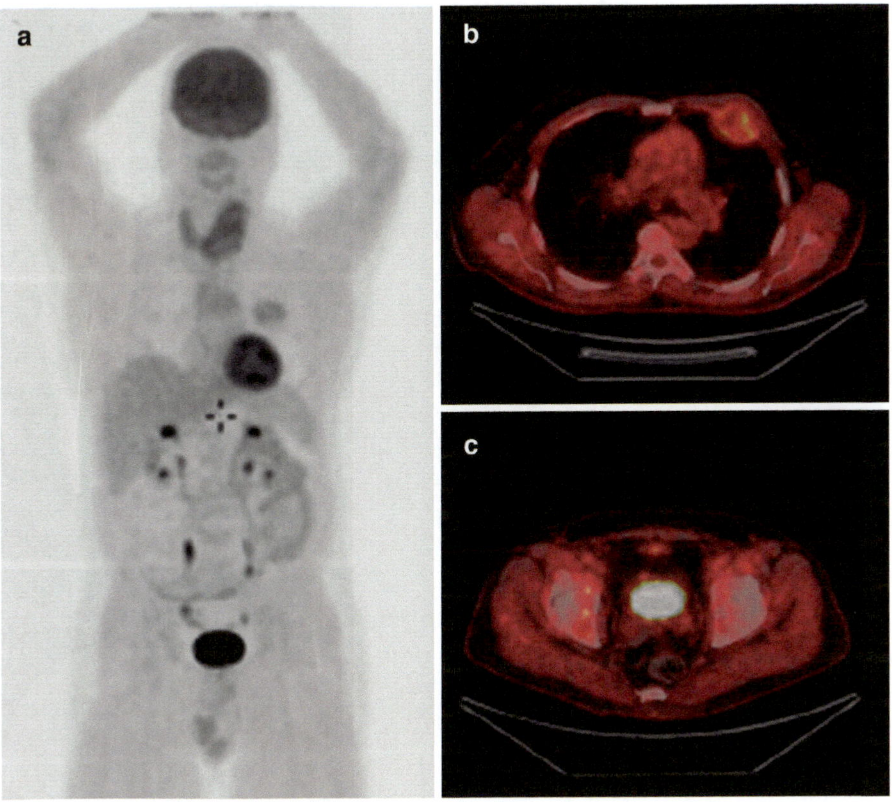

Fig. 31.1 ^{18}F-FDG PET/CT scan performed at initial staging. (**a**) ^{18}F-FDG PET/CT whole-body maximum intensity projection (MIP) showing uptake in 6 cm left lobe thyroid cancer (SUVmax: 6) and in the third left rib (SUVmax: 3.4) corresponding to a 4 cm lytic lesion. There was no significant ^{18}F-FDG uptake in multiple lung nodules of few millimeters' diameter. (**b**) Axial fusion image showing high ^{18}F-FDG uptake in the third left rib lesion. (**c**) Axial fusion image showing no significant ^{18}F-FDG uptake in the right ischial lesion

Assessment and Literature Review

Data from the Surveillance, Epidemiology, and End Results-9 (SEER-9) cancer registry program of the USA showed that the overall incidence of thyroid cancer from 1974 to 2013 increased 3% annually [1], representing approximately 2% of all tumors. Mostly of new diagnosed thyroid cancers are represented by indolent tumors, while metastatic disease represents only 4% of differentiated thyroid carcinoma patients (DTC) [1]. Distant metastases represent one of the most important prognostic factors together with patient age, histological subtype, radioactive iodine (^{131}I), and ^{18}F-FDG avidity and the leading cause of cancer-related death in DTC patients [2]. In fact, 5-year survival greatly varies on the basis of stage at diagnosis,

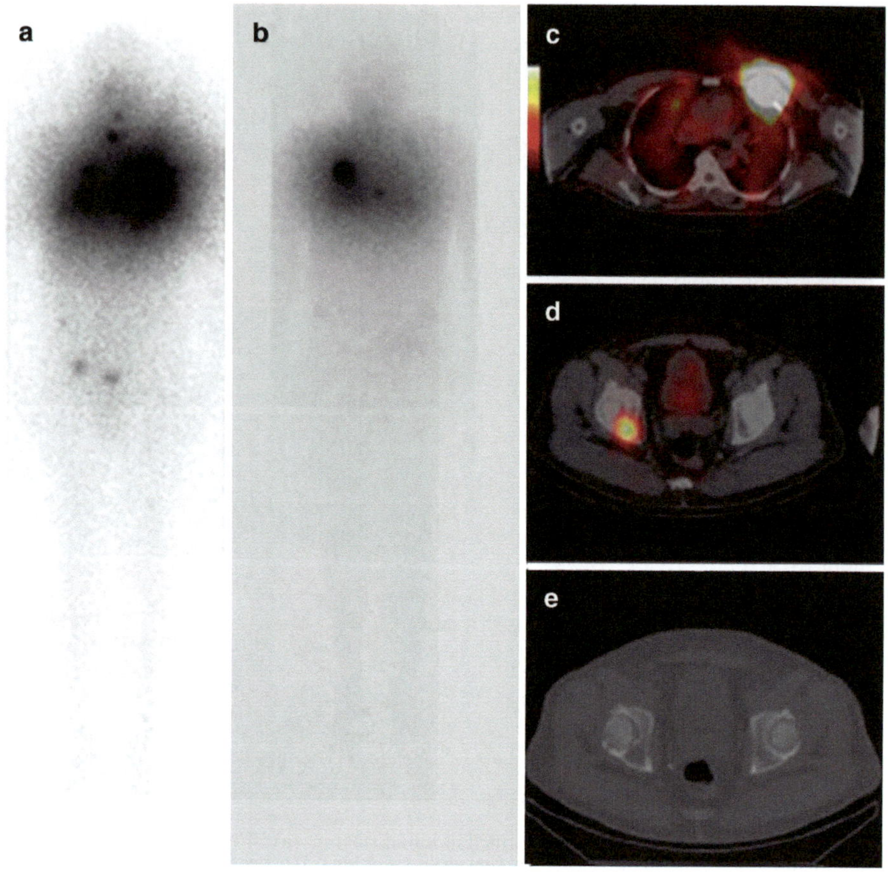

Fig. 31.2 ^{131}I post-therapy whole-body (WB) scan after administration of 100 mCi (3.7 GBq) after thyroid hormone withdrawal for 4 weeks. (**a**, **b**) Anterior and posterior view showing high ^{131}I uptake in the third left rib lesion, in the right ischial lesion, and in the spine T8 and a diffuse uptake in the lung. (**c**) Axial fusion image (SPECT/CT) showing high ^{131}I uptake in the third left rib. (**d**) Axial fusion image (SPECT/CT) showing high ^{131}I uptake in the right ischium. (**e**) Axial image of CT component of SPECT/CT showing a 23 mm lytic lesion in the right ischium

with rates ranging from 99.9% in case of localized thyroid cancer to 56.2% in case of distant metastases at diagnosis [3].

In this contest, bone metastases are the second most common sites of metastasis in thyroid cancer, after lung, and occur in less than 2–13% of patients according to different series. They are often a cause of morbidity for local pain, fracture risk, and neurological complications [4, 5].

In particular follicular histotype shows an increased incidence of bone metastases (7–28%), compared to the classic papillary thyroid cancer (1–7%), spreading hematogenously to distant sites more frequently than through lymphatic system [6].

In a recent study evaluating the prevalence of bone metastases in a cohort of 30.063 patients with thyroid cancer, Choksi et al. [7] identified bone events in 2457 patients (8.2%), of which 1173 (3.9%) developed bone metastasis; the occurrence of bone metastasis was 16.4%, 15.0%, 13.4%, 11.0%, and 6.9% for medullary, follicular, anaplastic, Hurthle cell and papillary thyroid cancer, respectively. Among patient with bone metastases, 372 patients (32%) developed a skeletal-related event (SRE), including pathological fracture (268 of 372, 23%) or a spinal cord compression due to the involvement of axial skeleton (the most frequent site of bone metastasis are the spine, the pelvis, and the ribs [8]).

Bone metastasis can occur as a first manifestation of unknown thyroid cancers or as incidental imaging findings after the first ^{131}I treatment or as a relapse of disease during follow-up; in all those three cases, the presence of multiple bone lesions and the occurrence of SRE is related to a poor quality of life and worse prognosis [9].

The median reported overall survival in case of bone metastases is 2–4 years after their diagnosis, but may range from 96% at 10 years in young patients (<45 years) without radiological abnormalities to less than 10% in older patients (>40 years) with multiple and macroscopic bone lesions associated with radiological abnormalities and frequently associated with macronodular lung metastases [4, 10–12]. In presence of ^{131}I avid metastases, ^{131}I is normally used as first-line treatment [3, 13].

Although ^{131}I may eradicate small metastases, it is poorly effective at treating large metastases, and, moreover, 60–70% of metastatic disease become refractory to radioactive iodine, with a significant negative impact on prognosis and a mean life expectancy of 3–5 years [14]. In patients with radioactive iodine refractory thyroid cancer, systemic treatments such as tyrosine-kinase inhibitors (TKi) are less effective in bone lesions compared to visceral metastases [13, 15–17]. In such cases, local treatment modalities such as external beam radiotherapy (EBRT), stereotactic EBRT, surgery, percutaneous interventional techniques (such as trans-arterial embolization, trans-arterial chemoembolization, radiofrequency, cryoablation), and consolidative techniques such as cementoplasty are becoming more and more important in the management of these patients. An appropriate multidisciplinary therapy approach, personalized to each patient, can prolong the patient survival [18, 19].

Literature data on the management of bone metastases from thyroid cancer are mainly focused on surgery or radiotherapy [20–23], but minimally invasive thermal ablation techniques are frequently used in patients with bone metastases for pain control, local tumor control, and lesion stabilization in case of risk of fractures [24–27]. During the time, additional studies have been carried out to determine the role of thermal ablation in patients with bone metastases from thyroid cancer [28–30].

Characteristics of Bone Lesions from Differentiated Thyroid Cancer

Bone lesions from thyroid cancer are often lytic and can be associated with extension into surrounding soft tissues [31]. The spine is the most frequent site, and spinal metastases can be the first manifestation of follicular thyroid cancer [31, 32].

The major risks are the cortical rupture and local complications, such as medullary compression or fracture [32]. Bone metastases are often vascular, and this pattern makes them accessible to embolization. In patients with bone metastases, one of the most important prognostic factors is the extent of the disease, considering the size and the number of lesions [4, 10].

Whole-body functional imaging can give important information on the patient's stage and prognosis and, recently, the "Martinique principles" – a joint statement by EANM, ATA, ETA, and SNMMI [33, 34] – defined the importance of use of high-resolution imaging. In fact, to evaluate the sodium-iodide symporter (NIS), expression on differentiated thyroid cancer cells is possible to use different iodine isotopes (^{123}I, ^{124}I, and ^{131}I) and acquisition modalities (planar vs. single-photon emission computed tomography [SPECT] vs. SPECT/CT vs. PET/CT) with varying sensitivity and specificity [34–37]. Furthermore, whole-body ^{131}I post-therapy scan can show radioactive iodine uptake in small lesions that are not visualized on cross-sectional imaging.

In particular, SPECT/CT provides much more functional and anatomic detail than planar imaging and it is mandatory to stage metastatic patient. Both ^{131}I post-therapy images and ^{18}F-FDG PET/CT are recommended to stage metastatic patients at the time of diagnosis, as they will provide important information for both prognosis and therapy. High ^{18}F-FDG uptake in distant metastases is a negative prognostic and predictive factor for response to radioactive iodine [8, 38–40]. Nevertheless, bone lesions even deriving from well-differentiated tumors are frequently ^{18}F-FDG avid due to their vascularity and concomitant inflammatory bone reaction, but this does not exclude ^{131}I avidity.

In addition to ^{131}I scan and ^{18}F-FDG/PET CT, magnetic resonance (MR) imaging is useful to evaluate the presence of local complications and medullary compression, which can help to plan radiotherapy.

Another important aspect in the evaluation of thyroid cancer is the role of molecular pathogenesis, and in particular BRAF, RAS, TERT, TP53, PIK3CA, and AKT1 mutations are related to worst prognosis [19, 41]; in a recent study, Malik et al. have demonstrated how TERT mutations, coexisting with RAS mutations, are related to the presence of bone metastasis in DTC, independently by the primary tumor size, and, moreover, this molecular mutations can predict a favorable response to radioiodine therapy [42].

Treating Bone Metastases with Radioactive Iodine

Radioactive iodine (RAI) administration is recommended to explore ^{131}I avidity of distant metastases, to stage the disease, and to treat ^{131}I-avid distant metastases [13]. In patients with RAI-avid metastatic disease, the best way to manage ^{131}I treatment to improve disease response and patient outcome is still a matter of debate. In particular, a great debate on the best approach between empiric and dosimetry-determined activities is still ongoing, after more than 60 years of RAI use for thyroid cancer. American Thyroid Association guidelines [3] stated that RAI activity to be administered can be chosen empirically or determined by dosimetry, both in case of lung metastases and bone metastases, and do not recommend an approach over the other. Usually high and repeated activities of at least 3.7–7.4 GBq of ^{131}I for lung and bone disease, respectively, are recommended.

Two-thirds of patients with distant metastases show radioactive iodine uptake, but complete response is achieved in around 40% of these cases with initial RAI therapy, especially in case of young patients with ^{131}I-avid micrometastases without correlates on cross-sectional imaging [4]. The prognostic value of radioactive iodine uptake in patients with bone metastases has been reported [21]. Young patients with small or single bone lesions or with bone ^{131}I uptake but with no lesion visualized on CT can be treated by repeated ^{131}I administrations [10, 43]. On the other hand, ^{131}I is not sufficient for large or multiple bone lesions and local treatment may be warranted.

According to different approaches for RAI treatment in metastatic disease, tumor response rates are very heterogeneous [44] and varies among the studies; the different studies are not comparable and a superiority of a specific method to the others cannot be defined. In the last years, two retrospective studies compared the impact on overall survival (OS) and progression-free survival (PFS) of dosimetric and empiric approach. In a retrospective analysis conducted on patients with locoregionally advanced DTC or metastatic DTC treated with either dosimetric approach ($n = 43$) or empiric approach ($n = 44$), Klubo-Gwiezdzinska et al. [45] demonstrated higher efficacy of maximum tolerated activity based on the dosimetric approach compared to the empiric approach in patient with locally advanced DTC with a similar safety profile. In particular, patients treated by dosimetric approach tended to 70% less likely to progress (odds ratio, 0.29; 95% confidence interval, 0.087–1.02; $p = 0.052$) and more likely to obtain complete response (CR) (odds ratio, 8.2; 95% confidence interval, 1.2–53.5; $p = 0.029$) with only a trend of association with longer PFS for dosimetry-based approach. On the other hand, there was not statistical differences in response rate and PFS in the subgroup of patients with distant metastases ($p = 0.422$). In 2017, Deandreis et al. [46] in a retrospective study found no differences in OS in patient with metastatic DTC treated with whole-body/-blood clearance (WB/BC) dosimetric approach compared to empiric approach based on the administration of fixed activities of 3.7 GBq. Patients treated according to dosimetric approach received a significantly higher median cumulative activity compared to patient treated with empiric approach (24.2 GBq vs 14.8 GBq, $p < 0.0001$). In particular, no statistical differences in OS, both at 5 and 10 years, were found stratifying patients for age and metastases extension (p = no significant) with the worst prognosis for older patients (>40 years), multiple bone and lung lesions. For dosimetric studies, it is possible to evaluated the absorbed dose to each lesion, and both isotopes ^{131}I or ^{124}I can be used to quantify the ^{131}I avidity of remnant disease and distant metastases; for this purpose, the use of ^{124}I PET/CT results extremely helpful, and in fact both the PET images and the longer half-life ($T_{1/2}$) of ^{124}I permit quantification with better results compared to ^{131}I SPECT/CT scan [47, 48]. Concerning specifically bone metastases, Jentzen et al. have shown low efficacy of

^{131}I treatment on bone metastasis even using a dosimetry-guided approach [49]. Moreover, the study showed also that a higher absorbed dose compared to soft tissue metastasis is needed to achieve an objective response with a great variation of response for each single bone metastasis depending by the heterogeneity uptake at ^{124}I PET/CT in the pre-therapy setting.

There are not available data at this moment of the impact of lesion dosimetry on metastatic patients' outcome. Once again, literature suggests the importance of the assessment of tumor heterogeneity with RAI imaging to predict ^{131}I refractory disease [44]. Unfortunately, the potential utility achieved by personalized dosimetry is not yet standardized, and future prospective studies are requested to integrate dosimetry into routine clinical care [34, 37, 44, 50, 51]. Moreover, in patients with distant metastases, ^{18}F-FDG PET/CT has to be correlated with ^{131}I treatment to complete the pre-therapy setting, especially at initial staging, to evaluate ^{18}F-FDG uptake in distant lesions and to predict response to therapy. Patients with ^{18}F-FDG-avid and no ^{131}I-avid distant metastases ("flip flop" phenomenon) have rapidly progressive disease. In contrast, patients with ^{131}I-avid and ^{18}F-FDG negative lesions have a much better prognosis. Patients with both ^{18}F-FDG and ^{131}I uptake in the same lesions or ^{18}F-FDG and ^{131}I uptake in different lesions represent a very heterogeneous group, but their prognosis seems similar to the group with only ^{18}F-FDG uptake [37]. These different scenarios help identify patients or single lesion that could be refractory to ^{131}I [34] and that can benefit from both local and systemic therapies. Moreover, ^{18}F-FDG PET/CT scan can also be used for the evaluation of the metabolic response by PERCIST, which could be more accurate than RECIST 1.1 and MDA criteria to assess the bone metastasis response to therapy [52, 53].

Finally, some studies are suggesting that a pretreatment with tyrosine-kinase inhibitor in ^{131}I-refractory thyroid cancer can restore iodine trapping in these tumors ("redifferentiation" agents), restoring radio-iodine avidity and, therefore, the efficacy of a radio-iodine therapy [14, 54, 55]. This approach could improve tumor response in selected patients.

Indications and Options of Local Treatment

In case of symptomatic lesions, fracture, local compression, or spinal neurological damage, surgery is the first therapeutic choice [22, 56]. If complete and curative surgery can be achieved, this may improve patient survival, especially in young patients [21–23].

External beam radiation therapy (EBRT) has been used for recurrent lymph node metastases, after surgery, and in bone metastases for pain palliation, in association with surgery [57, 58].

Some cases of vascular embolization by polyvinyl alcohol particles have also been reported with effective and immediate pain relief after treatment [59]. Vascular embolization is routinely performed before surgery to limit bleeding.

In cases of limited bone lesions without soft tissue involvement but symptomatic or at risk of fracture, local thermal ablation by radiofrequency ablation (RFA) or cryotherapy is currently used more and more frequently. These techniques are preferred to other local treatment modalities because they are well tolerated, they are minimally invasive, and they can be repeated in the same patient together with cementoplasty for lesion stabilization [27]. All local treatments can be used in association with systemic treatments, such as radioactive iodine, if the lesions are ^{131}I avid or TKIs in the case of radioactive iodine refractory cancer.

Principles and Definition of External Beam Radiation Therapy

External beam radiotherapy (EBRT) is based on the use of three types of particles (photons, protons, and electrons), which aim radiation in the lesions. Conventional EBRT is used to reduce pain and to avoid pathological fracture or spinal cord compression from bone metastasis [60], but it seems also that conventional EBRT is related to higher rates of relapse [61] and short-term reversible toxicity such as fatigue, mucositis, or bowel irritation [60].

On the other hand stereotactic radiotherapy is becoming a very promising technique in spinal lesions as a selective and curative treatment of bone metastases [20, 62], but also for brain metastases and very small lung metastasis, without the risk of radiation fibrosis and respiratory dysfunction [63].

A recent study of Ito et al. [64] showed how stereotactic radiotherapy for spine metastases leads to 1-year control in more than 80% of bone metastases, even for radioresistant tumors such as thyroid cancer. A recent study of Ishigaki et al. [65], focused on thyroid cancer, showed how stereotactic radiotherapy of locoregional recurrence reduce recurrence of DTC with 3-year local control rate of 84.6%. Another study of Ishigaki et al. [66] showed the efficacy of stereotactic radiotherapy using the Cyber Knife on 60 bone metastases from DTC in 13 patients, with 1-year local control rate of 97.1% and limited adverse events as the radiation to the spinal cord.

Finally, in a phase I-II trials [67] evaluating the use of stereotactic radiotherapy on spine metastases from DCT, the 2-year local control rate was of 88% and the 3-year local control rate was of 79%, without grade 3–5 toxicity following.

Principles and Definition of Thermal Ablation

The principle of thermal ablation action is coagulative tissue necrosis by heating a tumor with high temperature (radiofrequency ablation) or freezing it with pressurized gas (cryoablation) [68, 69]. The main effects are intracellular, vascular, and interstitial damage causing cell apoptosis. Radiofrequency ablation and cryoablation are currently the most frequently used percutaneous minimally invasive techniques, but other options such as high-intensity focused ultrasound (HIFU), irreversible electroporation, or laser ablation are evolving [70]. The selective action is achieved by inserting needles (RFA) or cryoprobes (cryoablation) under imaging guidance during the procedure. After thermal ablation of soft tissue lesions, progressive lesion shrinkage can be monitored with imaging (CT or MR) with a fibrotic scar as final result. In some patients, ^{18}F-FDG PET/CT can be more sensitive in the detection of persistent disease or disease relapse earlier than anatomical imaging [71]. In contrast, the response to thermal ablation in bone lesions is more difficult to evaluate because frequently there are no changes in size or volume of treated lesions on cross-sectional imaging. In patients with bone lesions at risk for fracture due to metastases in the spine or in femoral region, percutaneous cementoplasty with cement injection can be used together with thermal ablation to stabilize the bone and for an analgesic effect [72]. Moreover, screws can be also inserted percutaneously in lesions with high risk of fracture to consolidate the bone.

Finally, surgical treatment can be performed on a metastasis lesion after that the radiofrequency ablation had reduced the volume of the lesion [73].

Thermal Ablation for Treatment of Bone Metastases

Thermal ablation has been used for several years for treating benign bone tumors and for palliation of bone metastases. The first cases examining the feasibility of percutaneous ablation and cementoplasty efficacy in treating bone metastases were reported in 1995–2000 [74–76], showing a good safety and efficacy in reducing pain and in stabilizing lesion preventing skeletal events in bone metastases [24, 26, 27]. In particular, Deschamps et al. evaluated the rate of complete response to thermal ablation in 89 patients with 122 bone metastases from solid tumor. The 1-year complete treatment rate was 67%. Oligometastatic status, metachronous metastases, and small lesions without cortical bone erosion or surrounding neurological structures were all predictive factors on multivariate analysis [27]. In a brief report including three patients with bone metastases from differentiated thyroid cancer treated by RFA in association with radioactive iodine, two of three patients with lesions of 30 and 50 mm were free of disease in 44 and 53 months, respectively, after ablation [28]. In eight patients with symptomatic spinal metastases from thyroid cancer, treatment included a surgical approach in the case of spinal compression or percutaneous vertebroplasty associated with systemic treatment (radioactive iodine or chemotherapy). The authors confirmed that local treatment can improve patients' quality of life by reducing pain and prolonging time to skeletal events, especially spinal cord compression, and can delay initiation of systemic treatment. Finally, local treatment can improve patient survival, with a median survival reported in this paper of 50 months after treatment [30]. Lesion size is another important predictive value of response: in a recent study, specific on thyroid cancer, Deschamps et al. [77] showed how 1-year control rate are, respectively, of 85% for spinal metastases under 2 cm, 81% between 2 and 3 cm, and 40% for lesion over 3 cm.

Generally, in all studies, thermal ablation showed good local control with improvement of patient quality of life after the procedure. In addition to be a palliative treatment for symptomatic lesions, percutaneous ablation may also be curative in patients with localized lesions, with a favorable impact on patient survival. An important recent review including only thyroid cancer, Cazzato et al. [78] found, for bone metastases treated with thermal ablation, an overall survival of 71.6%, 66.8%, and 60.1% at 1, 2, and 3 years, respectively.

Finally, Barata et al. [79] demonstrated how thermal ablation therapy prevents the risk of vertebral-related events (VRE) in patient with DTC, with a hazard ratio of 0.135; this result highlight also the importance of postoperative imaging to identify residual disease after thermal ablation, which must be performed not before than 6 weeks after the therapy to avoid false-positive results correlated with inflammatory process. These and other results show that ^{18}F-FDG PET/CT scan can be a useful tool for treatment follow-up also in bone lesions [71]. The American Thyroid Association guidelines [3] indicate to use thermal ablation therapy for symptomatic metastases disease or, in case of complication risk, in association with systemic treatment or after systemic treatment for residual metastases.

Thermal Ablation on Metastatic Sites Other Than Bone

Thermal ablation can also be performed for liver and lung metastases. Clinical trials show high efficacy of RFA on liver lesions from solid tumors, with local control equivalent to surgical resection ranging from 40% to 80%, and a prolonged overall survival in treated patients [80, 81]. In neuroendocrine tumors, treatment of liver lesions by thermal ablation is now considered an alternative to surgery, especially when there is a small number of lesions with diameter < to 3 cm [82]. A few cases of liver metastases from thyroid cancer treated by thermal ablation have been reported and no more data are recently available. In three patients with liver metastases from thyroid cancer (two medullary thyroid cancer and one follicular thyroid cancer) treated by RFA, thermal ablation reduced local symptoms due to hepatic capsular compression [83].

In a clinical trial focused on lung lesions, RFA was both effective and well tolerated, with a high complete tumor control rate (93%) at 18 months in 100 analyzed lung lesions, including primary lung tumors and distant metastases from solid tumors [84]. Another multicenter prospective trial including 183 lung metastases showed again a high complete response rate (88%) at 1 year and an overall survival of 92% and 64% at 1 year and at 2 years, respectively [85]. In all clinical trials, lesion size and lesion location are reported as the most important predictive factors of response.

In particular, recurrence occurs more frequently in lesions >3 cm with soft tissue or mediastinal invasion and if the lesion is in contact with large vessels [84]. ^{18}F-FDG PET/CT is a useful tool to evaluate response to treatment and to detect early relapse of disease when the lesions have ^{18}F-FDG uptake on a baseline ^{18}F-FDG PET/CT [71].

Denosumab and Bisphosphonates

To treat bone lesions, some systemic specific bone agents such as bisphosphonates and more recently the anti-RANK agent denosumab have demonstrated efficacy in reducing skeletal events in patients with bone metastases from prostate or breast cancer [86–88]. A beneficial effect of these agents has also been reported in patients with lytic lesions from other solid tumors such as lung, renal cell, or myeloma due to inhibition of osteoclast action. In particular, a beneficial effect of zoledronic acid treatment in terms of fewer and delayed skeletal events has been reported in some patients with bone lesions from thyroid cancer, leading to consideration of this drug as a valid therapeutic option [89–92].

On the other hand, no data are available on denosumab's efficacy on bone lesions from thyroid cancer, although it is a promising and potentially more effective therapy than zoledronic acid in other tumors [93]. They both may be useful in the case of disseminated and progressive bone metastases.

In a recent study including 50 DTC patients, Andrade et al. [94] demonstrated how zoledronic acid reduces the incidence of SRE and possibly affects overall survival in DTC patient with bone metastasis.

Bisphosphonates and denosumab are administered monthly by intravenous or subcutaneous injection, respectively, with careful follow-up to monitor for jaw osteonecrosis, hypocalcemia, and renal failure that are the most common side effects. To avoid hypocalcemia, calcium and vitamin D therapy is recommended.

Bisphosphonates and denosumab are not curative therapies, but they can be used in association with local treatment for symptomatic lesions or lesions at risk or with other systemic treatments such as TKi agents.

Management of the Case

This case shows that multidisciplinary treatment is frequently needed to treat bone lesions from thyroid cancer and that bone lesions remain the most challenging site to treat. Efficacy of ^{131}I in multiple and macrometastases is limited and local disease control is particularly important [29]. Therapeutic choices may have an impact on patient quality of life and survival [10].

Radioactive Iodine Treatment

This patient presented with multiple radioiodine-avid bone lesions that were not seen on CT scan. In this situation, a favorable ^{131}I response could be expected [43, 95, 96]. Only the rib and the ischial lesions needed local treatment for their size, the pain management (for the rib lesion), and the fracture risk (ischial lesion). The use of local treatment was necessary to obtain a potential complete resolution of the lesions and to prevent skeletal events. Radioactive iodine alone would not have been efficient to treat these two larger lesions [46]. On the other hand, the patient also had lung micrometastases with significant ^{131}I uptake. Miliary lung disease such as this typically has a good response to ^{131}I treatment [4, 97]. For these reasons, the patient received a second dose of radioactive iodine [100 mCi (3.7 GBq) after THW] 4 months after cryoablation and 6 months after the first radioactive iodine treatment.

Serum thyroglobulin level decreased to 722 ng/ml with TSH level of 78 mIU/l and negative anti-Tg antibodies. The second ^{131}I post-therapy scan showed a reduction in lung uptake with a reduction in size of lung lesions on the CT component of SPECT/CT and the disappearance of ^{131}I uptake in C4, T8, and right and left iliac bone lesions, confirming the efficacy of radioactive iodine in treating small lesions without morphological radiologic changes [43]. The administration of higher activities than 3.7 GBq could be discussed to achieve a better response in the lesions with higher volume.

The post-therapy scan showed also the disappearance of rib uptake and an important reduction of ischium uptake, confirming the efficacy of local treatment of these lesions. Unfortunately, on the post-therapy scan, an increased uptake was reported in T10 and L1 with millimeter-sized lytic lesions on the CT component of the SPECT/CT. There were also two new areas of uptake in the sacrum and in the left femur without structural evidence on the CT component. Progression of disease in the bones, with appearance of new lesions, was confirmed on a third post-therapy scan after administration of 100 mCi (3.7 GBq) 6 months later, while the uptake in the lungs completely disappeared. The disease in the bones was then defined as refractory to radioactive iodine therapy due to the progression despite ^{131}I administration [13].

In our patient, ^{18}F-FDG PET/CT was performed at initial presentation and ^{18}F-FDG uptake was very heterogeneous. The lung metastases did not show significant ^{18}F-FDG uptake, and several bone lesions did not show any ^{18}F-FDG uptake and were detected only on ^{131}I WB scan. All these lesions showed a good response to ^{131}I. Only the rib lesion, the most aggressive and largest lesion, showed significant ^{18}F-FDG uptake. The patient was reevaluated by ^{18}F-FDG PET scan after the third ^{131}I treatment. No ^{18}F-FDG uptake was detected in the lung or in the lesions treated by cryoablation. This case showed that ^{18}F-FDG PET can be used to follow up bone lesions treated by thermal ablation as previously reported in liver and in lung lesions, but further studies are necessary to evaluate the impact of ^{18}F-FDG uptake in this field [71]. The other new bone ^{131}I refractory lesions showed moderate ^{18}F-FDG uptake, probably due to their small size. It was decided to evaluate disease progression with serial PET scans every 6 months, to monitor for disease progression, which might be an indication for additional local therapy or systemic treatment.

Cryoablation and Cementoplasty

This patient was a good candidate for local treatment in association with radioactive iodine. Patients who are candidates for thermal ablation are defined as follows: "(**a**) patients with limited painful metastatic disease who have failed conventional therapies or have refused conventional therapy; (**b**) patients at risk for further morbidity, with progression of a metastatic tumor that may be at risk for fracture or invasion of adjacent critical structures; and (**c**) patients with limited metastatic disease who are not surgical candidates" [70].

Our patient had limited metastatic disease without neurological compression, with at least two macrometastases (>1 cm) not treatable by ^{131}I alone: a painful lesion in the rib and a cortical lytic lesion with fracture risk in the ischium. Surgery was not indicated because of the absence of local compression. Lesion size and location were favorable for needle access and for good efficacy of thermal ablation [27].

The goal was reducing the local pain and the fracture risk, but also to obtain a local control of these lesions. Cryoablation was chosen over RFA and was performed under conscious sedation using special probes (IceRod, Galil Medical, Yokneam, Israel) inserted into the tumor under imaging (CT) guidance. The passage of pressurized gas (argon) through the probes rapidly freezes the lesion with no damage to surrounding tissues. The effect of ablation by "cold temperature" is the formation of the so-called iceball that can be seen and followed up by imaging during the procedure.

Cryotherapy is frequently preferred to RFA because it is less painful during and after the procedure, due to a more selective action on the target lesion and also because the "iceball" can be seen by unenhanced CT during the procedure to monitor the completeness of treatment of the target lesion [27].

Cementoplasty was performed after thermal ablation to consolidate the bone lytic lesion. The cement injection is normally performed in the same manner used to insert the cryoprobe in the bone lesion. Also, the cement is a dense material that can be easily visualized at imaging (Fig. 31.3). During the procedure, potential collateral effects such as pain or neurological symptoms are evaluated by the operator.

The risk of collateral effects is higher in case of lesions in the spine, and in this case the size of lesion is an important criterion to predict local tumor control [77].

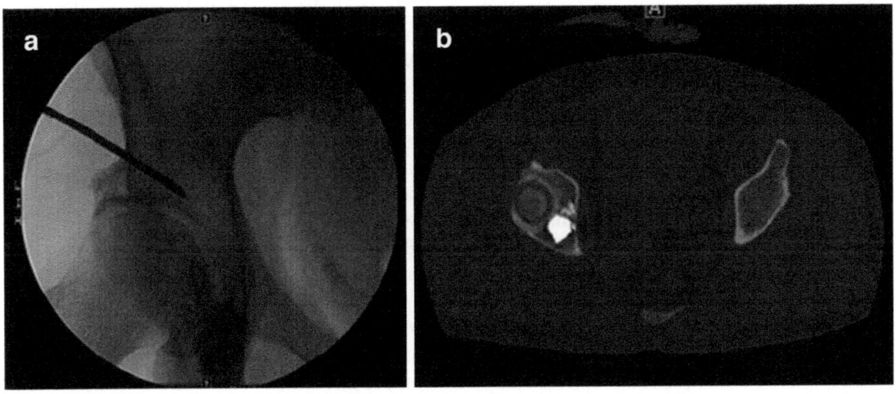

Fig. 31.3 Interventional radiology images during cementoplasty procedure in the right ischium lesion. (**a**) Fluoroscopy image showing cement injection in the right ischium lesion. (**b**) Axial CT image showing cement in the right ischium lesion

Clinical Pearls/Pitfalls

- In case of bone lesion from DTC, a multidisciplinary approach is necessary. A good response can be achieved with RAI in low-volume bone lesions without correlate on morphological imaging and ^{131}I avid.
- High-volume lesions should be selected for local treatment. The goal of local treatments is to reduce pain, to possibly cure the lesion, and to avoid local complications such as pathological fracture or medullary compression.
- Local treatments can also prolong patient survival and delay systemic treatment such as TKi.

References

1. Howlader N, Noone AM, Krapcho M et al. Cancer statistics review, 1975–2014 - SEER statistics. SEER Cancer Stat Rev - Bethesda Natl Cancer Inst [Internet]. 2011 [cited 2019 Dec 30];1975_2008. Available from: https://seer.cancer.gov/archive/csr/1975_2014/.
2. Cabanillas ME, McFadden DG, Durante C. Thyroid cancer. Lancet. Lancet Publishing Group. 2016;388:2783–95.
3. Haugen BR, Alexander EK, Bible KC, Doherty GM, Mandel SJ, Nikiforov YE, et al. 2015 American Thyroid Association management guidelines for adult patients with thyroid nodules and differentiated thyroid cancer: the American Thyroid Association guidelines task force on thyroid nodules and differentiated thyroid cancer. Thyroid. 2016;26(1):1–133.

4. Schlumberger M, Challeton C, De Vathaire F, Travagli JP, Gardet P, Lumbroso JD, et al. Radioactive iodine treatment and external radiotherapy for lung and bone metastases from thyroid carcinoma. J Nucl Med. 1996;37(4–6):598–605.
5. Muresan MM, Olivier P, Leclère J, Sirveaux F, Brunaud L, Klein M, et al. Bone metastases from differentiated thyroid carcinoma [Internet]. Endocr Relat Cancer. 2008 [cited 2019 Dec 30];15:37–49. Available from: http://www.ncbi.nlm.nih.gov/pubmed/18310274.
6. Kallel F, Hamza F, Charfeddine S, Amouri W, Jardak I, Ghorbel A, et al. Clinical features of bone metastasis for differentiated thyroid carcinoma: a study of 21 patients from a Tunisian center. Indian J Endocrinol Metab. 2014;18(2):185–90.
7. Choksi P, Papaleontiou M, Guo C, Worden F, Banerjee M, Haymart M. Skeletal complications and mortality in thyroid cancer: a population-based study. J Clin Endocrinol Metab. 2017;102(4):1254–60.
8. Robbins RJ, Wan Q, Grewal RK, Reibke R, Gonen M, Strauss HW, et al. Real-time prognosis for metastatic thyroid carcinoma based on 2-[18F] fluoro-2-deoxy-D-glucose-positron emission tomography scanning [Internet]. J Clin Endocrinol Metabol. 2006 [cited 2019 Dec 20];91:498–505. Available from: http://www.ncbi.nlm.nih.gov/pubmed/16303836.
9. Farooki A, Leung V, Tala H, Tuttle RM. Skeletal-related events due to bone metastases from differentiated thyroid cancer. J Clin Endocrinol Metab. 2012;97(7):2433–9.
10. Durante C, Haddy N, Baudin E, Leboulleux S, Hartl D, Travagli JP, et al. Long-term outcome of 444 patients with distant metastases from papillary and follicular thyroid carcinoma: benefits and limits of radioiodine therapy. J Clin Endocrinol Metab [Internet]. 2006 [cited 2019 Dec 20];91(8):2892–9. Available from: http://www.ncbi.nlm.nih.gov/pubmed/16684830.
11. Schlumberger M. Targeted therapy in refractory thyroid cancer. Eur J Cancer [Internet]. 2011 [cited 2019 Dec 27];47(SUPPL. 3):S328–9. Available from: http://www.ncbi.nlm.nih.gov/pubmed/21944002.
12. Choi YM, Kim WG, Kwon H, Jeon MJ, Lee JJ, Ryu JS, et al. Early prognostic factors at the time of diagnosis of bone metastasis in patients with bone metastases of differentiated thyroid carcinoma. Eur J Endocrinol. 2016;175(3):165–72.
13. Cooper DS, Doherty GM, Haugen BR, Kloos RT, Lee SL, Mandel SJ, et al. Revised American Thyroid Association management guidelines for patients with thyroid nodules and differentiated thyroid cancer [Internet]. Thyroid. 2009 [cited 2019 Dec 20];19:1167–214. Available from: http://www.ncbi.nlm.nih.gov/pubmed/19860577.
14. Fugazzola L, Elisei R, Fuhrer D, Jarzab B, Leboulleux S, Newbold K, et al. 2019 European Thyroid Association guidelines for the treatment and follow-up of advanced radioiodine-refractory thyroid cancer [Internet]. Eur Thyroid J. 2019 [cited 2020 Jan 3];8:227–45. Available from: https://www.karger.com/Article/FullText/502229.
15. Sheu NW, Jiang HJ, Wu CW, Chiang FY, Chiou HYC, Hsiao PJ. Lenvatinib complementary with radioiodine therapy for patients with advanced differentiated thyroid carcinoma: case reports and literature review. World J Surg Oncol [Internet]. 2019 [cited 2020 Jan 3];17(1):84. Available from: https://wjso.biomedcentral.com/articles/10.1186/s12957-019-1626-4.
16. Cooray SD, Topliss DJ. The management of metastatic radioiodine-refractory differentiated thyroid cancer requires an integrated approach including both directed and systemic therapies. Endocrinol Diabetes Metab Case Rep. 2017;2017:16-0089.
17. Ullmann TM, Gray KD, Moore MD, Zarnegar R, Fahey TJ. Current controversies and future directions in the diagnosis and management of differentiated thyroid cancers. Gland Surg. AME Publishing Company. 2018;7:473–86.
18. Tumino D, Frasca F, Newbold K. Updates on the management of advanced, metastatic, and radioiodine refractory differentiated thyroid cancer. Front Endocrinol. Frontiers Media S.A. 2017;8:312.
19. Khatami F, Larijani B, Nikfar S, Hasanzad M, Fendereski K, Tavangar SM. Personalized treatment options for thyroid cancer: current perspectives. Pharmgenomics Pers Med. Dove Medical Press Ltd. 2019;12:235–45.

20. Tubiana M, Haddad E, Schlumberger M, Hill C, Rougier P, Sarrazin D. External radiotherapy in thyroid cancers. Cancer. 1985;55(9 S):2062–71.
21. Bernier MO, Leenhardt L, Hoang C, Aurengo A, Mary JY, Menegaux F, et al. Survival and therapeutic modalities in patients with bone metastases of differentiated thyroid carcinomas. J Clin Endocrinol Metab [Internet]. 2001 [cited 2019 Dec 20];86(4):1568–73. Available from: http://www.ncbi.nlm.nih.gov/pubmed/11297585.
22. Zettinig G, Fueger BJ, Passler C, Kaserer K, Pirich C, Dudczak R, et al. Long-term follow-up of patients with bone metastases from differentiated thyroid carcinoma - surgery or conventional therapy? Clin Endocrinol (Oxf). 2002;56(3):377–82.
23. Kushchayeva YS, Kushchayev SV, Wexler JA, Carroll NM, Preul MC, Teytelboym OM, et al. Current treatment modalities for spinal metastases secondary to thyroid carcinoma. Thyroid [Internet]. 2014 [cited 2019 Dec 20];24(10):1443–55. Available from: http://www.ncbi.nlm.nih.gov/pubmed/24827757.
24. Goetz MP, Callstrom MR, Charboneau JW, Farrell MA, Mans TP, Welch TJ, et al. Percutaneous image-guided radiofrequency ablation of painful metastases involving bone: a multicenter study. J Clin Oncol [Internet]. 2004 [cited 2019 Dec 20];22(2):300–6. Available from: https://ascopubs.org/doi/full/10.1200/JCO.2004.03.097?url_ver=Z39.88-2003&rfr_id=ori:rid:crossref.org&rfr_dat=cr_pub%3Dpubmed.
25. Thanos L, Mylona S, Galani P, Tzavoulis D, Kalioras V, Tanteles S, et al. Radiofrequency ablation of osseous metastases for the palliation of pain. Skeletal Radiol [Internet]. 2008 [cited 2019 Dec 20];37(3):189–94. Available from: http://www.ncbi.nlm.nih.gov/pubmed/18030464.
26. Dupuy DE, Liu D, Hartfeil D, Hanna L, Blume JD, Ahrar K, et al. Percutaneous radiofrequency ablation of painful osseous metastases: a multicenter American College of Radiology Imaging Network trial. Cancer [Internet]. 2010 [cited 2019 Dec 20];116(4):989–97. Available from: http://onlinelibrary.wiley.com/doi/10.1002/cncr.24837/abstract.
27. Deschamps F, Farouil G, Ternes N, Gaudin A, Hakime A, Tselikas L, et al. Thermal ablation techniques: a curative treatment of bone metastases in selected patients? Eur Radiol [Internet]. 2014 [cited 2019 Dec 20];24(8):1971–80. Available from: http://www.ncbi.nlm.nih.gov/pubmed/24859596.
28. Monchik JM, Donatini G, Iannuccilli J, Dupuy DE. Radiofrequency ablation and percutaneous ethanol injection treatment for recurrent local and distant well-differentiated thyroid carcinoma. Ann Surg. 2006;244(2):296–304.
29. Sugitani I, Fujimoto Y, Yamamoto N. Papillary thyroid carcinoma with distant metastases: survival predictors and the importance of local control. Surgery [Internet]. 2008 [cited 2019 Dec 20];143(1):35–42. Available from: http://www.ncbi.nlm.nih.gov/pubmed/18154931.
30. Quan GMY, Pointillart V, Palussière J, Bonichon F. Multidisciplinary treatment and survival of patients with vertebral metastases from thyroid carcinoma. Thyroid. 2012;22:125–30.
31. Pittas AG, Adler M, Fazzari M, Tickoo S, Rosai J, Larson SM, et al. Bone metastases from thyroid carcinoma: clinical characteristics and prognostic variables in one hundred forty-six patients. Thyroid [Internet]. 2000 [cited 2019 Dec 20];10(3):261–8. Available from: http://www.ncbi.nlm.nih.gov/pubmed/10779141.
32. Kushchayeva YS, Kushchayev S V, Carroll NM, Felger EA, Links TP, Teytelboym OM, et al. Spinal metastases due to thyroid carcinoma: an analysis of 202 patients. Thyroid [Internet]. 2014 [cited 2019 Dec 20];24(10):1488–500. Available from: http://www.ncbi.nlm.nih.gov/pubmed/24921429.
33. Ahuja S, Avram AM, Dillehay G, Greenspan BS, Gulec S, Van Nostrand D. The Martinique principles. J Nucl Med. Society of Nuclear Medicine Inc. 2019;60:1334–5.
34. Michael Tuttle R, Ahuja S, Avram AM, Bernet VJ, Bourguet P, Daniels GH, et al. Controversies, consensus, and collaboration in the use of 131I therapy in differentiated thyroid cancer: a joint statement from the American Thyroid Association, the European Association of Nuclear Medicine, the Society of Nuclear Medicine and Molecular I. Thyroid [Internet]. 2019 [cited 2020 Jan 3];29(4):461–70. Available from: https://www.liebertpub.com/doi/10.1089/thy.2018.0597.

35. Lee SW. SPECT/CT in the treatment of differentiated thyroid cancer. Nucl Med Mol Imaging. Springer Verlag. 2017;51:297–303.
36. Lee CH, Jung JH, Son SH, Hong CM, Jeong JH, Jeong SY, et al. Risk factors for radioactive iodine-avid metastatic lymph nodes on post I-131 ablation SPECT/CT in low-or intermediate-risk groups of papillary thyroid cancer. PLoS One. 2018;13(8):e0202644.
37. Choudhury PS, Gupta M. Differentiated thyroid cancer theranostics: radioiodine and beyond. Br J Radiol. British Institute of Radiology. 2018;91:20180136.
38. Wang W, Larson SM, Fazzari M, Tickoo SK, Kolbert K, Sgouros G, et al. Prognostic value of [18 F]Fluorodeoxyglucose positron emission tomographic scanning in patients with thyroid cancer 1. J Clin Endocrinol Metab. 2000;85(3):1107–13.
39. Wang W, Larson SM, Tuttle RM, Kalaigian H, Kolbert K, Sonenberg M, et al. Resistance of [18F]-fluorodeoxyglucose - avid metastatic thyroid cancer lesions to treatment with high-dose radioactive iodine. Thyroid [Internet]. 2001 [cited 2019 Dec 27];11(12):1169–75. Available from: http://www.ncbi.nlm.nih.gov/pubmed/12186505.
40. Deandreis D, Al Ghuzlan A, Leboulleux S, Lacroix L, Garsi JP, Talbot M, et al. Do histological, immunohistochemical, and metabolic (radioiodine and fluorodeoxyglucose uptakes) patterns of metastatic thyroid cancer correlate with patient outcome? Endocr Relat Cancer [Internet]. 2011 [cited 2019 Dec 20];18(1):159–69. Available from: http://www.ncbi.nlm.nih.gov/pubmed/21118976.
41. Pozdeyev N, Gay LM, Sokol ES, Hartmaier R, Deaver KE, Davis S, et al. Genetic analysis of 779 advanced differentiated and anaplastic thyroid cancers. Clin Cancer Res [Internet]. 2018 [cited 2020 Jan 4];24(13):3059–68. Available from: http://www.ncbi.nlm.nih.gov/pubmed/29615459.
42. Malik N, Nikitski AV, Klam E, Hunt J, Witt B, Chadwick B, et al. Molecular profile and clinical outcomes in differentiated thyroid cancer patients presenting with bone metastasis. Endocr Pract. 2019;25:1255–62.
43. Robenshtok E, Farooki A, Grewal RK, Tuttle RM. Natural history of small radioiodine-avid bone metastases that have no structural correlate on imaging studies. Endocrine [Internet]. 2014 [cited 2019 Dec 20];47(1):266–72. Available from: http://www.ncbi.nlm.nih.gov/pubmed/24366637.
44. Finessi M, Liberini V, Deandreis D. Major limits of dosimetrically determined activities in advanced differentiated thyroid carcinoma. Q J Nucl Med Mol Imaging [Internet]. 2019 [cited 2019 Dec 11];63(3):258–66. Available from: http://www.minervamedica.it.
45. Klubo-Gwiezdzinska J, Van Nostrand D, Atkins F, Burman K, Jonklaas J, Mete M, et al. Efficacy of dosimetric versus empiric prescribed activity of 131I for therapy of differentiated thyroid cancer. J Clin Endocrinol Metab [Internet]. 2011 [cited 2020 Jan 5];96(10):3217–25. Available from: http://www.ncbi.nlm.nih.gov/pubmed/21849530.
46. Deandreis D, Rubino C, Tala H, Leboulleux S, Terroir M, Baudin E, et al. Comparison of empiric versus whole-body/-blood clearance dosimetry-based approach to radioactive iodine treatment in patients with metastases from differentiated thyroid cancer. J Nucl Med. 2017;58(5):717–22.
47. Wierts R, Brans B, Havekes B, Kemerink GJ, Halders SG, Schaper NN, et al. Dose-response relationship in differentiated thyroid cancer patients undergoing radioiodine treatment assessed by means of 124I PET/CT. J Nucl Med [Internet]. 2016 [cited 2020 Jan 5];57(7):1027–32. Available from: http://www.ncbi.nlm.nih.gov/pubmed/26917706.
48. Jentzen W, Hoppenbrouwers J, Van Leeuwen P, Van Der Velden D, Van De Kolk R, Poeppel TD, et al. Assessment of lesion response in the initial radioiodine treatment of differentiated thyroid cancer using 124I PET imaging. J Nucl Med. 2014;55(11):1759–65.
49. Jentzen W, Verschure F, Van Zon A, Van De Kolk R, Wierts R, Schmitz J, et al. 124I PET assessment of response of bone metastases to initial radioiodine treatment of differentiated thyroid cancer. J Nucl Med. 2016;57(10):1499–504.
50. Goldsmith SJ. Targeted radionuclide therapy: a historical and personal review. Semin Nucl Med. 2020;50(1):87–97.

51. Marti JL, Morris LGT, Ho AS. Selective use of radioactive iodine (RAI) in thyroid cancer: no longer "one size fits all". Eur J Surg Oncol. WB Saunders Ltd. 2018;44:348–56.
52. Castello A, Lopci E. Response assessment of bone metastatic disease: seeing the forest for the trees RECIST, PERCIST, iRECIST, and PCWG-2. Q J Nucl Med Mol imaging Off Publ Ital Assoc Nucl Med [and] Int Assoc Radiopharmacol (IAR), [and] Sect Soc of. 2019;63(2):150–8.
53. Costelloe CM, Chuang HH, Madewell JE, Ueno NT. Cancer response criteria and bone metastases: RECIST 1.1, MDA and PERCIST. J Cancer. Ivyspring International Publisher. 2010;1:80–92.
54. Leboulleux S, Dupuy C, Lacroix L, Attard M, Grimaldi S, Corre R, et al. Redifferentiation of a BRAFK601E-mutated poorly differentiated thyroid cancer patient with dabrafenib and trametinib treatment. Thyroid [Internet]. 2019 [cited 2020 Jan 5];29(5):735–42. Available from: https://www.liebertpub.com/doi/10.1089/thy.2018.0457.
55. Gild ML, Topliss DJ, Learoyd D, Parnis F, Tie J, Hughes B, et al. Clinical guidance for radioiodine refractory differentiated thyroid cancer [Internet]. Clin Endocrinol. 2018 [cited 2020 Jan 5];88:529–37. Available from: http://www.ncbi.nlm.nih.gov/pubmed/29095527.
56. Kato S, Murakami H, Demura S, Yoshioka K, Yokogawa N, Yonezawa N, et al. Kidney and thyroid cancer-specific treatment algorithm for spinal metastases: a validation study. World Neurosurg. 2019;122:e1305–11.
57. So K, Smith RE, Davis SR. Radiotherapy in well-differentiated thyroid cancer: is it underutilized? ANZ J Surg [Internet]. 2016 [cited 2020 Jan 5];86(9):696–700. Available from: http://www.ncbi.nlm.nih.gov/pubmed/26573999.
58. Chen PV, Osborne R, Ahn E, Avitia S, Juillard G. Adjuvant external-beam radiotherapy in patients with high-risk well-differentiated thyroid cancer. Ear Nose Throat J. 2009;88(7):E01.
59. Smit JWA, Vielvoye GJ, Goslings BM. Embolization for vertebral metastases of follicular thyroid carcinoma. J Clin Endocrinol Metab [Internet]. 2000 [cited 2019 Dec 20];85(3):989–94. Available from: http://www.ncbi.nlm.nih.gov/pubmed/10720028.
60. Gerszten PC, Mendel E, Yamada Y. Radiotherapy and radiosurgery for metastatic spine disease. Spine (Phila Pa 1976) [Internet]. 2009 [cited 2020 Jan 5];34(Supplement):S78–92. Available from: https://insights.ovid.com/crossref?an=00007632-200910151-00011.
61. Klekamp J, Samii H. Surgical results for spinal metastases. Acta Neurochir. 1998;140(9):957–67.
62. Lo SS, Fakiris AJ, Chang EL, Mayr NA, Wang JZ, Papiez L, et al. Stereotactic body radiation therapy: a novel treatment modality [Internet]. Nat Rev Clin Oncol. 2010 [cited 2019 Dec 20];7:44–54. Available from: http://www.ncbi.nlm.nih.gov/pubmed/19997074.
63. Dunne EM, Fraser IM, Liu M. Stereotactic body radiation therapy for lung, spine and oligometastatic disease: current evidence and future directions. Ann Transl Med [Internet]. 2018 [cited 2020 Jan 5];6(14):283–283. Available from: http://www.ncbi.nlm.nih.gov/pubmed/30105233.
64. Ito K, Ogawa H, Shimizuguchi T, Nihei K, Furuya T, Tanaka H, et al. Stereotactic body radiotherapy for spinal metastases: clinical experience in 134 cases from a single Japanese institution. Technol Cancer Res Treat [Internet]. 2018 [cited 2020 Jan 5];17:1533033818806472. Available from: http://www.ncbi.nlm.nih.gov/pubmed/30355246.
65. Ishigaki T, Uruno T, Tanaka T, Ogimi Y, Masaki C, Akaishi J, et al. Usefulness of stereotactic radiotherapy using the CyberKnife for patients with inoperable locoregional recurrences of differentiated thyroid cancer. World J Surg [Internet]. 2019 [cited 2020 Jan 5];43(2):513–8. Available from: http://link.springer.com/10.1007/s00268-018-4813-5.
66. Ishigaki T, Uruno T, Sugino K, Masaki C, Akaishi J, Hames KY, et al. Stereotactic radiotherapy using the CyberKnife is effective for local control of bone metastases from differentiated thyroid cancer. J Radiat Res [Internet]. 2019 [cited 2019 Dec 20];60(6):831–6. Available from: http://www.ncbi.nlm.nih.gov/pubmed/31423531.
67. Bernstein MB, Chang EL, Amini B, Pan H, Cabanillas M, Wang XA, et al. Spine stereotactic radiosurgery for patients with metastatic thyroid cancer: secondary analysis of phase I/II trials. In: Thyroid [Internet]. 2016 [cited 2020 Jan 5]. p. 1269–75. Available from: http://www.ncbi.nlm.nih.gov/pubmed/27334245.

68. Erinjeri JP, Clark TWI. Cryoablation: mechanism of action and devices [Internet]. J Vasc Interv Radiol. 2010 [cited 2019 Dec 20];21:S187–91. Available from: http://www.ncbi.nlm.nih.gov/pubmed/20656228.
69. Hong K, Georgiades C. Radiofrequency ablation: mechanism of action and devices [Internet]. J Vasc Interv Radiol. 2010 [cited 2019 Dec 20];21:S179–86. Available from: http://www.ncbi.nlm.nih.gov/pubmed/20656227.
70. Rosenthal D, Callstrom MR. Critical review and state of the art in interventional oncology: benign and metastatic disease involving bone [Internet]. Radiology. 2012 [cited 2019 Dec 20];262:765–80. Available from: http://pubs.rsna.org/doi/10.1148/radiol.11101384.
71. Deandreis D, Leboulleux S, Dromain C, Auperin A, Coulot J, Lumbroso J, et al. Role of FDG PET/CT and chest CT in the follow-up of lung lesions treated with radiofrequency ablation. Radiology [Internet]. 2011 [cited 2019 Dec 20];258(1):270–6. Available from: http://www.ncbi.nlm.nih.gov/pubmed/21045185.
72. Proschek D, Kurth A, Proschek P, Vogl TJ, Mack MG. Prospective pilot-study of combined bipolar radiofrequency ablation and application of bone cement in bone metastases. Anticancer Res [Internet]. 2009 [cited 2019 Dec 20];29(7):2787–92. Available from: http://www.ncbi.nlm.nih.gov/pubmed/19596962.
73. Mazzeo S, Cervelli R, Elisei R, Tarantini G, Cappelli C, Molinaro E, et al. mRECIST criteria to assess recurrent thyroid carcinoma treatment response after radiofrequency ablation: a prospective study. J Endocrinol Invest [Internet]. 2018 [cited 2020 Jan 6];41(12):1389–99. Available from: http://www.ncbi.nlm.nih.gov/pubmed/29687416.
74. Chiras J, Sola-Martinez MT, Weill A, Rose M, Cognard C, Martin-Duverneuil N. Vertébroplasties percutanées. La Rev Med interne [Internet]. 1995 [cited 2019 Dec 20];16(11):854–9. Available from: http://www.ncbi.nlm.nih.gov/pubmed/8570944.
75. Cotten A, Dewatre F, Cortet B, Assaker R, Leblond D, Duquesnoy B, et al. Percutaneous vertebroplasty for osteolytic metastases and myeloma: effects of the percentage of lesion filling and the leakage of methyl methacrylate at clinical follow-up. Radiology [Internet]. 1996 [cited 2019 Dec 20];200(2):525–30. Available from: http://www.ncbi.nlm.nih.gov/pubmed/8685351.
76. Fourney DR, Schomer DF, Nader R, Chlan-Fourney J, Suki D, Ahrar K, et al. Percutaneous vertebroplasty and kyphoplasty for painful vertebral body fractures in cancer patients. J Neurosurg. 2003;98(1):21–30.
77. Deschamps F, Farouil G, De Baere T. Percutaneous ablation of bone tumors. Diagn Interv Imaging. Elsevier Masson SAS. 2014;95:659–63.
78. Cazzato RL, Garnon J, Koch G, Shaygi B, Tsoumakidou G, Caudrelier J, et al. Current role of interventional radiology in the management of visceral and bone metastases from thyroid cancer [Internet]. Gland Surgery. 2018 [cited 2020 Jan 6];7:80–8. Available from: http://www.ncbi.nlm.nih.gov/pubmed/29770304.
79. Barat M, Tselikas L, de Baère T, Gravel G, Yevich S, Delpla A, et al. Thermal-ablation of vertebral metastases prevents adverse events in patients with differentiated thyroid carcinoma. Eur J Radiol. 2019;1:119.
80. De Baere T, Elias D, Dromain C, El Din MG, Kuoch V, Ducreux M, et al. Radiofrequency ablation of 100 metastases with a mean follow-up of more than 1 year. Am J Roentgenol [Internet]. 2000 [cited 2019 Dec 20];175(6):1619–25. Available from: http://www.ncbi.nlm.nih.gov/pubmed/11090390.
81. Solbiati L, Livraghi T, Goldberg SN, Ierace T, Meloni F, Dellanoce M, et al. Percutaneous radio-frequency ablation of hepatic metastases from colorectal cancer: long-term results in 117 patients. Radiology [Internet]. 2001 [cited 2019 Dec 20];221(1):159–66. Available from: http://www.ncbi.nlm.nih.gov/pubmed/11568334.
82. De Baere T, Deschamps F, Tselikas L, Ducreux M, Planchard D, Pearson E, et al. GEP-NETs update: interventional radiology: role in the treatment of liver metastases from GEP-NETs [Internet]. Eur J Endocrinol. 2015 [cited 2019 Dec 20];172:R151–66. Available from: http://www.ncbi.nlm.nih.gov/pubmed/25385817.

83. Wertenbroek MWJLAE, Links TP, Prins TR, Plukker JTM, Van Der Jagt EJ, De Jong KP. Radiofrequency ablation of hepatic metastases from thyroid carcinoma. Thyroid [Internet]. 2008 [cited 2019 Dec 20];18(10):1105–10. Available from: https://www.liebertpub.com/doi/10.1089/thy.2008.0080.
84. De Baère T, Palussière J, Aupérin A, Hakime A, Abdel-Rehim M, Kind M, et al. Midterm local efficacy and survival after radiofrequency ablation of lung tumors with minimum follow-up of 1 year: prospective evaluation. Radiology [Internet]. 2006 [cited 2019 Dec 20];240(2):587–96. Available from: http://www.ncbi.nlm.nih.gov/pubmed/16864679.
85. Lencioni R, Crocetti L, Cioni R, Suh R, Glenn D, Regge D, et al. Response to radiofrequency ablation of pulmonary tumours: a prospective, intention-to-treat, multicentre clinical trial (the RAPTURE study). Lancet Oncol. 2008;9(7):621–8.
86. Coleman R, Body JJ, Aapro M, Hadji P, Herrstedt J. Bone health in cancer patients: ESMO clinical practice guidelines. Ann Oncol. 2014;25:124–37.
87. Rosen LS, Gordon D, Tchekmedyian NS, Yanagihara R, Hirsh V, Krzakowski M, et al. Long-term efficacy and safety of zoledronic acid in the treatment of skeletal metastases in patients with nonsmall cell lung carcinoma and other solid tumors: a randomized, phase III, double-blind, placebo-controlled trial. Cancer [Internet]. 2004 [cited 2020 Jan 6];100(12):2613–21. Available from: http://www.ncbi.nlm.nih.gov/pubmed/15197804.
88. Hortobagyi GN, Van Poznak C, Harker WG, Gradishar WJ, Chew H, Dakhil SR, et al. Continued treatment effect of zoledronic acid dosing every 12 vs 4 weeks in women with breast cancer metastatic to bone: the OPTIMIZE-2 randomized clinical trial. JAMA Oncol [Internet]. 2017 [cited 2020 Jan 6];3(7):906–12. Available from: http://www.ncbi.nlm.nih.gov/pubmed/28125763.
89. Orita Y, Sugitani I, Toda K, Manabe J, Fujimoto Y. Zoledronic acid in the treatment of bone metastases from differentiated thyroid carcinoma. Thyroid [Internet]. 2011 [cited 2019 Dec 20];21(1):31–5. Available from: http://www.ncbi.nlm.nih.gov/pubmed/21058881.
90. Orita Y, Sugitani I, Toda K, Manabe J, Fujimoto Y. Zoledronic acid in the treatment of bone metastases from differentiated thyroid carcinoma. Thyroid. 2011;21(1):31–5.
91. Orita Y, Sugitani I, Takao S, Toda K, Manabe J, Miyata S. Prospective evaluation of zoledronic acid in the treatment of bone metastases from differentiated thyroid carcinoma. Ann Surg Oncol. 2015;22(12):4008–13.
92. Choksi P, Papaleontiou M, Guo C, Worden F, Banerjee M, Haymart M. Skeletal complications and mortality in thyroid cancer: a population-based study. J Clin Endocrinol Metab [Internet]. 2017 [cited 2020 Jan 6];102(4):1254–60. Available from: http://www.ncbi.nlm.nih.gov/pubmed/28324052.
93. Fizazi K, Carducci M, Smith M, Damião R, Brown J, Karsh L, et al. Denosumab versus zoledronic acid for treatment of bone metastases in men with castration-resistant prostate cancer: a randomised, double-blind study. Lancet [Internet]. 2011 [cited 2019 Dec 20];377(9768):813–22. Available from: http://www.ncbi.nlm.nih.gov/pubmed/21353695.
94. Andrade F, Probstner D, Decnop M, Bulzico D, Momesso D, Corbo R, et al. The impact of zoledronic acid and radioactive iodine therapy on morbi-mortality of patients with bone metastases of thyroid cancer derived from follicular cells. Eur Thyroid J. 2019;8(1):46–55.
95. Proye CAG, Dromer DHR, Carnaille BM, Gontier AJP, Goropoulos A, Carpentier P, et al. Is it still worthwhile to treat bone metastases from differentiated thyroid carcinoma with radioactive iodine? World J Surg. 1992;16(4):640–5.
96. Petrich T, Widjaja A, Musholt TJ, Hofmann M, Brunkhorst T, Ehrenheim C, et al. Outcome after radioiodine therapy in 107 patients with differentiated thyroid carcinoma and initial bone metastases: side-effects and influence of age. Eur J Nucl Med [Internet]. 2001 [cited 2019 Dec 20];28(2):203–8. Available from: http://www.ncbi.nlm.nih.gov/pubmed/11303891.
97. Ilgan S, Karacalioglu AO, Atac GK, Arslan N, Ozturk E, Gunalp B, et al. Iodine-131 treatment and high-resolution CT: results in patients with lung metastases from differentiated thyroid carcinoma. Eur J Nucl Med Mol Imaging [Internet]. 2004 [cited 2019 Dec 20];31(6):825–30. Available from: http://www.ncbi.nlm.nih.gov/pubmed/14762699.

Chapter 32
Differentiated Thyroid Cancer and Brain Metastases

Steven I. Sherman

Case Presentation

A 70-year-old woman presented to her primary care physician with acute onset of persistent dizziness, without headache or motor difficulties. Her past history was notable for papillary thyroid carcinoma, diagnosed 49 years previously that had initially been treated with thyroidectomy. No adjuvant therapy had been administered, and she had been followed by primary care physicians without specific monitoring for her thyroid carcinoma. Her past history was also notable for type II diabetes mellitus, hypertension, and obesity. On presentation, cerebrovascular disease was initially suspected as the cause of her dizziness. A computed tomography (CT) angiogram demonstrated no evidence of vascular disease or stroke, but magnetic resonance imaging (MRI) instead showed a 2.7 × 2.5 × 2.6 cm multilobulated cystic mass in the right frontal lobe involving the cingulate gyrus, without surrounding edema (Fig. 32.1). Dexamethasone, 8 mg twice daily, and levetiracetam, 500 mg twice daily, were given to prevent seizures. The clinical impression was a low-grade glioma versus metastatic tumor, and she underwent right frontotemporal craniotomy with gross total excision of the tumor. Surgical pathology demonstrated metastatic papillary thyroid carcinoma, with immunohistochemical staining intensely positive for both thyroglobulin and TTF-1. Two weeks after surgery, she presented with acute shortness of breath, leading to CT scan of the chest that showed bilateral pulmonary emboli with signs of right heart strain. She began systemic anticoagulation and was transferred to a tertiary referral center. Steroids and anti-seizure medications were successfully weaned. A follow-up MRI showed enhancement along the inferior resection cavity and possibly involving the right optic nerve, suggesting residual tumor. Whole body tomographic imaging showed no evidence of other sites

S. I. Sherman (✉)
University of Texas M.D. Anderson Cancer Center, Houston, TX, USA
e-mail: sisherma@mdanderson.org

G. Grani et al. (eds.), *Thyroid Cancer*,
https://doi.org/10.1007/978-3-030-61919-0_32

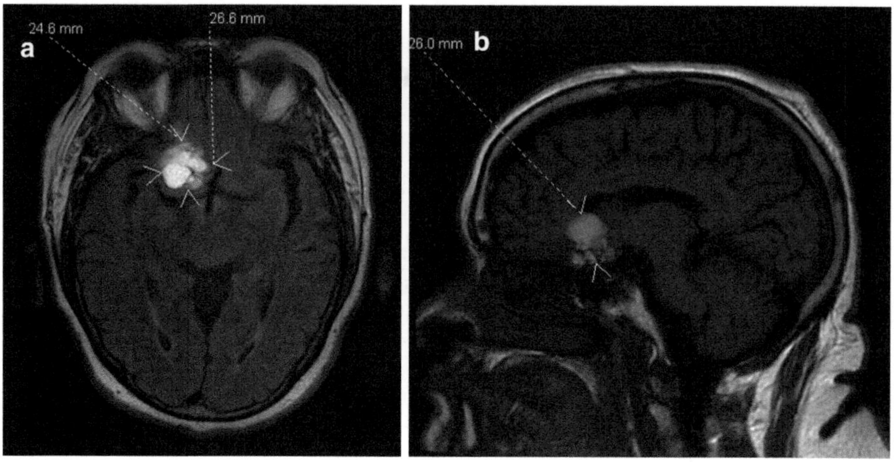

Fig. 32.1 Magnetic resonance imaging, axial T2 imaging (**a**) and sagittal T1 imaging (**b**) of patient with metastatic differentiated thyroid carcinoma to the right frontal lobe. Tumor was successfully resected followed by adjuvant stereotactic radiosurgery, rendering her disease-free

of metastatic disease. Intensity modulated radiotherapy, 30 Gy in 10 fractions, was administered to the resection cavity. Although serum thyroglobulin had always been undetectable, her levels of anti-thyroglobulin antibodies quickly fell to nearly undetectable as well. She experienced an uncomplicated full recovery from these events, and 2 years after treatment, she had no gross evidence remaining of metastatic tumor.

Literature Review

Brain metastases from differentiated thyroid carcinoma are uncommon, reported in up to 2% of all patients [1–5]. They are typically identified in older patients, with the median age of detection of brain metastases in these recent reports about 60 years, and the median time interval between initial cancer diagnosis and brain metastasis ranges from 4 to 10 years. Although most cases have been reported arising from papillary carcinomas, there may be a particular predisposition for the oxyphilic or Hürthle cell variant [1]. Usually, patients have had evidence of distant metastatic disease detected previously, though some patients may present with symptomatic brain metastasis at their initial diagnosis. A majority of patients are initially identified with oligometastatic brain disease, with three or fewer lesions detected by imaging [1, 3–5]. Historically, imaging to detect these lesions was triggered by symptoms; however, with the introduction of systemic therapy options for patients with distant metastases and more sensitive imaging modalities for comprehensive disease staging, up to half of patients may now be identified with brain metastases at an earlier, presymptomatic phase [3–5].

Compared with most patients with differentiated thyroid carcinoma, the prognosis of patients with brain metastases is poor. Median overall survival after the diagnosis of brain metastases has been reported as between 6 and 21 months [2–5], with almost all patients dying of complications of metastatic disease and/or treatment. Prognostic factors for prolonged survival may include age under 60 years, papillary histology, disease amenable to localized intervention such as surgical excision or stereotactic radiosurgery (which is likely to be oligometastatic), and good performance status [1–5]. Median survival for patients with Karnofsky performance status at least 70 was 31 months in one series, and for patients with WHO performance status of zero or one was 27 months in another [2, 3].

Treatment options for patients with brain metastases include surgical resection, various modalities of radiotherapy including radioactive iodine, TSH-suppressive thyroid hormone therapy, and systemic therapy. Supportive care must also be considered, particularly for patients with poor performance status and/or widespread intracranial disease [6]. Of note, there have been no randomized clinical trials specifically devoted to treatment of brain metastases from differentiated thyroid carcinoma, and thus recommendations rely primarily upon trials that included patients with various solid tumors or retrospective case series of thyroid patients (with their inherent risk for treatment bias).

Surgical excision is the traditional approach to treatment for solitary or oligometastatic brain lesions and has been associated with improved survival. In one series, median overall survival was nearly five times longer (16.7 versus 3.4 months) for patients who underwent surgical excision of one or more intracranial lesions compared with those who did not [1]. Resection may be preferred for patients whose metastatic tumors are greater than 3 cm in diameter [7]. Surgical excision can provide diagnostic information when there is uncertainty about the histologic diagnosis (e.g., patients with another primary malignancy as well as thyroid) and can be beneficial for relief of acute intracranial swelling if high-dose glucocorticoids are insufficiently effective. On the other hand, surgery requires time for recovery both before and after hospital discharge, carries a degree of risk, and may not be appropriate for patients with an expected short survival time due to rapidly progressive systemic metastases or poor performance status. Postoperative adjuvant stereotactic radiosurgery (SRS) is increasingly recommended, based on greater than 50% improvement in local recurrence-free survival in randomized studies despite lack of prolonged overall survival. Postoperative whole brain radiotherapy (WBRT) may be associated with worse neurocognitive performance than SRS [8].

SRS provides an attractive option for patients with multiple small intracerebral metastases by allowing the delivery of a highly focused radiation dose to the tumors while minimizing radiation damage to surrounding uninvolved brain tissue [7]. In one series of thyroid cancer patients, median overall survival was 37.4 months after SRS [2], and in a more recent publication, median overall survival was prolonged more than eightfold after SRS [4]. Multiple lesions can be treated simultaneously with a limited number of outpatient treatment sessions, and recovery can be rapid. SRS is most appropriate for patients with tumors up to 3 cm in diameter, minimal intracerebral shift as evidence of mass effect, and good performance status [7]. Due to the highly focused radiation dosimetry of SRS, necrosis of surrounding brain tissue is uncommon and typically asymptomatic. Like surgery, there is no evidence to support an overall survival advantage by adding WBRT after SRS for metastases from solid tumors, although intracerebral recurrence-free survival may be enhanced by the combination [7].

WBRT can be of benefit in the local control of multifocal brain metastases in patients who are not candidates for surgery or SRS [8]. A standard treatment approach to deliver 3000 cGy in ten fractions is commonly employed. Studies in other solid tumors have failed to demonstrate a significant advantage to the use of altered dosing strategies or concomitant radiosensitizers [6]. Combining WBRT with subsequent SRS or using WBRT following either surgery or SRS has been associated with improved intracerebral recurrence-free survival, but overall survival has not been improved in multiple trials for either oligometastatic or widely metastatic disease [6, 9]. Unfortunately, eventual development of broad cognitive decline has been associated with WBRT, limiting the benefit of this intervention in patients anticipated to have longer survival.

Radioiodine has a potential role unique to treating metastases from differentiated thyroid carcinoma. In one report, only 17% of patients scanned with radioiodine had visible uptake concentrated in a brain metastasis, which may be expected given the older age of these patients and their advanced disease [1]. In those cases, surgical resection combined with high administered activities of radioiodine was employed successfully for intracerebral disease control. The use of exogenous recombinant human TSH to stimulate radioiodine uptake instead of endogenous TSH elevation following thyroid hormone withdrawal may be theoretically preferable to minimize the period of excessive thyrotropin stimulation to tumor growth [1]. Dexamethasone should also be given prophylactically to minimize risk for peritumoral edema or hemorrhage following recombinant human TSH or therapy with radioiodine [1].

Systemic therapy with kinase inhibitors and immunotherapy have significantly improved outcomes of some patients with brain metastases, such as those with melanoma, but reports for thyroid carcinoma patients are limited [8, 10]. In one retrospective series of patients with brain metastases from differentiated thyroid carcinoma, 12 were treated with various tyrosine kinase inhibitors, often in addition to local therapy [4]. Overall survival was fivefold longer in patients treated with a kinase inhibitor regimen compared with those without any systemic therapy, but multivariate analysis was not performed to try to isolate the effect of the systemic therapy itself. Newer agents such as mutation-selective inhibitors selpercatinib and dabrafenib appear to be effective in brain metastases from RET-fusion lung carcinoma and BRAF-mutated melanoma, respectively, and may have a role in differentiated thyroid cancer patients whose tumors bear those mutations as well.

High-dose glucocorticoids may be helpful in the control of cerebral edema that often accompanies brain metastases from solid malignancies. In the presence of neurologic symptoms but without impending herniation, starting doses of dexamethasone of 4 or 8 mg daily followed by rapid tapering appear to provide optimal symptomatic relief while minimizing Cushingoid toxicities associated with higher doses [8]. Conversely, in the setting of severe neurologic compromise or risk for herniation, higher daily doses of dexamethasone may be warranted. It is reasonable to use thyroid hormone to suppress TSH levels, given the stimulatory effect reported from high levels of TSH on tumor growth, but data are lacking regarding actual efficacy of this approach. Anti-seizure medications are warranted in the presence of seizure activity or in the immediate postoperative period, but have not been shown to be of value when given prophylactically.

Management of the Case

The patient presented decades after her initial treatment for thyroid carcinoma with a symptomatic, solitary brain metastasis in the absence of any other site of distant disease. Despite comorbidities, her good performance status suggested that she would benefit from aggressive local therapy. Surgical resection was followed by adjuvant radiotherapy to try to reduce the likelihood of recurrence in the surgical cavity. Although prolonged anti-seizure medication would not typically be recommended, her acute need for anticoagulation for deep venous thrombosis and pulmonary emboli necessitated caution to minimize risk of further neurologic complication. Fortunately, she fully recovered without sequelae and remains without evidence of disease more than 2 years from presentation with solitary metastasis.

Clinical Pearls

- Brain metastases are an uncommon, late event in differentiated thyroid carcinoma.
- Prognosis is poor, similar to other solid tumors that metastasize to the brain.
- Selected patients with oligometastatic disease and good performance status may benefit from either surgical excision or SRS.
- Radioiodine uptake occasionally permits additional intervention with this modality.
- Supportive care with judiciously administered dexamethasone can help provide symptomatic relief while minimizing symptoms of glucocorticoid excess.
- Future studies are required to evaluate the role of systemic therapy options for brain metastases from thyroid carcinoma.

References

1. Chiu AC, Delpassand ES, Sherman SI. Prognosis and treatment of brain metastases in thyroid carcinoma. J Clin Endocrinol Metab. 1997;82(11):3637–42.
2. Bernad DM, Sperduto PW, Souhami L, Jensen AW, Roberge D. Stereotactic radiosurgery in the management of brain metastases from primary thyroid cancers. J Neurooncol. 2010;98(2):249–52.
3. Henriques de Figueiredo B, Godbert Y, Soubeyran I, Carrat X, Lagarde P, Cazeau AL, et al. Brain metastases from thyroid carcinoma: a retrospective study of 21 patients. Thyroid. 2014;24(2):270–6.
4. Gomes-Lima CJ, Wu D, Rao SN, Punukollu S, Hritani R, Zeymo A, et al. Brain metastases from differentiated thyroid carcinoma: prevalence, current therapies, and outcomes. J Endocr Soc. 2019;3(2):359–71.
5. Choi J, Kim JW, Keum YS, Lee IJ. The largest known survival analysis of patients with brain metastasis from thyroid cancer based on prognostic groups. PLoS One. 2016;11(4):e0154739.
6. Tsao MN, Lloyd N, Wong R, Chow E, Rakovitch E, Laperriere N. Whole brain radiotherapy for the treatment of multiple brain metastases. Cochrane Database Syst Rev. 2006;(3):CD003869.
7. Linskey M, Andrews D, Asher A, Burri S, Kondziolka D, Robinson P, et al. The role of stereotactic radiosurgery in the management of patients with newly diagnosed brain metastases: a systematic review and evidence-based clinical practice guideline. Journal of Neuro-Oncology. 2010;96(1):45–68.
8. Moravan MJ, Fecci PE, Anders CK, Clarke JM, Salama AKS, Adamson JD, et al. Current multidisciplinary management of brain metastases. Cancer. 2020;126(7):1390–406.
9. Gaspar L, Mehta M, Patchell R, Burri S, Robinson P, Morris R, et al. The role of whole brain radiation therapy in the management of newly diagnosed brain metastases: a systematic review and evidence-based clinical practice guideline. Journal of Neuro-Oncology. 2010;96(1):17–32.
10. Soffietti R, Trevisan E, Ruda R. Targeted therapy in brain metastasis. Curr Opin Oncol. 2012;24(6):679–86.

Chapter 33
RAI-Refractory, Advanced Differentiated Thyroid Cancer Receiving Kinase Inhibitor Treatment: Checking for Drug-Drug Interactions

Steven I. Sherman

Case Presentation

A 67-year-old man presented to his local emergency room with complaints of lightheadedness and an intermittently irregular heart rhythm, without chest pain or shortness of breath. His past medical history was notable for diagnosis of papillary thyroid carcinoma 5 years previously, treated initially with total thyroidectomy, bilateral modified neck dissection, and adjuvant radioiodine. His post-therapy scan showed minimal uptake in the neck, but a TSH-stimulated thyroglobulin level of 524 ng/mL had subsequently prompted tomographic imaging that revealed bilateral lung lesions compatible with metastatic thyroid carcinoma. With progressive radiographic enlargement over the succeeding 12 months, and repeat radioiodine imaging that was negative, he was started on oral therapy with sorafenib for radioiodine-refractory progressive metastases. He initially responded well, but with subsequent progression, his therapy was switched 14 months prior to this emergency room visit to sunitinib. Treatment was complicated by adverse events, including hypertension, diarrhea, and hypomagnesemia. Two weeks before his emergency room visit, he presented to his local primary care physician with acute bronchitis, and antibiotic therapy with clarithromycin was initiated. He returned to his physician 4 days later complaining of worsening diarrhea and was found to have a blood pressure of 170/100 mm Hg and a pulse of 96 beats per minute. Verapamil was added to his chronic valsartan therapy, along with an increase in his dosing of diphenoxylate/atropine for his diarrhea. On examination in the emergency room, his pulse was 52 beats per minute and blood pressure 126/62 mm Hg. An electrocardiogram revealed sinus bradycardia, with a prolonged QT_c of 520 msec. His serum magnesium level was low, 0.9 mg/dL. While preparing an intravenous magnesium infusion, his heart rate was noted to increase acutely to 140 beats per minute, and a

S. I. Sherman (✉)
University of Texas M.D. Anderson Cancer Center, Houston, TX, USA
e-mail: sisherma@mdanderson.org

G. Grani et al. (eds.), *Thyroid Cancer*,
https://doi.org/10.1007/978-3-030-61919-0_33

transient episode of torsades de pointes was identified on his cardiac monitoring. An infusion of magnesium, 16 meq, was initiated, and subsequent monitoring demonstrated improvement in the QT_c to 470 msec and resolution of his tachyarrhythmia to baseline sinus bradycardia.

Literature Review

Most available KIs used for treating thyroid carcinoma are dosed once or twice per day, with long half-lives that facilitate such dosing schedules [3]. With slow metabolic clearance, often active metabolites and narrow therapeutic windows, the blood concentration of KIs can be significantly altered by other agents that interact with the enzymes metabolizing their clearance, thus potentially contributing to concentration-related toxicities. Most KIs are primarily metabolized through hepatic cytochrome P450s, such as CYP3A4 or CYP2C8, and by UDP-glucuronosyltransferases [3]. Thus, drugs that activate one of these enzymes might reduce the therapeutic effectiveness of a KI by enhancing its metabolic clearance, whereas drugs that inhibit the metabolic enzyme might be anticipated to increase susceptibility to toxic side effects. On the other hand, gastric acid suppressants, which commonly reduce enteric absorption of many oral therapies, have minor effects on absorption and drug levels for the KIs used commonly for thyroid carcinoma. Further, some KIs carry the potential to inhibit other drug metabolizing enzymes, thus introducing the potential for the KI to interfere with metabolism of other therapies. Finally, occasionally combining a KI with another drug with similar toxicity can yield pharmacodynamic interaction that intensifies the risk for that particular side effect even if neither drug by itself would be considered toxic.

The potential to prolong the QT interval and increase risk for torsades de pointes has been a key focus for studies of drug-drug interactions for multitargeted KIs relevant to thyroid carcinoma [4]. The interval, defined as the time between the beginning of the QRS complex and the end of the T wave, is highly sensitive to inhibition of the myocyte potassium channel associated with human ether-a-go-go (hERG) that mediates ventricular repolarization during phase II–III of the action potential [5]. No single mechanism has emerged to explain the ability of multitargeted KIs to inhibit the hERG, and it appears to vary among the different KIs themselves. However, alterations in the function of numerous intracellular protein kinases including PI3K, AKT, and protein kinase A that function downstream from the tyrosine kinases affected by KIs have all been implicated to contribute [5]. Electrolyte abnormalities, such as hypokalemia and hypomagnesemia which can commonly result from KI-induced diarrhea, may also independently contribute to a risk of QT prolongation and torsades de pointes.

The magnitude of the effect of KIs on significant QT prolongation was evaluated in a trial-level meta-analysis of placebo-controlled studies that included EKG monitoring while on therapy with any of the following drugs: sunitinib, sorafenib, pazopanib, axitinib, vandetanib, cabozantinib, ponatinib, and regorafenib; note that all of the first six drugs have been formally studied in phase II or phase III trials in radioiodine-refractory differentiated thyroid cancer, and sorafenib is FDA-approved for treating thyroid cancer [4]. More than 4% of patients experienced any grade of prolongation of the QT interval during therapy with a multitargeted KI, in contrast with 0.25% for those untreated, and high-grade prolongation was 2.7-fold more likely in the KI-treated patients. The risks were highest for patients treated with sunitinib or vandetanib, and importantly a significant correlation was noted between drug dosing and frequency of QT prolongation.

The dose-response effect on QT intervals suggests that the risk for pro-arrhythmic adverse effect from the KI can be enhanced by concomitant drugs that increase KI levels by inhibiting KI metabolism though CYP3A4. Unfortunately, many drugs that might be used during supportive care of oncology patients have the potential to inhibit CYP3A4, including macrolide and azole antibiotics and calcium-channel blockers. Ketoconazole, for example, increases plasma levels of sunitinib by 51%, which could be expected to have a major effect on the QT interval, whereas the effect on sorafenib concentrations is only 11% [3, 6].

An alternative concern results from concomitant use of drugs that stimulate CYP3A4 activity, thereby accelerating the clearance of KIs and potentially reducing their oncologic effectiveness. For example, rifampin, a potent inducer of CYP3A4, reduces sunitinib plasma levels by nearly 50%, but the impact on lenvatinib levels is negligible [3, 7]. Complementary and alternative medicines may also interact. Both St. John's wort (*Hypericum perforatum*) and *Echinacea*, which are available as over-the-counter medicinal herbs, induce CYP3A4 and have been implicated in altering KI pharmacokinetics [6].

Overall, lenvatinib and sorafenib, both FDA-approved for treatment of radioiodine-refractory differentiated thyroid carcinoma, are thought to have only minor risk for drug-drug interactions due to alteration of KI metabolism. Strong inhibitors or inducers of CYP3A4 or CYP2C8 should be avoided, however, in patients treated with less commonly used KIs for this disease, such as cabozantinib, cobimetinib, dabrafenib, pazopanib, sunitinib, or vandetanib; KI dose reduction should be empirically considered if strong cytochrome inhibitors are required [3].

Less commonly, KIs themselves create drug-drug interactions that alter the effectiveness of other medications. Most relevant to patients with thyroid carcinoma is the common effect of all KIs to contribute to rising TSH levels [2]. Although some KIs, most notably sunitinib, cause hypothyroidism when used to treat other malignancies in patients with baseline normal thyroid function, the mechanism of this effect likely differs in postthyroidectomy patients. Inadequate thyroid hormone absorption and accelerated thyroid hormone metabolism are likely to contribute to loss of TSH suppression in thyroid carcinoma patients treated with multitargeted KIs like lenvatinib or sorafenib, necessitating careful monitoring of TSH levels and frequent increases in hormone dosing [1]. A similar effect of KIs is postulated to contribute to a need for increased vitamin D dosing in postthyroidectomy patients with decreased parathyroid function or frank hypoparathyroidism [1]. Non-cytochrome mediated pathways of drug clearance can secondarily be affected by KIs, altering drug exposure of other medications and predisposing to drug toxicity.

For example, sorafenib partially inhibits several UDP-glucuronosyltransferases (such as UGT1A9 and UGT1A1), which can lead to slower clearance of acetaminophen and increased risk for hepatotoxicity [6].

The frequency of coadministration of medications that could lead to drug-drug interactions is surprisingly high. In one study of patients treated with KIs at the Mayo Clinic, the rate of coadministration of medications that could increase KI-induced toxicity ranged from 25% for sunitinib to 75% for pazopanib [8]. In a second study in renal cell carcinoma, 47% of sunitinib-treated patients were coadministered medications that would inhibit CYP3A4 and potentiate sunitinib concentration-dependent toxicities [9]. Unfortunately, the widespread use of electronic health records has had only a modest effect on reducing hospital-based risk for drug-drug interactions.

With the plethora of possible drug-drug interactions that could increase KI drug levels and risk for KI-induced toxicities, or otherwise alter the effectiveness or tolerance of KI therapy for metastatic thyroid carcinoma, it is imperative that a patient's medications be reconciled at multiple key points in their clinical care to identify potential problems that could emerge [1]. At baseline, before a patient is initiated on KI therapy, the clinician should review and reconcile the medication list including all over-the-counter nonprescription drugs as well as complementary or alternative medications that the patient may be obtaining from other sources. If potential drug-drug interactions are identified, the clinician can proactively change one of the offending medications or alter drug dosing so as to minimize the impact of the anticipated interaction. Similarly, such medication reconciliation should take place whenever a new concomitant drug is added to the patient's therapies. The difficulty, as demonstrated in this case, is that multiple providers may all be involved in the patient's care, introducing greater risk from polypharmacy and the potential for drug-drug interactions. Thus, there is also a need for thorough communication among all providers for the patient, such that awareness of all medications being prescribed is universal. Perhaps most critical, the patient must be educated and reminded by the provider team prescribing the KI of the risk for drug-drug interactions and of the importance of medication review by each prescribing provider to minimize that risk. This should certainly be a component of the initial informed consent process prior to starting a KI, as well as a part of each subsequent follow-up visit [1].

Several tools are available online that simplify the ability to screen for significant drug-drug interactions, in addition to those that exist within electronic health record and medication prescribing software. The risk for life-threatening arrhythmia due to QT interval prolongation can be assessed using the website http://crediblemeds.org/healthcare-providers/drug-drug-interaction/, which provides the most up-to-date and well-annotated summary of information. For more general information and to search for other types of interactions, websites such as http://www.webmd.com/interaction-checker/default.htm and http://healthinfo.uclahealth.org/Library/DrugReference/DrugInteraction/ provide useful information, including interactions with commonly used herbal and over-the-counter supplements. Apps for mobile devices have also become available, including a powerful interaction checker in the commonly used app Epocrates.

Management of the Case

The patient experienced a combination of events that led to heightened risk for cardiac arrhythmia. In addition to the potential for QT prolongation by sunitinib, the patient developed significant electrolyte loss due to drug-induced diarrhea. With the onset of bronchitis, he was given clarithromycin, a recognized inhibitor of CYP3A4, which likely led to increased sunitinib concentrations. Regardless of whether the worsening diarrhea was secondary to higher sunitinib levels or was antibiotic induced, his electrolyte loss worsened, and he developed even greater risk for QT prolongation due to severe hypomagnesemia. Exacerbation of hypertension led to addition of a calcium-channel antagonist that likely altered the QT interval even further, eventually leading to a typical acquired torsades de pointes that fortunately was self-limited and did not degenerate into ventricular tachycardia or fibrillation. By treating the hypomagnesemia, the acute risk was averted, and gradual clearance of the interacting medications allowed eventual restoration of sunitinib therapy.

Clinical Pearls

- Drug-drug interactions are common with the use of KI therapy.
- Interactions can markedly increase risk for drug toxicity, particularly life-threatening complications such as torsades de pointes and other cardiac arrhythmias.
- Loss of KI efficacy and alteration in the effectiveness and toxicities of other concomitant medications can also result from unanticipated drug-drug interactions, including effect on levothyroxine and vitamin D therapy.
- All involved providers and most critically the patient must be made aware of the risk for drug-drug interactions throughout the course of KI therapy.

References

1. Carhill AA, Cabanillas ME, Jimenez C, Waguespack SG, Habra MA, Hu M, et al. The non-investigational use of tyrosine kinase inhibitors in thyroid cancer: establishing a standard for patient safety and monitoring. J Clin Endocrinol Metab. 2013;98(1):31–42.
2. Cabanillas ME, Ryder M, Jimenez C. Targeted therapy for advanced thyroid cancer: kinase inhibitors and beyond. Endocr Rev. 2019;40(6):1573–604.
3. Hussaarts K, Veerman GDM, Jansman FGA, van Gelder T, Mathijssen RHJ, van Leeuwen RWF. Clinically relevant drug interactions with multikinase inhibitors: a review. Ther Adv Med Oncol. 2019;11:1758835918818347.
4. Ghatalia P, Je Y, Kaymakcalan MD, Sonpavde G, Choueiri TK. QTc interval prolongation with vascular endothelial growth factor receptor tyrosine kinase inhibitors. Br J Cancer. 2015;112:296–305.
5. Shah RR, Morganroth J, Shah DR. Cardiovascular safety of tyrosine kinase inhibitors: with a special focus on cardiac repolarisation (QT interval). Drug Saf. 2013;36(5):295–316.

6. Thomas-Schoemann A, Blanchet B, Bardin C, Noe G, Boudou-Rouquette P, Vidal M, et al. Drug interactions with solid tumour-targeted therapies. Crit Rev Oncol Hematol. 2014;89(1):179–96.
7. van Erp NP, Gelderblom H, Guchelaar HJ. Clinical pharmacokinetics of tyrosine kinase inhibitors. Cancer Treat Rev. 2009;35(8):692–706.
8. Bowlin SJ, Xia F, Wang W, Robinson KD, Stanek EJ. Twelve-month frequency of drug-metabolizing enzyme and transporter-based drug-drug interaction potential in patients receiving oral enzyme-targeted kinase inhibitor antineoplastic agents. Mayo Clin Proc. 2013;88(2):139–48.
9. Kruse V, Somers A, Van Bortel L, De Both A, Van Belle S, Rottey S. Sunitinib for metastatic renal cell cancer patients: observational study highlighting the risk of important drug-drug interactions. J Clin Pharm Ther. 2014;39(3):259–65.

Part VI
Medullary Thyroid Cancer

Chapter 34
Management of Postoperative Hypercalcitoninemia in Medullary Thyroid Carcinoma

Douglas W. Ball

Abbreviations

DOTATATE	DOTA-(Tyr^3)-octreotate
MEN 2	Multiple endocrine neoplasia type 2
MTC	Medullary thyroid cancer
RET	Oncogene, rearranged during transfection
SEER	Surveillance, Epidemiology, and End Results

Case Presentation

A 25-year-old man noted a painless left neck mass. CT of the neck showed left cervical adenopathy. On thyroid ultrasound, the left lobe was largely replaced by a 5 cm lobulated mass. Neck ultrasound showed sonographically suspicious left level 3 and 4 nodes measuring up to 5.2 cm, with smaller bilateral level 6 nodes. FNA of the thyroid mass, left level 3 node, and a left level 6 node were all positive for medullary thyroid cancer. Preoperative calcitonin was 9203 pg/mL and CEA 85.1 ng/mL. In addition to the neck mass, the patient also noted significant diarrhea. Plasma metanephrines, calcium, and PTH were normal. Family history was negative for MTC and tumors related to MEN 2. Germline RET gene testing was negative for exons 10, 11, and 13–16. CT of the chest abdomen and pelvis, including an arterial phase contrast liver examination, showed a 2.5 cm left paratracheal node in low left level 6. The lungs, liver, adrenals, and the visualized skeleton were normal.

D. W. Ball (✉)
Division of Endocrinology, Diabetes, and Metabolism, and Department of Oncology, Johns Hopkins University School of Medicine, Baltimore, MD, USA
e-mail: dball@jhmi.edu

G. Grani et al. (eds.), *Thyroid Cancer*,
https://doi.org/10.1007/978-3-030-61919-0_34

He underwent total thyroidectomy, bilateral central neck dissection, and left modified neck dissection including levels 2–5. Surgical pathology showed a 3.8 cm focus of medullary thyroid cancer in the left lobe and a smaller 3 mm focus in the isthmus. Anterior and posterior surgical margins were focally positive. Altogether, 19 of 47 lymph nodes were positive for MTC, including a 4.5 cm left level 6 node and a 5.5 cm left level 3 node. Extranodal extension was not definitively seen. RET mutation analysis of tumor DNA revealed the high-risk M918T allele.

The postoperative calcitonin nadir was 114 pg/mL and CEA nadir was 2.0 ng/mL, and the diarrhea resolved. Follow-up measurements every 3 months showed a calculated calcitonin doubling time of 3.0 months. Five months after surgery, his diarrhea recurred. Fifteen months after surgery, Ga^{68}-DOTATATE PET-CT showed abnormal uptake in left level 2A and left paratracheal nodes. He underwent resection of a 1.2 cm L level 2A and 4 mm left paratracheal node, accessed through the neck. His calcitonin continued to rise to over 3600 pg/mL, 2 years after the initial surgery. Repeat Ga^{68}-DOTATATE PET-CT showed an increased number of paratracheal mediastinal nodes. After median sternotomy, level 7 resection showed two of six nodes positive, the largest focus 7 mm. A liver wedge biopsy and thymectomy performed during that procedure were negative for malignancy.

Postoperatively the calcitonin was 6422 pg/mL and CEA 9.3 ng/mL. He felt well except for ongoing diarrhea despite maximal doses of loperamide. Repeat CT imaging showed a growing left upper paratracheal nodal mass, now 2.6 cm. Small lung nodules up to 3 mm were newly noted. Based on inoperable progressive MTC and a pathogenic RET mutation, he was referred to a clinical trial of a highly selective RET inhibitor, Loxo292, now known as selpercatinib (Retevmo®). On 160 mg twice daily, his calcitonin progressively fell to <2 pg/mL at his latest follow-up, 17 months after initiation. CT of the chest showed stable subcentimeter paratracheal nodularity, likely representing treated lymph nodes.

Assessment and Literature Review

This patient presented with locally extensive, nonfamilial MTC at age 25. Despite aggressive surgical management, he had local neck recurrences and difficult-to-manage paratracheal nodes above and below the thoracic inlet.

Medullary thyroid cancer accounts for only 1–3% of thyroid cancers. MTC derives from calcitonin-producing parafollicular C-cells. Although older literature proposed a neural crest origin for C-cells, a more contemporary lineage-tracing study conclusively showed derivation from foregut endoderm [1]. Twenty-five percent of MTC cases are familial, stemming from germline RET gene mutations. Inherited disease was initially suspected in this patient but germline RET testing was negative. Tumoral (somatic) RET mutation is present in ~40% of nonfamilial patients [2]. Mutations in RAS genes are seen in ~30% of the remaining sporadic tumors [3].

Clinical presentations of MTC are heterogeneous. Cervical lymph node metastases are identified in 25–82% of patients [4–6]. Distant metastases are detectable at presentation in approximately 15% of patients and are rare when the preoperative calcitonin is less than 500 pg/mL [7]. The principal metastatic sites are the lung, liver, and bone. Liver and bone metastases may be challenging to detect with conventional imaging. Symptomatic presentations with diarrhea or flushing are seen in patients with advanced disease.

Postoperative Staging of MTC Patients

TNM staging of MTC is illustrated in the accompanying box. In general, MTC staging resembles differentiated thyroid cancer (DTC) staging of patients over 55 years old. Younger age in MTC does not carry the marked prognostic advantage seen in cases of DTC.

From a practical perspective, the postoperative calcitonin and CEA levels are very important. Surgically cured individuals have an undetectable basal calcitonin (and pentagastrin-stimulated calcitonin, if performed). Persistently detectable calcitonin levels, even in the normal range for an individual with an intact thyroid, indicate persistent disease. Our practice, consistent with ATA guidelines, is to follow individuals with low-level postoperative calcitonin elevations with neck ultrasound [8]. Calcitonin levels greater than 150 pg/mL prompt cross-sectional imaging. Giraudet et al. proposed an imaging set including neck ultrasound, CT of the chest, and liver MRI or arterial phase CT, plus skeletal imaging [9]. In patients with advanced MTC, bone metastases are very common. MRI of the axial skeleton (with arterial phase contrast) and or DOTATATE PET-CT are relatively effective means of detecting these sites [9, 10]. Early detection of liver metastases remains an unmet clinical need.

Prognosis of Postoperative Patients

Overall 10-year disease-specific survival in MTC patients is approximately 75% [11]. Key prognostic features include TNM stage, calcitonin doubling time, and somatic RET mutation status. For stage I, II, III, and IV, the 10-year disease-specific survival is 100%, 93%, 71%, and 21%, respectively [12]. In US SEER (Surveillance, Epidemiology, and End Results) data, the 10-year survival for patients with distant metastases at the time of diagnosis is 40% [13]. These results predate effective oral chemotherapy for MTC. Subtotal thyroidectomy or no thyroid surgery versus total thyroidectomy has also been associated with decreased survival [13].

Box: TNM Classification of MTC (American Joint Committee on Cancer)

Primary tumor (T)

- *T0*—No evidence of primary tumor
- *T1*—Tumor 2 cm or less in greatest dimension limited to the thyroid (T1a, tumor 1 cm or less; T1b, tumor more than 1 cm but not more than 2 cm)
- *T2*—Tumor more than 2 cm, but not more than 4 cm, in greatest dimension limited to the thyroid
- *T3*—Tumor more than 4 cm in greatest dimension limited to the thyroid or any tumor with minimal extrathyroidal extension (e.g., extension to sternothyroid muscle or perithyroid soft tissues)
- *T4a*—Tumor of any size extending beyond the thyroid capsule to invade subcutaneous soft tissues, larynx, trachea, esophagus, or recurrent laryngeal nerve
- *T4b*—Tumor invades prevertebral fascia or encases carotid artery or mediastinal vessels

*Regional lymph nodes (N)**

- *NX*—Regional lymph nodes cannot be assessed
- *N0*—No regional lymph node metastases
- *N1*—Regional lymph node metastases
  - *N1a*—Metastasis to level VI (pretracheal, paratracheal, and prelaryngeal/delphian lymph nodes)
  - *N1b*—Metastasis to unilateral, bilateral, or contralateral cervical or superior mediastinal lymph nodes

*Central compartment, lateral cervical and upper mediastinal lymph nodes

Distant metastases (M)

- *MX*—Distant metastasis cannot be assessed
- *M0*—No distant metastasis
- *M1*—Distant metastasis

Stage

Stage I: T1, N0, M0

- *Stage II*: T2, N0, M0
- *Stage III*: T3, N0, M0 T1, N1a, M0T2, N1a, M0T3, N1a, M0
- *Stage IVA*: T4a, N0, M0T4a, N1a, M0T1, N1b, M0T2, N1b, M0T3, N1b, M0T4a, N1b, M0
- *Stage IVB*: T4b, any N, M0
- *Stage IVC*: Any T, any N, M1

Calcitonin doubling time has an important impact on survival and is an especially useful indicator in the first year following surgery [14]. In the study of Barbet et al., calcitonin doubling time provided prognostic information that complimented tumor stage, allowing identification of higher-risk stage III patients similar to this case. Patients with calcitonin doubling time less than 6 months had a median survival of only 2.5 years. In contrast, no disease-related deaths were recorded in the patient cohort with a doubling time greater than 2 years [14]. Measurement of calcitonin (and CEA) at 3-month intervals over the first postoperative year is useful to detect higher-risk individuals.

In the context of nonfamilial MTC, tumoral or somatic mutations in the RET gene are an important prognostic marker. Elisei and colleagues identified somatic RET mutations in 43% of sporadic cases. Seventy-nine percent of these were RET M918T, similar to this case. RET mutation correlated with persistent calcitonin elevation, nodal and distant metastases, and worsened overall survival. Fifty-six percent of mutation-negative patients were free of disease at follow-up vs. 17% mutation-positive patients [2]. Patients with tumoral RET mutations need to undergo germline RET mutation testing (if not already done) to make sure the mutation is not a heritable germline finding.

Treatment

Initial Surgical Approach to Patients with Clinically Apparent MTC

Standard surgical management of MTC includes total thyroidectomy and a variable degree of lymph node dissection. Exclusion of pheochromocytoma and hyperparathyroidism is mandatory prior to MTC surgery. Patients with associated pheochromocytoma should undergo appropriate adrenal surgery prior to neck surgery.

The optimal extent of lymph node dissection in MTC patients is controversial. Current American Thyroid Association guidelines recommend bilateral central neck dissection as the typical baseline operation, with therapeutic lateral neck dissection as directed by preoperative neck ultrasound and FNA [8]. A minority of panelists recommended prophylactic ipsilateral neck dissection. The argument in favor of prophylactic neck dissection is fueled by the significant correlation between central and lateral compartment involvement [7]. Against prophylactic lateral neck dissection is the observation that even bilateral central and lateral dissections rarely lead to surgical cure when >5 affected nodes are present. The majority of surgically cured patients have zero affected nodes [7]. Patients with substantial preoperative calcitonin burdens have strong suspicion for distant metastases and should have preoperative imaging that assesses the chest, liver, and the axial skeleton.

Surgical Approach to Patients with Persistent or Recurrent MTC

The majority of patients with persistent calcitonin elevations after initial surgery are asymptomatic. A watchful-waiting approach may be justified in asymptomatic patients in the absence of high volume or progressive metastatic disease. Palliative repeat neck surgery is sometimes warranted, in order to forestall complications such as tracheal invasion, recurrent laryngeal nerve injury, or neck pain. Repeat neck surgery with curative intent has a more limited role. Moley and colleagues reported a 38% chance of undetectable postoperative calcitonin after second surgery in a selected series of patients [15]. A significant fraction of these patients did have recurrent calcitonin elevation at a later point. Other series have pointed to lower rates of calcitonin undetectability following reoperation with curative intent [16]. The role of adjuvant external beam radiation after initial or repeat surgery is uncertain. An older series from the University of Toronto suggested improved locoregional control without impact on overall survival, in patients selected to have highest risk of local recurrence [17]. Indeed, patients selected for external beam radiation had adverse prognosis in the SEER population [13]. External beam radiation often makes subsequent surgery challenging, with a higher risk of complications.

Role of Somatic RET Mutation Testing in Selection of Patients for Targeted Oral Chemotherapy

The 2015 American Thyroid Association guidelines recommended germline RET mutation testing in the majority of family history negative cases while recommending neither for or against somatic RET mutation testing [8]. Arguments in favor of somatic RET testing include (1) prognostic information cited above, (2) predictive information for likelihood of response to approved multikinase inhibitors vandetanib and cabozantinib, and (3) eligibility for treatment with second-generation highly selective RET inhibitors such as selpercatinib. Both vandetanib and cabozantinib achieve higher partial response rates and improved progression-free survival rates in patients bearing a RET M918T mutation [18, 19]. In the case of cabozantinib, this tumor genotype was the only one to clearly show improved overall survival compared with assignment to placebo [20]. In the phase III vandetanib trial, a provision for patient crossover from placebo to active drug at progression probably hindered the detection of any impact of genotype on overall survival.

Selpercatinib is a highly selective RET inhibitor studied in the LIBRETTO-001 phase I/II trial in RET-mutated MTC, RET-rearranged DTC, and RET-rearranged lung cancer. Favorable efficacy and tolerability data from this study led to FDA approval in May 2020 for three indications including adult and pediatric patients $\geq$12 years of age with advanced or metastatic RET-mutant medullary thyroid cancer (MTC) who require systemic therapy.

Management of the Case

Striking features of this case include the locally extensive disease, the relatively young age despite negative germline testing, the aggressive local recurrence, and rapidly rising calcitonin despite aggressive surgical management. The availability of the selpercatinib clinical trial allowed a dramatic improvement in his imaging and tumor markers with excellent drug toleration.

Clinical Pearls

- MTC prognosis depends on tumor stage, calcitonin doubling time, and RET mutation status.
- A rapid calcitonin doubling time is an important adverse prognostic indicator even in patients with stage III disease or with a relatively favorable post-op calcitonin nadir level.
- Somatic RET mutation testing in nonfamilial patients who are not surgically cured can be a highly useful prognostic and predictive marker.
- Highly selective RET inhibitors offer a promising approach to inoperable and metastatic RET-mutant MTC.

References

1. Johansson E, Andersson L, Ornros J, et al. Revising the embryonic origin of thyroid C cells in mice and humans. Development. 2015;142:3519–28.
2. Elisei R, Cosci B, Romei C, et al. Mutations in sporadic medullary thyroid cancer: a 10-year follow-up study. J Clin Endocrinol Metab. 2008;93:682–7.
3. Agrawal N, Jiao Y, Sausen M, et al. Exomic sequencing of medullary thyroid cancer reveals dominant and mutually exclusive oncogenic mutations in RET and RAS. J Clin Endocrinol Metab. 2013;98:E364–9.
4. Raue F, Kotzerke J, Reinwein D, et al. Prognostic factors in medullary thyroid carcinoma: evaluation of 741 patients from the German medullary thyroid carcinoma register. Clin Investig. 1993;71:7–12.
5. Rossi RL, Cady B, Meissner WA, et al. Non familial medullary thyroid carcinoma. Am J Surg. 1980;139:554–60.
6. Moley JF, De Benedetti MK. Patterns of nodal metastases in palpable medullary thyroid carcinoma: recommendations for extent of node dissection. Ann Surg. 1999;229:880–7.
7. Machens A, Dralle H. Biomarker-based risk stratification for previously untreated medullary thyroid cancer. J Clin Endocrinol Metab. 2010;95:2655–63.
8. Wells SA Jr, Asa SL, Dralle H, et al. Revised American Thyroid Association guidelines for the management of medullary thyroid carcinoma. Thyroid. 2015;25:567–610.
9. Giraudet AL, Vanel D, Leboulleux S, et al. Imaging medullary thyroid carcinoma with persistent elevated calcitonin levels. J Clin Endocrinol Metab. 2007;92:4185–90.
10. Castroneves LA, Coura Filho G, de Freitas RMC, et al. Comparison of 68Ga PET/CT to other imaging studies in medullary thyroid cancer: superiority in detecting bone metastases. J Clin Endocrinol Metab. 2018;103:3250–9.

11. Hundahl SA, Fleming ID, Fremgen AM, Menck HR. A National Cancer Data Base report on 53,856 cases of thyroid carcinoma treated in the U.S., 1985–1995. Cancer. 1998;83:2638–48.
12. Modigliani E, Cohen R, Campos JM, et al. Prognostic factors for survival and for biochemical cure in medullary thyroid carcinoma: results in 899 patients. The GETC Study Group. Clin Endocrinol (Oxf). 1998;48:265–73.
13. Roman S, Lin R, Sosa JA. Prognosis of medullary thyroid carcinoma: demographic, clinical, and pathologic predictors of survival in 1252 cases. Cancer. 2006;107(9):2134–42.
14. Barbet J, Campion L, Kraeber-Bodéré F, Chatal JF, GTE Study Group. Prognostic impact of serum calcitonin and carcinoembryonic antigen doubling-times in patients with medullary thyroid carcinoma. J Clin Endocrinol Metab. 2005;90(11):6077–84.
15. Fialkowski E, DeBenedetti M, Moley J. Long-term outcome of reoperations for medullary thyroid carcinoma. World J Surg. 2008;32(5):754–65.
16. Kebebew E, Kikuchi S, Duh QY, Clark OH. Longterm results of reoperation and localizing studies in patients with persistent or recurrent medullary thyroid cancer. Arch Surg. 2000;135:895–901.
17. Brierley J, Tsang R, Simpson WJ, et al. Medullary thyroid cancer: analyses of survival and prognostic factors and the role of radiation therapy in local control. Thyroid. 1996;6:305–10.
18. Wells SA Jr, Robinson BG, Gagel RF, et al. Vandetanib in patients with locally advanced or metastatic medullary thyroid cancer: a randomized, double-blind phase III trial. J Clin Oncol. 2012;30:134–41.
19. Elisei R, Schlumberger MJ, Müller SP, et al. Cabozantinib in progressive medullary thyroid cancer. J Clin Oncol. 2013;31:3639–46.
20. Schlumberger M, Elisei R, Müller S, et al. Overall survival analysis of EXAM, a phase III trial of cabozantinib in patients with radiographically progressive medullary thyroid carcinoma. Ann Oncol. 2017;28:2813–9.

Chapter 35
Tumor Related- and Non-tumor-Related Diarrhea in a Medullary Thyroid Cancer Patient

Rosa Falcone, Valeria Ramundo, and Giorgio Grani

Case Presentation

A 37-year-old man presented to the emergency department with a 1-month history of dysphonia and a painful, progressively enlarging neck mass. He had no relevant previous medical or family history, except for a 2-year history of chronic diarrhea with three to four loose, watery stools per day, without mucus or blood. The frequency of the diarrhea had recently increased. He denied nausea, vomiting, or fever but had occasional mild abdominal cramping. These symptoms were not related to meals, and the diarrhea did not improve despite a lactose-free diet. Stool analysis was negative for bacteria, fungi, and parasites. Colonoscopy and gastroscopy were normal. Laryngoscopy performed in the emergency room revealed a left vocal cord paralysis. A neck and chest computed tomography (CT) scan showed an intrathoracic goiter with multiple suspicious central and left neck nodes and suspicious bilateral axillary and mediastinal nodes, as well as vertebral metastases. The patient was referred to the endocrinology department. Thyroid ultrasound confirmed an enlarged thyroid gland with multiple nodules, the most significant measuring 3.6 × 2.8 × 1.7 cm in the left lobe, and multiple sonographically suspicious ipsilateral lymph nodes. Fine needle aspiration (FNA) cytology of the dominant thyroid nodule and one left neck lymph node was interpreted as suspicious for thyroid carcinoma (Bethesda class V) and was suggestive of medullary thyroid carcinoma (MTC). Serum calcitonin was 16,639 pg/ml (reference range, < 10 pg/ml), and serum carcinoembryonic antigen (CEA) was 29 ng/ml (reference range, < 3.4 ng/ml). Catecholamines and metanephrines in urine were requested to rule out a pheochromocytoma in the context of a possible genetic syndrome and were normal.

R. Falcone · V. Ramundo · G. Grani (✉)
Department of Translational and Precision Medicine, Sapienza University of Rome, Rome, Italy
e-mail: giorgio.grani@uniroma1.it

G. Grani et al. (eds.), *Thyroid Cancer*,
https://doi.org/10.1007/978-3-030-61919-0_35

The patient underwent a total thyroidectomy with central and bilateral lateral neck dissections. The surgical pathology revealed multifocal medullary thyroid cancer, involving the resection margin, with lymphatic and vascular invasion. Metastases were found in 22 of 31 lymph nodes in the lateral and central neck (pT4a pN1b R1 cM1, stage IVC, AJCC TNM staging system, eighth edition). A germline RET mutation was ruled out, while a somatic T918M somatic RET mutation was identified. Two months after surgery, calcitonin increased to 24,000 pg/ml and diarrhea persisted. He was started on symptomatic treatment with loperamide, with improvement (two stools per day). Three months later, a total body CT scan showed progressive disease on the mediastinum and bone, and serum calcitonin had increased to 28,694 pg/ml with stable CEA levels. The multidisciplinary endocrine tumors team decided to initiate systemic treatment for rapidly progressive metastatic MTC. Cabozantinib was started at a dose of 140 mg daily. The patient experienced grade (G) 2 hypertension and G2 weight loss during the first 2 months of treatment, with stable disease as the best response (−16% at CT scan according to RECIST 1.1 criteria). Starting from the third month of cabozantinib, diarrhea, which never disappeared, worsened to G2 (six stools per day), and loperamide was not able to provide relief (Table 35.1). The dose of cabozantinib was reduced twice without benefit: diarrhea worsened to G3. The patient required hospitalization for hydration therapy, and octreotide was added as symptomatic treatment and cabozantinib was held. At that time, CT scan showed stable disease with a mild increase in mediastinal nodes. Cabozantinib was permanently discontinued because the patient needed more than 1 month to recover, and the multiple toxicities were considered unacceptable for the patient (G3 diarrhea, G3 weight loss, G3 asthenia, G2 hypertension, G2 hand foot syndrome, G2 bleeding). After 2 months of a treatment holiday, the patient recovered completely. He was occasionally taking loperamide for G1 diarrhea and no other medications. His weight improved but the serum calcitonin was increasing, and chest CT scan showed a pleural effusion with progression in the mediastinal nodes. At that point, treatment with vandetanib 300 mg daily was started and is ongoing after 7 months with stable disease as the best objective response according to RECIST 1.1. criteria. Tolerability of vandetanib has been acceptable with G1 skin

Table 35.1 Classification of the drug-related diarrhea according to common terminology criteria for adverse events (CTCAE) v5.0

	Diarrhea
Grade 1	Increased of <4 stools per day over baseline, mild increase in ostomy output compared to baseline
Grade 2	Increased of 4–6 stools per day over baseline, moderate increase in ostomy output compared to baseline. Limiting instrumental ADL
Grade 3	Increased of ≥7 stools per day over baseline, hospitalization indicated, severe increase in ostomy output compared with baseline. Limiting self-care ADL
Grade 4	Life-threatening consequence. Urgent intervention indicated
Grade 5	Death

ADL Activities of daily living

rash (papules and pustules covering <10% body surface area, without pruritus or tenderness) and G1 hypertension. Since starting vandetanib, his diarrhea has completely resolved.

Diarrhea in MTC

When faced with a patient with chronic diarrhea (lasting for more than 4–6 weeks), neuroendocrine tumors should always be considered in the differential diagnosis [1]. Clues should be sought in the clinical history, physical examination, laboratory tests, and complementary studies [2]. They can help rule out more common causes of chronic diarrhea such as infections, drug use, chronic inflammatory diseases, cathartic agent use, and diabetic diarrhea. Symptoms associated with carcinoid syndrome diarrhea are watery stools and large stool volume (>1 L/day), not affected by fasting, occurring during daytime and nighttime, with stool frequency ranging from 2 to >20/day [2].

Diarrhea has been described in 10–30% of patients with MTC, with an increased rate in advanced, metastatic disease [3, 4]. Two pathophysiological mechanisms have been postulated to explain diarrhea in MTC: (1) a secretory process induced by hyper-calcitoninemia or small molecules such as prostaglandins and (2) dysfunction of the colon, probably secondary to the marked shortening of transit time in this organ [5].

In the past, diarrhea was considered to result from a secretory process induced by raised circulating calcitonin: indeed, an acute intravenous infusion of calcitonin induces small bowel (i.e., jejunal and ileal) secretion of water and electrolytes in normal man. In addition, pathophysiological studies of two cases of MTC with diarrhea confirmed that the increased fecal output of water and electrolytes was caused by the impairment of small intestine function [6, 7]. Other evidence suggested that circulating prostaglandins E2 and F2a, serotonin, and substance P can be increased in patients with MTC [8] and act synergistically with calcitonin. For instance, excess serotonin increases peristalsis, which results in reduced absorption of water and electrolytes, leading to diarrhea. Prostaglandins activate the adenylyl cyclase/cAMP mechanism, leading to net intestinal fluid secretion. However, some patients with MTC and diarrhea have normal circulating concentrations of these biologically active agents [5]. Other findings do not support the hypothesis of the increased fecal output of water and electrolytes caused by the impairment of small intestine function and propose an insufficient net absorption in the colon, secondary to a motor disturbance [5]. The humoral agent responsible for this motility disorder remains to be discovered.

Regardless of diarrhea pathogenesis (an imbalance between secretion and absorption of water and electrolytes in small bowel and colon), adequate symptomatic control is needed because chronic diarrhea impairs the quality of life of these patients. Diarrhea has a particularly noticeable adverse impact on physical, emotional, and social well-being [9]. Interventions to improve individual daily activities and productivity can improve health-related QoL and reduce stress.

Management of Diarrhea in MTC

The optimal management of diarrhea in advanced MTC is critical to improving the quality of life of these patients (Table 35.2). There is more clinical experience with patients suffering from secretory neuroendocrine tumors (NET) rather than MTC. However, since diarrhea is a symptom/sign in both groups, it is usual to apply the same management of diarrhea in NET to MTC [2]. The initial treatment approach is based on antimotility agents such as loperamide, diphenoxylate with atropine, and tincture of deodorized opium. The treatment should begin with loperamide because of its low potential for abuse and dependence. Deodorized tincture of opium is very potent and is useful in severe cases but can induce drug dependence.

Somatostatin analogs (SSA) are a cornerstone in the management of carcinoid syndrome-related diarrhea. Both long- and short-acting SSAs (octreotide, lanreotide) effectively control the symptom. There is a clinical benefit of using somatostatin analogs, but the mechanism is uncertain since a reduction in calcitonin concentrations has not been demonstrated with those agents. SSAs are generally well tolerated but have some side effects such as nausea, abdominal discomfort, bloating, diarrhea, hyperglycemia, and fat malabsorption within the first weeks of treatment. One of the most important is the reduction of gallbladder contractility and delay in postprandial gallbladder emptying; up to 25% of patients develop asymptomatic cholesterol gallstones during the first 18 months of treatment. In 2017, the FDA approved telotristat ethyl, a tryptophan hydroxylase inhibitor that decreases serotonin production, in combination with SSA therapy for the treatment of adults with carcinoid syndrome diarrhea that SSA therapy alone has inadequately controlled [10]. In refractory cases, patients may obtain relief of symptoms with therapies that reduce tumor burden, such as tumor ablation (chemoembolization, radioembolization, radiofrequency) or surgical debulking. Unfortunately, symptoms reappear with disease recurrence or progression.

Although dietary modifications for management of carcinoid syndrome diarrhea are recommended through patient websites and healthcare provider interviews, there is no clear evidence that demonstrates their efficacy, and neither of the main treatment guidelines provide dietary advice [11, 12]. Anecdotal evidence for symptom improvement has been observed by physicians in their clinical practice recommending frequent small meals and avoidance of aged cheeses, fermented foods with high amine content, drinks that contain caffeine, and sugar-rich beverages. Hydration is always recommended. On the whole, it is essential to maintain adequate hydration with electrolyte replacement and antispasmodic and analgesic treatment to control cramps. If an infection is suspected, appropriate antibiotics should be administered (Table 35.2).

Table 35.2 Supportive treatment for the management of diarrhea in patients with medullary thyroid cancer (MTC)

Fluidotherapy	Hydration; electrolytes and water replacement
Antidiarrheal drugs	Loperamide 4 mg followed by 2 mg/4 h (maximal dose 16 mg/day)
Somatostatin analogs	Lanreotide (90–120 mg SC every 4 weeks) Octreotide (150–250 mcg SC TID) Octreotide LAR (20–30 mg IM every 4 weeks)
Antibiotics	Metronidazole, quinolones
Analgesia	Spasmolytic drugs

Diarrhea as an Adverse Event of Novel Targeted Agents in MTC

Vandetanib and cabozantinib are drugs approved by the Food and Drug Administration and the European Medicines Agency to treat unresectable, late-stage, metastatic MTC. These agents may be effective in treating advanced MTC, also controlling carcinoid syndrome symptoms (i.e., diarrhea, flushing), but, at the same time, these systemic therapies may cause diarrhea as a side effect.

Vandetanib is a multikinase inhibitor (MKI) targeting RET, VEGFR, and EGFR signaling. In the randomized, placebo-controlled, double-blind, phase III ZETA trial, diarrhea (any grade) was observed in 56% of patients ($N = 130$) in the vandetanib arm compared to 26% of patients ($N = 26$) in the placebo arm [13]. Severe diarrhea (>G3) occurred in 11% ($N = 25$) of patients in the vandetanib group and in 2% ($N = 2$) in the control arm. Final recommendations for vandetanib use in patients with MTC require close monitoring of diarrhea that can be related either to the disease or to an adverse drug reaction. In case of diarrhea, the presence of dehydration, electrolyte imbalance, and/or impaired renal function may increase the risk of prolonging the QTc interval and predispose to malignant cardiac arrhythmias. Therefore, close ECG monitoring is mandatory. It is also important to maintain normal serum potassium, magnesium, and calcium levels as well as renal function during treatment with vandetanib.

Cabozantinib was the second drug approved for the treatment of MTC patients. It is a MKI that targets three relevant pathways: MET, VEGFR2, and RET. In the double-blind, phase III trial comparing cabozantinib (140 mg daily) with placebo, diarrhea (all grade) was reported in 63.1% ($N = 135$) of patients treated with cabozantinib compared to 33% ($N = 36$) in the control group. Diarrhea (≥G3) was seen in 15.9% of patients in cabozantinib group versus 1.8% in the placebo group [14].

Optimal management of MKIs is required to obtain the maximum therapeutic effect with an acceptable tolerability profile. In clinical trials, diarrhea-related adverse events were managed with antidiarrheal medications, hydration, drug dose reduction, or drug suspension/discontinuation, based on the severity of toxicity. If severe diarrhea is identified (grade 3 according to the common terminology criteria for adverse events), the MKI should be discontinued until the patient recovers and diarrhea reduces to G1 or less. Hospitalization is recommended for hydration, monitoring of electrolyte imbalance, renal function, QT status, and management of symptoms. Once diarrhea reduces to grade 1 or less, vandetanib or cabozantinib could be reintroduced at a reduced dose. If life-threatening G4 diarrhea occurs and it is recognized as a treatment-related side effect, hospitalization is mandatory, and MKI discontinuation is recommended.

Back to the Patient

Symptomatic Management of the Case

Our patient had advanced sporadic MTC, with metastases to distant nodes and bone at the time of diagnosis. He required two courses of systemic MKI to control progressive disease.

In particular, diarrhea was the presenting manifestation of MTC as well as a side effect of cabozantinib. Drug-related diarrhea was managed with loperamide and somatostatin analog therapy, dose reduction, and, finally, drug discontinuation. Ultimately, the diarrhea resolved with the radiological response to vandetanib.

Clinical Pearls

- Diarrhea is a nonspecific symptom, and a delay in MTC diagnosis is common.
- Chronic diarrhea in MTC has been related to a secretory process induced by hyper-calcitoninemia and/or to insufficient net absorption in the colon, secondary to a possible motor disturbance (marked shortening of transit time in this organ). The humoral agent responsible for this motility disorder remains unknown.
- The treatment of diarrhea in a patient with MTC includes fluid and electrolyte replacement, antidiarrheal drugs, and somatostatin analogs. Antidiarrheal drugs, slowing intestinal motility, can be effectively used as first-line therapies. In more severe cases, somatostatin analogs may be useful. In refractory patients, tumor burden-reducing techniques represent a more aggressive strategy that should be considered.
- It is important to differentiate MKI-related diarrhea from MTC-related diarrhea, or diarrhea caused by other complications (such as infection), in order to provide the most specific and effective treatment.
- Control of disease-related symptoms and side effects in patients with MTC is essential to provide an optimal quality of life to affected patients.

Bibliography

1. Ernaga Lorea A, Migueliz Bermejo I, Eguílaz Esparza N, Hernández Morhain MC, Pineda Arribas J. Chronic diarrhea: the first symptom of a metastatic medullary thyroid carcinoma. Gastroenterol Hepatol. 2018;41(2):105–7.
2. Naraev BG, Halland M, Halperin DM, Purvis AJ, O'Dorisio TM, Halfdanarson TR. Management of diarrhea in patients with carcinoid syndrome. Pancreas. 2019;48(8):961–72.
3. Williams ED. Diarrhoea and thyroid carcinoma. Proc R Soc Med. 1966;59(7):602–3.
4. Kebebew E, Ituarte PH, Siperstein AE, Duh QY, Clark OH. Medullary thyroid carcinoma: clinical characteristics, treatment, prognostic factors, and a comparison of staging systems. Cancer. 2000;88(5):1139–48.
5. Rambaud JC, Jian R, Flourié B, Hautefeuille M, Salmeron M, Thuillier F, et al. Pathophysiological study of diarrhoea in a patient with medullary thyroid carcinoma. Evidence against a secretory mechanism and for the role of shortened colonic transit time. Gut. 1988;29(4):537–43.
6. Isaacs P, Whittaker SM, Turnberg LA. Diarrhea associated with medullary carcinoma of the thyroid. Studies of intestinal function in a patient. Gastroenterology. 1974;67(3):521–6.
7. Cox TM, Fagan EA, Hillyard CJ, Allison DJ, Chadwick VS. Rôle of calcitonin in diarrhoea associated with medullary carcinoma of the thyroid. Gut. 1979;20(7):629–33.
8. Skrabanek P, Cannon D, Dempsey J, Kirrane J, Neligan M, Powell D. Substance P in medullary carcinoma of the thyroid. Experientia. 1979;35(9):1259–60.
9. Fröjd C, Larsson G, Lampic C, von Essen L. Health related quality of life and psychosocial function among patients with carcinoid tumours. A longitudinal, prospective, and comparative study. Health Qual Life Outcomes. 2007;5:18.
10. Kulke MH, Hörsch D, Caplin ME, Anthony LB, Bergsland E, Öberg K, et al. Telotristat ethyl, a tryptophan hydroxylase inhibitor for the treatment of carcinoid syndrome. J Clin Oncol. 2017;35(1):14–23.
11. Wells SA Jr, Asa SL, Dralle H, Elisei R, Evans DB, Gagel RF, et al. Revised American Thyroid Association guidelines for the management of medullary thyroid carcinoma. Thyroid. 2015;25(6):567–610.
12. Filetti S, Durante C, Hartl D, Leboulleux S, Locati LD, Newbold K, et al. Thyroid cancer: ESMO clinical practice guidelines for diagnosis, treatment and follow-up. Ann Oncol. 2019;30:1856–83.
13. Wells SA, Robinson BG, Gagel RF, Dralle H, Fagin JA, Santoro M, et al. Vandetanib in patients with locally advanced or metastatic medullary thyroid cancer: a randomized, double-blind phase III trial. J Clin Oncol. 2012;30(2):134–41.
14. Elisei R, Schlumberger MJ, Müller SP, Schöffski P, Brose MS, Shah MH, et al. Cabozantinib in progressive medullary thyroid cancer. J Clin Oncol. 2013;31(29):3639–46.

Chapter 36
Clinical Management of a Patient with a Locally Recurrent Medullary Thyroid Cancer and Asymptomatic Slowly Progressing Distant Metastases

Virginia Cappagli, Valeria Bottici, and Rossella Elisei

Case Presentation

On May 1994, a 21-year-old woman with a 3.5 cm left thyroid nodule underwent total thyroidectomy mainly for aesthetic reasons. Paratracheal lymph nodes were also removed because they were found to be enlarged and suspicious by the surgeon. The histology identified a 3.2 cm medullary thyroid cancer (MTC) with three metastases out of six paratracheal lymph nodes (T2N1aM0). No information about presurgical functional thyroid status or serum calcitonin (Ct) levels were available. Fine-needle aspiration cytology (FNAC) was indeterminate showing a microfollicular cell pattern that could be nowadays included in the category III of Bethesda cytological classification.

In October 1994, the patient arrived at our center for consultation: serum Ct was 118 pg/ml (normal <14 pg/ml), and neck ultrasound showed the presence of a post-surgical remnant thyroid tissue in the thyroid bed with no evidence of suspicious lymph nodes in the neck. The screening for germline *RET* mutations was negative.

In the subsequent 2 years, serum Ct progressively, but slowly, increased with no evidence of structural disease on neck ultrasound or computerized tomography (CT). In November 1996, a suspicious left laterocervical lymph node measuring 1.2 cm was found on neck ultrasound; at that time, serum Ct was 736 pg/ml; the cytology of the lymph node and the high values of Ct in the washout of the needle used for the aspiration (1648 pg/ml) confirmed an MTC lymph node metastasis. In February 1997 [serum Ct, 1360 pg/ml, and carcinogenic embryonic antigen (CEA), 46.3 ng/ml], the patient underwent bilateral and central compartment nodal dissections. However, out of 32 lymph nodes that were removed, only the left

V. Cappagli · V. Bottici · R. Elisei (✉)
Endocrine Unit, Department of Clinical and Experimental Medicine, University Hospital of Pisa, Pisa, Italy
e-mail: rossella.elisei@med.unipi.it

G. Grani et al. (eds.), *Thyroid Cancer*,
https://doi.org/10.1007/978-3-030-61919-0_36

laterocervical lymph node, corresponding to the one observed on neck ultrasound, was metastatic.

Two months after surgery, serum Ct was still elevated (1048 pg/ml) and increasing up to 2240 pg/ml in July 1997; a neck CT scan performed in September 1997 showed a left paratracheal/mediastinal nodule of 19 × 23 × 32 mm, with a suspicious cytology and Ct in the needle washout >2400 pg/ml. Because a total body (TB) CT scan did not show any other lesion in extracervical sites, we decided to proceed with local therapy. In November 1997, the patient underwent a diathermy ablation of the lesion with a 40% reduction in its volume. Eighteen months later, at the end of April 1999, the lesion measured at neck ultrasound was even bigger than before (19 × 28 × 32 mm) (Fig. 36.1); total body CT scans confirmed that this was the only lesion, and we performed a surgical paratracheal dissection. The histology showed that the removed tissue was a recurrence of the primary tumor, since only medullary cancer cells and no lymphoid elements were present. The tissue analysis for somatic *RET* mutation showed the presence of a somatic M918T mutation. The postsurgical serum Ct progressively dropped and become <14 pg/ml (Fig. 36.2). Neck ultrasound and CT scan were negative in follow-up.

In 2001, basal Ct was still <14 pg/ml but a pentagastrin stimulation test showed a peak Ct of 88 pg/ml. At this time, both neck ultrasound and total body CT scan were still negative.

From 2001 to 2005, the patient, by her choice, did not undergo any biochemical or radiological assessment. In February 2005, she returned to our center, and at that time, serum Ct was 21 pg/ml; neck ultrasound and neck CT scan showed subcentimeter lymph nodes that were not clearly metastatic. No distant metastases were present, and a total body bone scan was negative. We continued to follow our patient with clinical, biochemical, and imaging assessment every 12 months, and from 2005 to 2009, the disease was stable.

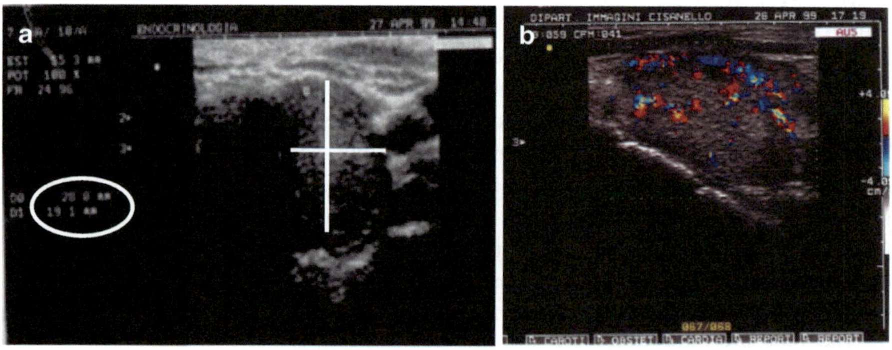

Fig. 36.1 Neck ultrasound of the *left* paratracheal lesion in April 1999, before the surgical excision, the histology of which demonstrated a medullary thyroid cancer local recurrence. (Panel **a**) Standard neck ultrasound transverse section with the anteroposterior (28.0 mm) and latero-lateral (19.1 mm) diameters of the paratracheal lesion. (Panel **b**) Color-Doppler imaging of the paratracheal lesion showing the intralesion irregular hypervascularity (sagittal section, 32 mm)

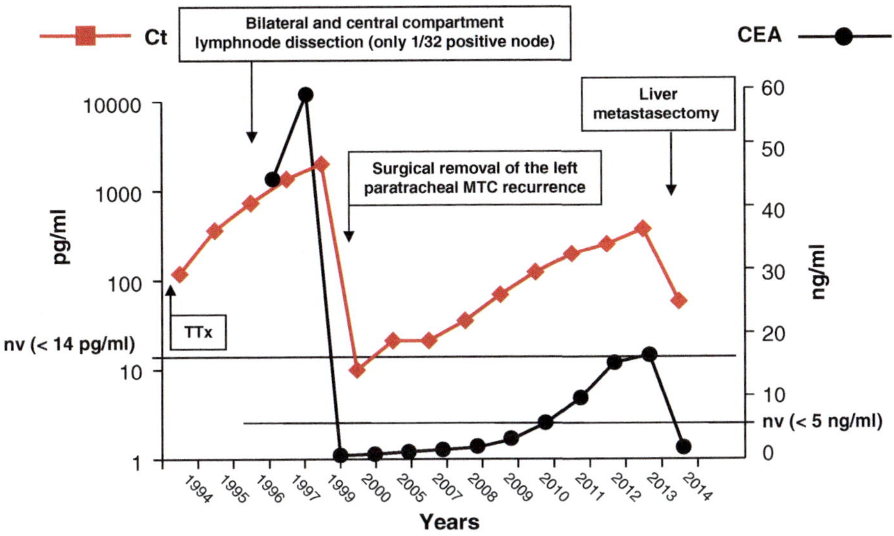

Fig. 36.2 Serum Ct and CEA variations during the follow-up of the patient: a correlation between the two markers is evident as well as a correlation with therapeutic interventions

In June 2009, the total body CT scan showed the persistence of small lymph nodes in the neck, the appearance of micronodules in the lung, and three new hepatic lesions (largest was 12 mm) with radiographic characteristics suspicious for metastatic lesions. Serum Ct levels had slowly increased up to 69 pg/ml while serum CEA was in the normal range (<5 ng/ml). We decided to not recommend active therapies but to follow the strategy of "wait and see."

During the following 3 years, radiological assessments showed the progression of the hepatic metastases; in particular, the one that had been 12 mm in 2009 grew to 14 mm in 2010, 15 mm in 2011, and 17 mm in September 2012 (Fig. 36.3, Panel a) with a mean size increase of 20% per year. In parallel, serum Ct increased from 69 pg/ml on June 2009 to 314 pg/ml on September 2012 and CEA levels from 3.12 ng/ml on June 2009 to 15.6 ng/ml on September 2012 (Fig. 36.2). At this moment, the doubling time of both Ct and CEA was 1.5 years.

In January 2013, the total body CT scan confirmed that the only growing lesion was the hepatic one which was now 19 mm. At this point, we explored the possibility of performing locoregional percutaneous thermoablation, but because of its close relationship with the gallbladder and the risk for unsuccessful treatment, we agreed on a surgical approach and the patient underwent hepatic metastasectomy.

One year later, the radiological assessments confirmed the stability of small cervical lymph nodes, small lung nodules, and the other two subcentimeter hepatic lesions, in the absence of new metastatic or suspicious lesions (Fig. 36.3, Panel b). The serum Ct dropped very rapidly, and for several years it remained stable, as well as all the micrometastatic lesions in the lung and the liver.

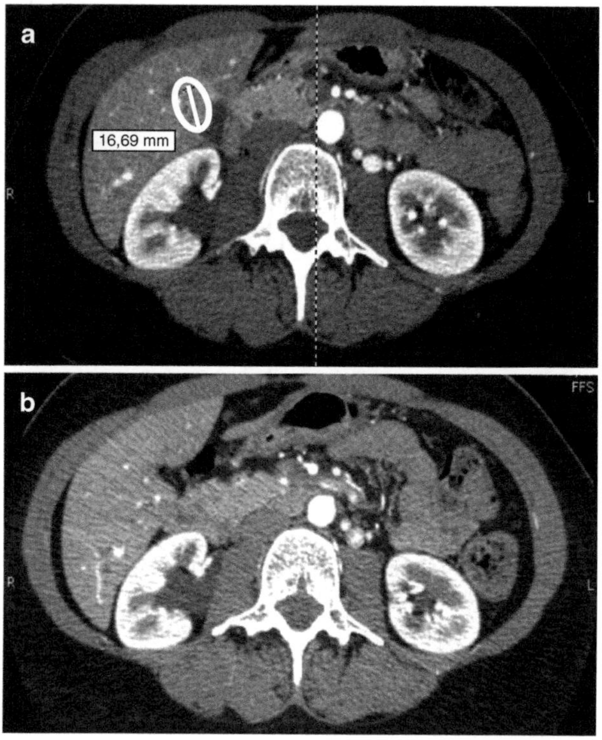

Fig. 36.3 (Panel **a**) CT scan of the hepatic metastases, with the largest one located very close to the gallbladder and measuring 17 mm in September 2012. (Panel **b**) Patient's liver CT scan 12 months after metastasectomy in 2014: no recurrence of the largest lesion was visible

Five years later, in 2018 some of the liver microlesions started to grow and a transarterial radioembolization (TARE) was performed with success (Fig. 36.4). The patient is now 47 years old; her general health and quality of life are still very good after 26 years from the diagnosis.

Diagnosis/Assessment

This case offers the opportunity to discuss several still controversial issues related to the diagnosis and treatment of metastatic disease in MTC patients.

MTC is a rare thyroid tumor representing only 5–7% of all thyroid malignancies. It can be sporadic (80%) or familial (20%). Its pathogenesis is related to a molecular alteration of *RET* oncogene that can be present at the germline level in familial cases or at somatic level in sporadic cases [1]. MTC prognosis is strongly related to the presence of metastatic disease outside the neck, with a survival rate of about 30–35% at 10 years when distant metastases are present at the time of diagnosis [2]. Also the presence of a somatic *RET* mutation has been demonstrated to be correlated to an advanced stage and a lower survival [3–5]. The detection of a somatic *RET* mutation in the paratracheal tissue of the patient is suggestive of a more aggressive

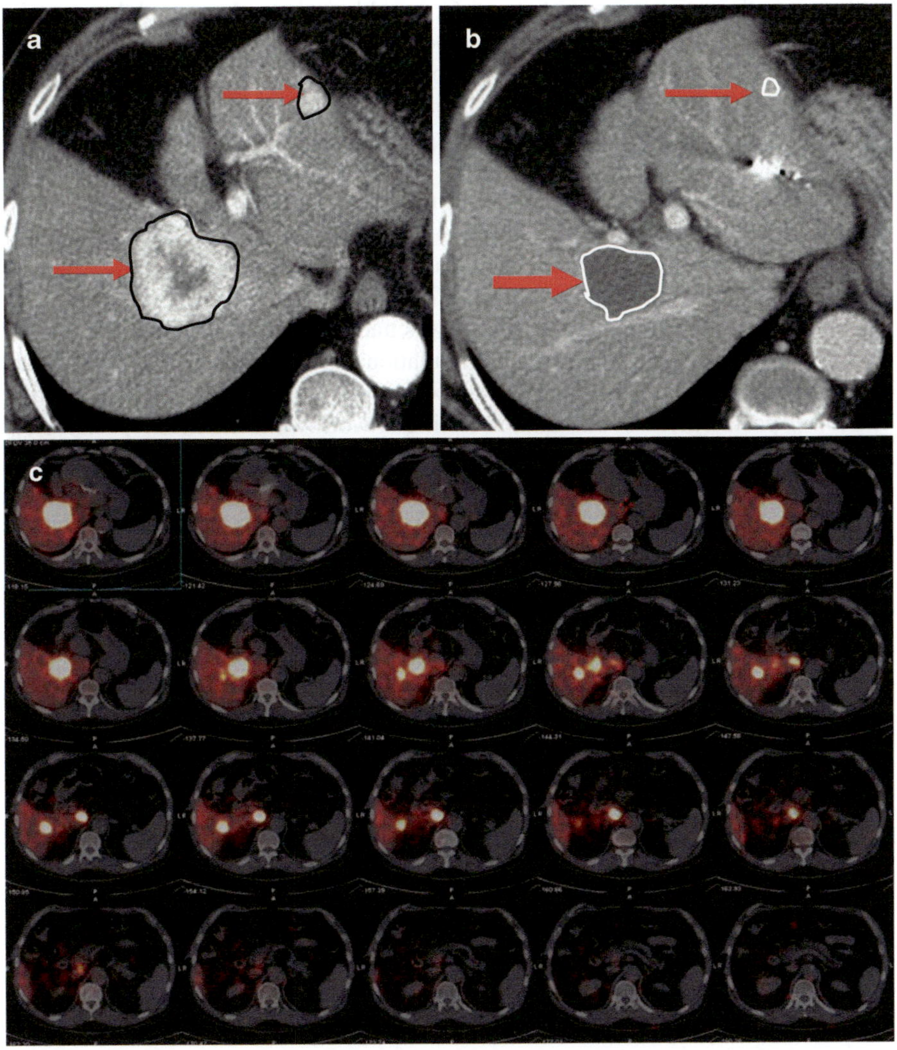

Fig. 36.4 The CT scan images of the liver metastasis of the patient before (Panel **a**) and after (Panel **b**) the YTTRIUM-90 TARE treatment. Panel **c** shows the images of the hepatic angioscintigraphy with microaggregated albumin labeled with 99mTC that must be performed before TARE to verify the presence of contraindications

phenotype, with a higher risk of disease-related mortality even though the absence of distant metastases at the time of diagnosis likely reduces this risk [6, 7].

This is a typical case in which the presurgical diagnosis of MTC was missed since the serum Ct was not measured and the cytological diagnosis of the nodule was indeterminate, as it can sometimes happen in MTC. An international and multicenter study recently demonstrated that the FNAC was able to identify only 46% of 245 sporadic MTCs evaluated in 12 centers across 7 nations in 4 continents [8].

In this case, the measurement of serum Ct could have helped to avoid this mistake and allowed the appropriate surgical procedure to have been performed, which would possibly have changed the long-term outcome.

The measurement of Ct in the washout of the needle used for aspiration is of great help in the diagnosis of both primary MTC and lymph node metastases [9]. This procedure is particularly useful when the cytology is unclear or undefined and the serum Ct is borderline. Sometimes, if the serum Ct levels are very high, blood contamination can lead to a false-positive result, but the identification of a cutoff above which metastatic disease is likely can solve this problem [10].

At a certain point during the follow-up of this patient, she could have been considered to be "cured" since the serum Ct was undetectable (<14 pg/ml) from 1999 to 2001. However, the pentagastrin stimulation test demonstrated a peak Ct of 88 pg/ml suggesting that residual disease was still present. It is still a matter of discussion if postsurgical Ct stimulation testing is worthwhile when the postsurgical basal serum Ct is undetectable or in the normal range. There are studies showing that MTC patients with a basal Ct lower than the upper limit of the reference range have a risk of recurrence of 10%, and therefore they can be considered to be cured, and their follow-up can be less intensive [11]. However, this percentage is reduced to 3% in patients with negative Ct stimulation test [10], and thus, we believe that at least one stimulation Ct test after surgery can be useful to better identify patients who have a higher probability of being free of disease [12].

Management

Newly diagnosed patients with MTC are usually 45–50 years old at the time of the diagnosis, and thus our patient was rather young. However, age at presentation is not a risk factor neither for the progression of the disease nor survival. However, younger age can impact on the choice of therapy. For example, after the third surgery, external radiotherapy (ERT) might have been considered, but the patient was only 25 years old, and her young age was a relative contraindication to ERT [13, 14]. Nevertheless, no further recurrence in the neck has been observed thus far, after 15 years from the last surgery.

The choice to repeat surgery in the neck was made because of the evidence that the disease was locally metastatic without distant metastases. There is a general agreement among experts [14] that when MTC is characterized by a single metastatic lesion or several but subcentimeter lesions and not progressive, a local treatment is preferred, thus delaying systemic therapy, especially in young patients. The rationale underlying this concept is related to two major factors: the slow growth that characterizes the biological behavior of many MTCs and the multiplicity of adverse effects of systemic therapy. As far as the degree of progression is concerned, only a progression rate of the target lesion(s) greater than 20% in at least 12–14 months is considered sufficiently worrisome to consider initiation of systemic therapy [15]. If the growth rate is slower, it is better to wait and see with periodical imaging controls. The doubling times of both serum Ct and CEA are good indicators of progression [16–17] and are very helpful in planning the follow-up schedule: if the doubling time is shorter than 6–12 months, the patient must be revaluated at shorter time intervals, and it is likely that at one of these assessments cross-sectional imaging will demonstrate a significant increase of one or more lesions. In contrast, if the doubling time is greater than 12–24 months, the patient can be monitored less frequently, e.g., every 12–18 months, because of a lower risk of significant progression on imaging. Our patient had a Ct and CEA doubling time of 1.5 years, and for this reason, we monitored her once a year. However, since one of her several distant micrometastases was growing and because it was very close to the gallbladder, we decided to treat the patient surgically rather than with systemic therapy. Few years later, some of the liver lesions, but not the others, started to grow and we decided to treat the patient with an "organ" local therapy such as TARE. This mini-invasive therapy performed by introducing selective internal radiation (YTTRIUM-90) microspheres is commonly used for neuroendocrine liver metastases [18] and can also be used in MTC liver metastases, especially if small, disseminated, and well vascularized. A hepatic artery angiography [19], for diagnostic evaluation of liver metastases, and to exclude a pulmonary shunt, which represents a contraindication to TARE, should always be performed before TARE (Fig. 36.4, panel C).

Outcome

This is a very typical intermediate-risk MTC patient with a long survival from the time of the diagnosis (i.e., 26 years, at present), with a good quality of life and a low relative risk of death from the disease. All together she has had four surgical treatments in 26 years, with many years of good health between procedures. If, during her follow-up, we had decided to initiate systemic therapy, only standard chemotherapy would have been available until 2005. Several regimens have been proposed over the years, but none of them has been demonstrated to be clinically effective despite having high levels of toxicity [20]. After 2005, several clinical trials with new targeted therapies were initiated, based on the ability of some of these drugs to inhibit tyrosine kinase receptors (TKIs) which are frequently involved in tumor transformation and progression. One of these receptors is coded by *RET* oncogene that is frequently altered in MTC, which is the rationale for such therapy in this condition. Unfortunately, these therapies have a lot of adverse reactions, including life-threatening events that, if not controlled or limited, can greatly affect the quality of life of treated patients and potentially even cause mortality [21, 22]. This was the reason we postponed for as long as possible the initiation of systemic therapy in our young patient even when one of the liver metastases started to grow. Since the lymph node and lung metastases were substantially stable, we preferred to treat the patient with a specific "organ" local therapy such as TARE that was able to stop the growth of, and even reduce, the liver lesions. With this therapy we further postponed the need to start a systemic therapy following the suggestions of experts [23].

In accord with the natural history of MTC and the fact that a somatic *RET* mutation was present in the tumor tissue, we can anticipate progression of the metastatic lesions that have already been detected or the appearance of new lesions within a few years. At that time, together with the patient, we will decide if it will be the right time to start systemic therapy or if there will still be a role for another local treatment. In the meantime, she is continuing to have a good quality of life after 26 years from the diagnosis.

Conclusions

This case represents a typical MTC case in which the combination of local treatments and "wait-and-see" strategy allowed the patient to have a relatively normal life with no other medication other than levothyroxine therapy.

Clinical Pearls/Pitfalls

- Serum Ct measurement may be a useful test in the initial evaluation of thyroid nodules, especially in those cases who are scheduled for surgery.
- The serum Ct and CEA doubling time can predict the growth rate of metastatic lesions, thus being a valuable tool for planning the schedule of follow-up controls and imaging and biochemical testing.
- Single metastatic lesions should be treated, if necessary, with local therapies.
- Systemic therapy should be reserved for MTC patients with multiple distant metastases or unresectable local disease with a clear evidence of progression on imaging.
- MTC patients with somatic *RET* mutations typically have more aggressive disease.

References

1. Ciampi R, et al. Genetic landscape of somatic mutations in a large cohort of sporadic medullary thyroid carcinomas studied by next-generation targeted sequencing. iScience. 2019;20:324–36.
2. Gharib H, et al. Medullary thyroid carcinoma: clinicopathologic features and long-term follow-up of 65 patients treated during 1946 through 1970. Mayo Clin Proc. 1992;67(10):934–40.
3. Elisei R, et al. Prognostic significance of somatic RET oncogene mutations in sporadic medullary thyroid cancer: a 10-year follow-up study. J Clin Endocrinol Metab. 2008;93(3):682–7.
4. Mian C, et al. Combined RET and Ki-67 assessment in sporadic medullary thyroid carcinoma: a useful tool for patient risk stratification. Eur J Endocrinol. 2011;164(6):971–6.
5. Moura MM, et al. Correlation of RET somatic mutations with clinicopathological features in sporadic medullary thyroid carcinomas. Br J Cancer. 2009;100(11):1777–83.

6. Romei C, Ciampi R, Elisei R. A comprehensive overview of the role of the RET proto-oncogene in thyroid carcinoma. Nat Rev Endocrinol. 2016;12(4):192–202.
7. Romei C, et al. New insights in the molecular signature of advanced medullary thyroid cancer: evidence of a bad outcome of cases with double <i>RET</i> mutations. J Med Genet. 2016;53(11):729–34.
8. Essig GF Jr, et al. Fine needle aspiration and medullary thyroid carcinoma: the risk of inadequate preoperative evaluation and initial surgery when relying upon FNAB cytology alone. Endocr Pract. 2013;19(6):920–7.
9. Boi F, et al. Calcitonin measurement in wash-out fluid from fine needle aspiration of neck masses in patients with primary and metastatic medullary thyroid carcinoma. J Clin Endocrinol Metab. 2007;92(6):2115–8.
10. Trimboli P, et al. Calcitonin measurement in aspiration needle washout fluids has higher sensitivity than cytology in detecting medullary thyroid cancer: a retrospective multicentre study. Clin Endocrinol (Oxf). 2014;80(1):135–40.
11. Pellegriti G, et al. Long-term outcome of medullary thyroid carcinoma in patients with normal postoperative medical imaging. Br J Cancer. 2003;88(10):1537–42.
12. Franc S, et al. Complete surgical lymph node resection does not prevent authentic recurrences of medullary thyroid carcinoma. Clin Endocrinol (Oxf). 2001;55(3):403–9.
13. Sun XS, et al. Indications of external beam radiation therapy in non-anaplastic thyroid cancer and impact of innovative radiation techniques. Crit Rev Oncol Hematol. 2013;86(1):52–68.
14. Schlumberger M, et al. European thyroid association guidelines for metastatic medullary thyroid cancer. Eur Thyroid J. 2012;1(1):5–14.
15. Eisenhauer EA, et al. New response evaluation criteria in solid tumours: revised RECIST guideline (version 1.1). Eur J Cancer. 2009;45(2):228–47.
16. Meijer JA, et al. Calcitonin and carcinoembryonic antigen doubling times as prognostic factors in medullary thyroid carcinoma: a structured meta-analysis. Clin Endocrinol (Oxf). 2010;72(4):534–42.
17. Laure Giraudet A, et al. Progression of medullary thyroid carcinoma: assessment with calcitonin and carcinoembryonic antigen doubling times. Eur J Endocrinol. 2008;158(2):239–46.
18. King J, et al. Radioembolization with selective internal radiation microspheres for neuroendocrine liver metastases. Cancer. 2008;113(5):921–9.
19. Mirka H, et al. Contribution of computed tomographic angiography to pretreatment planning of radio-embolization of liver tumors. Anticancer Res. 2018;38(7):3825–9.
20. Orlandi F, et al. Treatment of medullary thyroid carcinoma: an update. Endocr Relat Cancer. 2001;8(2):135–47.
21. Elisei R, et al. Cabozantinib in progressive medullary thyroid cancer. J Clin Oncol. 2013;31(29):3639–46.
22. Wells SA Jr, et al. Vandetanib in patients with locally advanced or metastatic medullary thyroid cancer: a randomized, double-blind phase III trial. J Clin Oncol. 2012;30(2):134–41.
23. Schlumberger M, et al. Definition and management of radioactive iodine-refractory differentiated thyroid cancer. Lancet Diabetes Endocrinol. 2014;2(5):356–8.

Chapter 37
A Patient with an Advanced Medullary Thyroid Cancer and Progressive, Symptomatic Distant Metastases: When to Start Systemic Therapy

Carlotta Giani, Antonio Matrone, and Rossella Elisei

Case Presentation

A 39-year-old man was diagnosed with a multinodular goiter after a neck ultrasound was performed because of familial thyroid disease. Neck ultrasound (US) showed the presence of a solid hypoechoic nodule measuring 3.8 cm in the left lobe and an anechoic nodule measuring 1.2 cm in the right lobe. Laboratory findings showed a TSH of 1.2 mU/l, negative TgAb and TPOAb, and normal values of both FT3 and FT4. A fine-needle aspiration cytology (FNAC) of the biggest nodule revealed a microfollicular lesion (Bethesda class III) and surgical treatment was suggested.

In April 2003, the patient was referred to our institution for a second opinion. A neck US performed in our center confirmed the presence of the two thyroid nodules but also showed three right hypoechoic laterocervical nodules with microcalcifications that were highly suspicious for lymph node metastases. Serum calcitonin (Ct) was markedly elevated at 3654 pg/ml (normal <10 pg/ml). Fine-needle aspiration cytology of the 3.8 cm thyroid nodule was positive for medullary thyroid cancer (MTC), and cytology of a 1.4 cm right laterocervical lymph node was positive for MTC as well. We performed germline *RET* mutational testing and a Ser891Ala mutation was found, thus converting the case from apparently sporadic to a hereditary form of MTC. Thereafter, the screening of his first-degree relatives (parents and siblings) was started, and several of them were found to be positive. A program of clinical and biochemical (i.e., basal and stimulated Ct) screening was initiated. The patient was submitted to clinical and biochemical evaluations to verify the presence of other endocrine neoplasia such as multiple adenomatosis of parathyroid glands and pheochromocytoma, but he was negative for both of them.

C. Giani · A. Matrone · R. Elisei (✉)
Endocrine Unit, Department of Clinical and Experimental Medicine, University Hospital of Pisa, Pisa, Italy
e-mail: rossella.elisei@med.unipi.it

G. Grani et al. (eds.), *Thyroid Cancer*,
https://doi.org/10.1007/978-3-030-61919-0_37

In May 2003, the patient underwent a total thyroidectomy with central and right laterocervical compartmental lymph node dissections. The histological examination showed an MTC of 2.9 cm with metastatic lymph nodes of the central (5/8) and right laterocervical (4/10) compartments (pT2N1bMx). Four months after surgery (September 2003), a neck ultrasound was performed that showed the presence of 4 new suspicious left laterocervical lymph nodes. The largest, measuring 1.2 cm, was biopsied and its metastatic nature was confirmed with Ct on the needle washout fluid >10,000 pg/ml; at this time, serum Ct was 1000 pg/ml and carcinoembryonic antigen (CEA) was 20 ng/ml (normal <5.0 ng/ml). Computerized tomography (CT) scan of the neck, mediastinum, and thorax confirmed the presence of metastatic lymph nodes in the neck and also revealed the presence of two suspicious metastatic lymph nodes in the mediastinum and some subcentimeter lung lesions which were too small to be better characterized; there were no other suspicious lesions.

At this point, we decided to perform a left laterocervical lymph node dissection with the simultaneous removal of the lymph nodes in the mediastinum. Histological examination confirmed the metastatic nature of the laterocervical (4/5) and mediastinal (2/2) MTC lymph nodes.

The first clinical follow-up visit after this second neck surgery was performed 6 months later (April 2004). Serum Ct was 650 pg/ml, CT scan confirmed the presence of unchanged lung micronodules, and neck US was negative for suspicious lymph nodes.

During the following annual visits and biochemical assessments, serum Ct slightly but progressively increased over the years (Fig. 37.1), but the chest CT scan

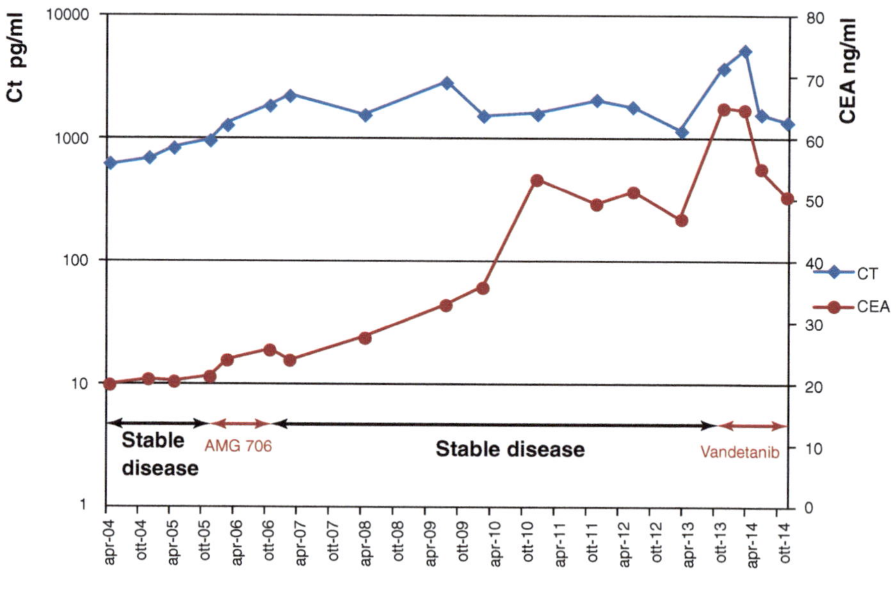

Fig. 37.1 Serum calcitonin (Ct) and carcinoembryonic antigen (CEA) during the years of follow-up of the patient: a more significant increase of both markers was observed just before the starting point of the TKI therapies just anticipating the imaging evidence of a significant increase of the size of the metastatic lesions

showed a stable disease. After 2 years of stable disease, the patient started to complain about diarrhea. The diarrhea was well controlled with medication (loperamide 2 mg, until eight tablets daily), but because of the progressive increase in serum Ct and the symptomatic disease (diarrhea), the patient was enrolled in the first experimental clinical trial with the tyrosine kinase inhibitor AMG 706 (i.e., motesanib) in February 2006. After 3 weeks of treatment, his diarrhea was completely controlled with no more need for loperamide, and his Ct levels remained substantially stable, with no evidence of progressive disease on the chest CT scan. In January 2007, despite the stable disease, motesanib was discontinued due to the development of hydrops of the gallbladder, one of the most common side effects of this drug. In February 2007, serum Ct was 824 pg/ml, CEA was 24 ng/ml, neck US was negative for lymph node metastases, and CT scan showed the stability of the microlesions of the lung.

From January 2007 to April 2010, no clinical, biochemical, and radiological findings of progression of MTC were observed; the diarrhea was under control with loperamide, and our patient had an acceptable quality of life. In October 2010, we found a slight increase of serum Ct and CEA with a relatively short and concerning doubling time (i.e., 1.4 year); the total body (TB) CT scan showed the presence of at least four mediastinal suspicious but subcentimeter lymph nodes and confirmed the stable lung microlesions. At this time, we decided upon a *wait-and-see* strategy, because of no evidence of significant radiological progression of the disease. The patient's clinical status remained stable until November 2013, when a rising serum Ct value was observed, with a doubling time <0.5 years (i.e., 3797 pg/ml vs. 1180 pg/ml of March 2013); similarly, an increase in CEA was found with a doubling time of 1.4 years (65 ng/ml vs. 47 ng/ml of March 2013). The neck US revealed the presence of a new 11 mm lymph node in the right paratracheal area. The CT scan showed a new metastatic lymph node in the right hilum measuring 24 mm and a 116% increase of the largest diameter of a mediastinal lymph node (from 12 mm to 26 mm in 6 months). In this period, the diarrhea was no longer well controlled despite regular therapy with loperamide.

Because of clear progression of the disease, in July 2014, we decided to initiate therapy with the TKI vandetanib (which became available for prescription in our country in June 2014 with the commercial name Caprelsa) with a starting dose of 300 mg daily. The severity of diarrhea immediately improved, but 6 weeks after the initiation of vandetanib, the patient developed a severe and extensive papular rash on the face, hands, and head (Fig. 37.2). This adverse event (AE) was considered to be grade 3 (i.e., very severe) and required the suspension of the TKI therapy until its complete resolution. In the meantime, topical and oral glucocorticoids, antihistamines, and antibiotics to prevent microbial superinfection were administered. After the resolution of this AE, we restarted vandetanib but at a reduced daily dose (100 mg daily).

On November 2014 (after 3 months of vandetanib therapy at 100 mg daily), the patient presented for follow-up in good clinical condition, without diarrhea or the need for antidiarrheal medication. His ECG showed a normal QTc interval, and serum electrolytes were in the normal range as were thyroid function tests after a levothyroxine dose adjustment performed in September 2014 because of an elevated

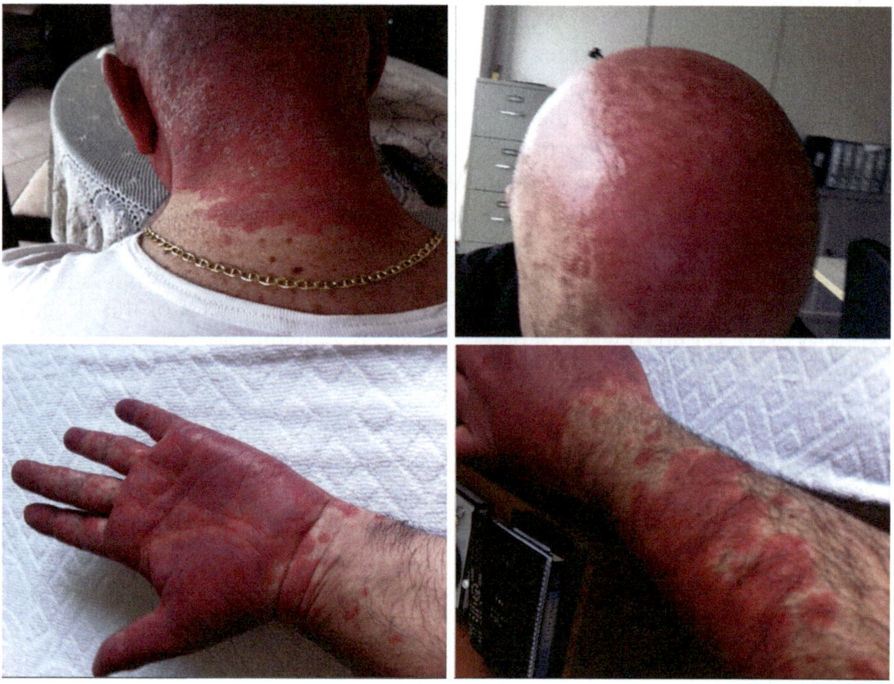

Fig. 37.2 The patient developed a severe erythroderma a few weeks after the start of the vandetanib therapy, mainly involving the sunlight-exposed areas of the body

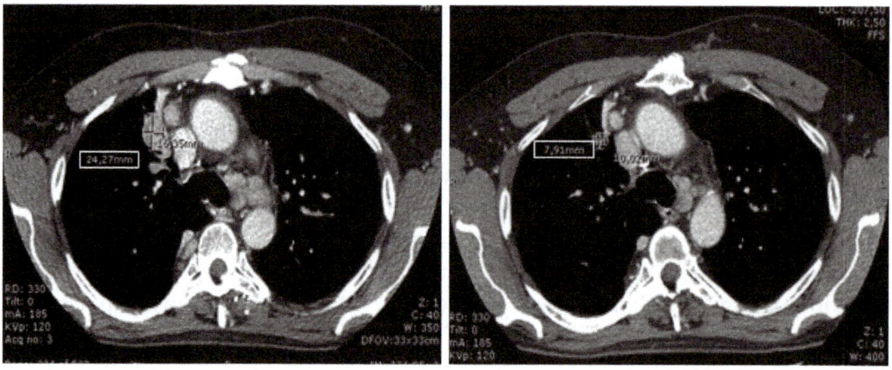

Fig. 37.3 CT scan of the lung performed 6 months after the vandetanib treatment (Panel **a**) showed a significant reduction of the metastatic lesions and in particular of the lymph node of the hilum with respect to the CT scan performed before starting vandetanib (10 mm vs. 24 mm: −58%) (Panel **b**)

serum TSH. TB CT scan showed a slight reduction of the right paratracheal lymph node (10 mm vs. 11 mm) and a significant reduction of the lesions in the mediastinum (20 mm vs. 26 mm) and in the hilum (10 mm vs. 24 mm) (Fig. 37.3); the microlesions in the lung remained stable.

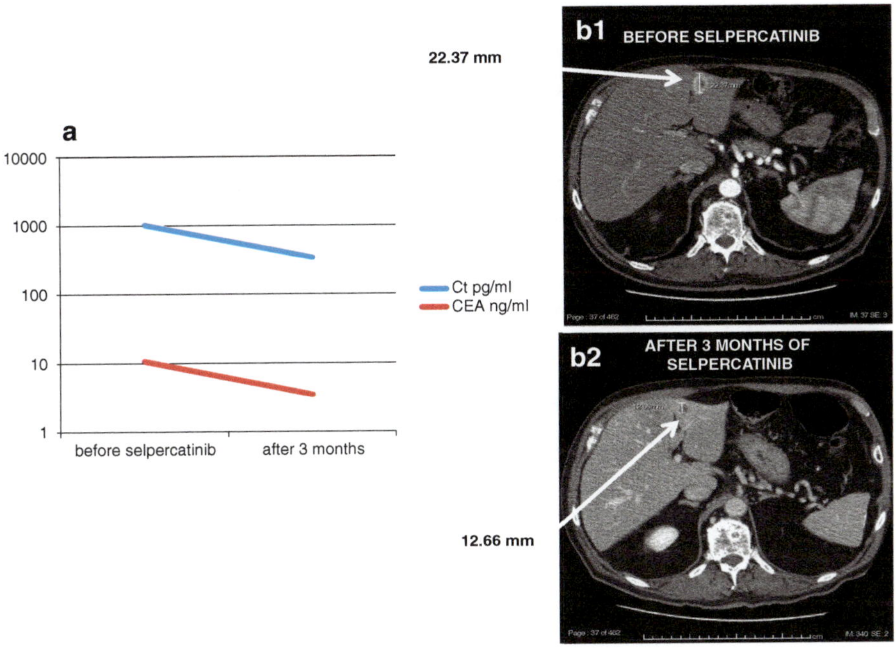

Fig. 37.4 Serum calcitonin (Ct) and carcinoembryonic antigen (CEA) before and 3 months after starting selpercatinib: a significant reduction of both markers was observed (Panel **A**) corresponding to a significant reduction of liver lesions one of which was 22.37 mm before selpercatinib (Panel **B1**) and became 12.66 mm after 3 months of therapy (Panel **B2**)

After almost 6 years of therapy with vandetanib that maintained a substantial stable disease, new liver metastasis were found at the CT scan control, and a new target therapy (i.e., selpercatinib), almost specifically directed against *RET* alterations, was started. The patient was included in an expanded access program, and after 3 months of therapy, the serum levels of Ct and CEA were 3 times lower and liver lesions significantly reduced (Fig. 37.4).

Diagnosis/Assessment

This case offers the opportunity to discuss some issues related to the diagnosis and treatment of advanced and metastatic disease in MTC patients. It is known that MTC can be sporadic (80%) or familial (20%), and the latter condition can be isolated (i.e., familial medullary thyroid cancer, FMTC) or associated with other endocrine neoplasia (i.e., multiple endocrine neoplasia type 2, MEN 2) [1]. In both cases, sporadic and familial, the pathogenesis of MTC is associated with the presence of a somatic or germline *RET* oncogene mutation, respectively [2]. This case had an apparently sporadic MTC without any familial history of MTC or any other associated endocrine neoplasia. However, *RET* mutational screening revealed a germline

RET Ser891Ala mutation consistent with familial MTC. This finding is not unexpected since 6–7% of apparently sporadic MTCs are positive for a *RET* germline mutation when the genetic screening is performed [3, 4]. The case illustrates the importance of performing *RET* genetic screening in all MTC cases, regardless of the clinical presentation. The finding of a germline *RET* mutation does not have any impact on the clinical management of the MTC of index case, but at variance, it is of great relevance for the first-degree relatives, who gain the knowledge of either having or not having the inherited *RET* mutation [5]. The *RET*-positive cases (i.e., gene carriers) require further investigation because they are at high risk of developing the MEN 2 syndrome. A prophylactic thyroidectomy potentially allows a definitive cure of these individuals, who probably would have had the diagnosis made too late if the *RET* screening was not performed. The timing of thyroidectomy and the modalities of follow-up should be personalized according to the specific *RET* mutation and the levels of serum Ct [6, 7].

Management

As previously stated, the finding of a germline *RET* mutation does not change the therapeutic strategy of MTC for this patient, who has been managed according to the biochemical and imaging results obtained during his follow-up. The disease was not cured by the first surgery, but this is consistent with the evidence that when MTC is already extrathyroidal and associated to neck lymph node metastases, the possibility of a definitive cure is rare [8]. This is the rationale for making an early diagnosis of MTC, either by measuring serum Ct in patients with thyroid nodules [9] or performing *RET* screening in hereditary forms [10]. In 2006, the patient was enrolled in a clinical trial with motesanib because of the development of diarrhea, which is a common symptom in advanced MTC with very high levels of serum Ct. The clinical trial was of interest because motesanib was the first tyrosine kinase inhibitor (TKI) employed in thyroid cancer and in particular in MTC [11]. Tyrosine kinase inhibitors are multitargeted therapies, which mainly block the activation of vascular endothelial growth factor receptors (mainly type 2) but also interfere with the function of other tyrosine kinase receptors including, in some cases, the one coded by the *RET* oncogene. The patient had a clinical benefit from treatment, including full control of diarrhea, but unfortunately, a severe side effect such as the hydrops of the gallbladder required the discontinuation of the drug.

Thereafter, the patient was followed up for 7 years without any specific therapy, except for loperamide that was again necessary to control diarrhea. He went into an active surveillance with clinical and biochemical controls every 6–8 months. This is the strategy recommended by many experts since MTC is, in the majority of cases, a slowly progressive cancer, and systemic therapy with TKI should be initiated only when the disease is progressive according to RECIST, thus showing an increase of the metastatic target lesions of at least 20% over 12–14 months [12]. Changes in serum markers alone, such as Ct and CEA, are not indications to start TKI. However, both serum Ct and CEA, and in particular their doubling times, are important to help define the schedule of follow-up visits and imaging [13].

Although it has been recently demonstrated that patients treated with vandetanib at younger age and for symptoms more than for progression are those with a longer progression-free survival time [14, 15], according to the experts' opinions and RECIST, TKI therapy should be started when there are multiple metastases, larger than 2 cm and whose largest diameter has increased by more than 20% over 12–14 months or less [16]. Therefore, in 2014, when the lung metastases and some lymph node metastases began to enlarge rapidly, we decided that it was time to begin therapy with another TKI. At that time, vandetanib had become available and had been demonstrated to significantly increase the time interval of progression-free survival and to reduce many of the symptoms related to the disease [17].

Unfortunately, vandetanib commonly causes severe cutaneous side effects mainly related to sun exposure, and although we informed the patient about this possible risk, he spent time in the sunlight. A few days later, he developed severe erythema (Fig. 37.2) that required the temporary suspension of the drug. The erythema was treated with steroids and antihistamines; few weeks later, when the erythema had almost completely resolved, the drug was restarted but at a lower daily dose (i.e., 100 mg/day). No side effects developed with this dose and the quality of life of our patient has been good. The control of side effects through the reduction of the daily dose or by using personalized protocols for drug administration is a validated method for managing patients on TKIs, since it has been demonstrated that they can continue to have a positive control on tumor growth even at lower doses [14].

Several other side effects can be caused by vandetanib, including hypertension, QTc interval prolongation, fatigue, anorexia, and diarrhea. Whenever possible, the introduction of specific drugs such as calcium channel blockers to control blood pressure or loperamide to control diarrhea can be effective and allow continued use of the TKI. At the present time, vandetanib (commercial name Caprelsa) and cabozantinib (commercial name Cometriq), another multitarget TKI with the specificity to act against *MET*, in addition to *RET* and VEGFR, are the only drugs approved by the Food and Drug Administration (i.e., FDA) and European Medicines Agency (i.e., EMA) for the treatment of MTC. However, we know that after a median period of 14 months, almost all patients develop a kind of resistance to therapy, and the disease begins to progress. Fortunately, other TKIs that may stop MTC growth are currently under development and some are in clinical trials. Indeed, it has been shown that cabozantinib can be effective in patients who have been treated with other TKIs and developed progressive disease [18].

New selective *RET* inhibitors selpercatinib and pralsetinib are demonstrating high activities, greater response rates, and less severe toxicity profiles in early clinical trials [19]. Selpercatinib inhibits wild-type *RET* and multiple mutated *RET* isoforms as well as VEGFR1, VEGFR3, and FGFR 1, 2. However, in cellular assays, selpercatinib inhibited *RET* at approximately 60-fold lower concentrations than FGFR and approximately 8-fold lower concentration than VEGFR. Thus, it can be considered *RET* specific. Recently selpercatinib has been approved with the name RETEMVO by Food and Drug Administration (FDA), specifically for people with

RET gene altered cancer [20]. Pralsetinib, is another investigational selective inhibitor of *RET* fusions and mutations, recently showing very interesting results in the phase 1/2 ARROW study (NCT03037385) in patients with *RET* fusion or *RET* point mutated–positive solid tumors. Pralsetinib, mainly still known as BLUE-667, is under FDA evaluation for approval [21]. Both of them showed great clinical benefits in advanced MTC and other RET altered tumors both if naïve or previously treated with other TKI [22, 23].

Outcome

The quality of life of our patient is, at the present, rather good: he can work and perform his usual practice physical activities. Diarrhea and erythema were both well controlled by reducing the daily dose of vandetanib that was continued until the evidence of clinical benefit. The escape phenomenon, due to the development of a resistance to the drug, commonly occurs with TKI treatment, regardless of tumor type. This is likely due to the method of action of TKIs, which are cytostatic and not cytotoxic drugs, and for this reason, surviving cells can develop resistance to the drug and then start to grow. Being cytostatic drugs, they should not be discontinued until there is evidence of disease progression. In some cases, if the progression is relatively limited, it could be clinically reasonable to continue the drug until the possibility of substitution with another drug. Both cabozantinib and the new selective drugs (i.e., selpercatinib and pralsetinib) are active also in patients previously treated with other TKIs who entered into progression after months or years of treatment. This is a very confortable information since advanced MTC patients have, at this moment, at least three to four lines of possible successful treatment.

Conclusions

MTCs that are already metastatic to the cervical nodes or extrathyroidal at the time of diagnosis have a low probability of cure with surgery alone. Patients can maintain a good quality of life, and the disease can grow rather slowly. However, when MTC metastases are multiple and rapidly growing, systemic therapy with a TKI should be considered. The management of patients with MTC who is receiving TKI therapy should be done in tertiary care centers where there is experience in managing the frequent side effects of these drugs that often are the major limitation to this type of therapy. When side effects interfere with the quality of life of patients, the best initial strategy is to reduce the daily dose of the drug before the side effect becomes too severe or, in the latter situation, to stop the treatment until the recovery, possibly without any unnecessary prolonged interruption, to restart with a lower dose. TKI should not be interrupted if there are no other therapeutic options; however, nowadays, at least three to four different types of TKi, more or less selective, are available and can be used for the control of the disease.

Clinical Pearls/Pitfalls

- *RET* genetic screening allows the identification of hereditary cases (approximately 7%) that are initially diagnosed as apparently sporadic cases.
- The screening of first-degree relatives is strongly recommended if there is a *RET* mutation.
- The serum Ct and CEA doubling time can predict the growth rate of metastatic lesions but should not be used for the decision to start TKI therapy.
- Multimetastatic and progressive MTC should be treated with systemic therapy when progression is defined according to RECIST or if the patient develops symptoms.
- TKIs represent the first-line systemic therapy: adverse events should be managed by experts to avoid interruption of therapy.
- New selective TKIs, selpercatinib and pralsetinib, are under evaluation which may provide improved efficacy and a better side effect profile than vandetanib or cabozantinib.

References

1. Romei C, et al. Genetic and clinical features of multiple endocrine neoplasia types 1 and 2. J Oncol. 2012;2012:705036.
2. Eng C, et al. The relationship between specific RET proto-oncogene mutations and disease phenotype in multiple endocrine neoplasia type 2. International RET mutation consortium analysis. JAMA. 1996;276(19):1575–9.
3. Romei C, et al. Twenty years of lesson learning: how does the ret genetic screening test impact the clinical management of medullary thyroid cancer? Clin Endocrinol (Oxf). 2014;82(6):892–9.
4. Elisei R, et al. Twenty-five years experience on RET genetic screening on hereditary MTC: an update on the prevalence of germline RET mutations. Genes (Basel). 2019;10(9):698.
5. Elisei R, et al. Clinical utility of genetic diagnosis for sporadic and hereditary medullary thyroid carcinoma. Ann Endocrinol (Paris). 2019;80(3):187–90.
6. Elisei R, et al. The timing of total thyroidectomy in RET gene mutation carriers could be personalized and safely planned on the basis of serum calcitonin: 18 years experience at one single center. J Clin Endocrinol Metab. 2012;97(2):426–35.
7. Wells S, et al. American Thyroid Association guidelines task force on medullary thyroid carcinoma. Revised American Thyroid Association guidelines for the management of medullary thyroid carcinoma. Thyroid. 2015;25(6):567–610.
8. Machens A, et al. Prospects of remission in medullary thyroid carcinoma according to basal calcitonin level. J Clin Endocrinol Metab. 2005;90(4):2029–34.
9. Pacini F, et al. Routine measurement of serum calcitonin in nodular thyroid diseases allows the preoperative diagnosis of unsuspected sporadic medullary thyroid carcinoma. J Clin Endocrinol Metab. 1994;78(4):826–9.

10. Pacini F, et al. Early treatment of hereditary medullary thyroid carcinoma after attribution of multiple endocrine neoplasia type 2 gene carrier status by screening for ret gene mutations. Surgery. 1995;118(6):1031–5.
11. Schlumberger MJ, et al. Phase II study of safety and efficacy of motesanib in patients with progressive or symptomatic, advanced or metastatic medullary thyroid cancer. J Clin Oncol. 2009;27(23):3794–801.
12. Eisenhauer EA, et al. New response evaluation criteria in solid tumours: revised RECIST guideline (version 1.1). Eur J Cancer. 2009;45(2):228–47.
13. Meijer JA, et al. Calcitonin and carcinoembryonic antigen doubling times as prognostic factors in medullary thyroid carcinoma: a structured meta-analysis. Clin Endocrinol (Oxf). 2010;72(4):534–42.
14. Valerio L, et al. Medullary thyroid cancer treated with vandetanib: predictors of a longer and durable response. Endocr Relat Cancer. 2020;27(2):97–110.
15. Kreissl MC, et al. Efficacy and safety of vandetanib in progressive and symptomatic medullary thyroid cancer: post hoc analysis from the ZETA trial. J Clin Oncol. 2020;25:JCO1902790.
16. Fugazzola L, et al. 2019 European thyroid association guidelines for the treatment and follow-up of advanced radioiodine-refractory thyroid cancer. Eur Thyroid J. 2019;8(5):227–45.
17. Wells SA Jr, et al. Vandetanib in patients with locally advanced or metastatic medullary thyroid cancer: a randomized, double-blind phase III trial. J Clin Oncol. 2012;30(2):134–41.
18. Elisei R, et al. Cabozantinib in progressive medullary thyroid cancer. J Clin Oncol. 2013;31(29):3639–46.
19. Belli C, et al. Progresses toward precision medicine in RET-altered solid tumors. Clin Cancer Res. 2020. https://doi.org/10.1158/1078-0432.CCR-20-1587. Epub ahead of print.
20. Markham A. Selpercatinib: first approval. Drugs. 2020;80(11):1119–24.
21. FDA approves selpercatinib; pralsetinib may soon follow. Cancer Discov. 2020;10(7):OF1. Epub 2020 Jun 3.
22. Shah MH, et al. Selpercatinib (LOXO-292) in patients with *RET*-mutant medullary thyroid cancer. J Clin Oncol. 2020;38:3594. (suppl; ASCO abstr 3594).
23. Subbiah V, et al. Clinical activity of the RET inhibitor pralsetinib (BLU-667) in patients with RET fusion+ solid tumors. Clin Oncol. 2020;38:109. (suppl; ASCO abstr 109).

Chapter 38
Medical Treatment Decision-Making for Advanced Medullary Thyroid Cancer

Ramona Dadu and Mimi I. Hu

Introduction

There are currently two multikinase inhibitors (MKIs) (vandetanib and cabozantinib) approved by the US Food and Drug Administration (FDA) and the European Medicines Agency and one selective RET inhibitor (selpercatinib) approved by the FDA for the treatment of advanced, progressive, or symptomatic medullary thyroid cancer (MTC). The National Comprehensive Cancer Network Cancer Practice Guidelines for MTC recommends consideration of one of these three agents with unresectable disease that is symptomatic or structurally progressive [1]. The approval of these agents has created new opportunities and challenges for clinicians treating patients with advanced MTC, necessitating a rethinking of how to integrate these treatments into existing surgical and radiotherapeutic approaches to management. A great deal of clinical judgment needs to be applied toward identifying which patients to treat and with which agent; providers should not treat patients with these agents simply because they are available.

An integration of these new agents into the management schema of MTC requires an understanding of the natural history of MTC. The detection of tumor markers, serum calcitonin (Ctn) and carcinoembryonic antigen (CEA), alerts the clinician of the presence of disease long before it may be clinically meaningful. As none of the current therapeutic approaches, other than surgical removal, is curative, it is important for the clinician to create a clear expectation that systemic therapy will be recommended only when there is a likelihood of benefit without added

R. Dadu · M. I. Hu (✉)
Department of Endocrine Neoplasia and Hormonal Disorders, The University of Texas MD Anderson Cancer Center, Houston, TX, USA
e-mail: mhu@mdanderson.org

G. Grani et al. (eds.), *Thyroid Cancer*,
https://doi.org/10.1007/978-3-030-61919-0_38

harm, usually years or even decades after the first appearance of an abnormal tumor marker. Active surveillance, or the "watch-and-wait" approach, is an important component in the care of MTC patients as they can enjoy a good quality of life for many years without requiring systemic therapy. As available systemic therapies are not curative, have side effects (some of which can be fatal), are administered chronically to control disease, and have not yet been shown to prolong overall survival, it is important to balance risk against benefit when considering initiating systemic therapy.

In contrast, patients with rapidly progressive and/or symptomatic disease or disease in areas that are potentially life threatening require a more aggressive approach. Treatment selection for these patients depends on the site of disease, tumor burden, and mutation status. Local therapy (such as surgical resection, radiotherapy, or embolization) could be employed when the disease burden is confined to one area and threatening quality of life or combined with systemic therapy when there is widespread, progressive disease. Understanding the molecular genetics of MTC may inform prognosis and the decision of systemic therapeutic approaches. A constitutively activated RET receptor due to a germline or somatic *RET* mutation is seen in >60% of all MTC patients. Mutually exclusive *RAS* mutations occur in approximately 14% of patients [2].

The discussion in this chapter will use a case-based approach to understanding the elements involved in medical decision-making for patients with advanced MTC.

Case 1: Active Surveillance

A 57-year-old man presented at an outside institution with progressive back pain and was found to have a destructive bone lesion at the L3 spine. A laminectomy with excision identified metastatic MTC to the bone. Staging studies noted a 2.8 cm mass in the left lobe of the thyroid with left lateral cervical adenopathy and metastatic lesions in the liver (up to 3.5 cm) but no pulmonary metastases; biopsies of the thyroid mass and a lymph node confirmed MTC. Baseline Ctn was 4723 pg/mL and CEA was 15.3 ng/mL. Germline *RET* was negative. The patient underwent external beam radiotherapy to the third lumbar surgical bed followed by total thyroidectomy, bilateral central lymph node dissection, and left level III and IV lateral neck dissection. His excised tumors were positive for *RET* M918T somatic mutation by next-generation sequencing (NGS) platform. Thereafter, active surveillance was recommended. After 9 years, the patient remains asymptomatic with no demonstrable evidence of progression nor new lesions by periodic neck ultrasound and other imaging studies [Fig. 38.1]. Serum Ctn and CEA doubling times are 10.6 years and 14.9 years, respectively [Fig. 38.2].

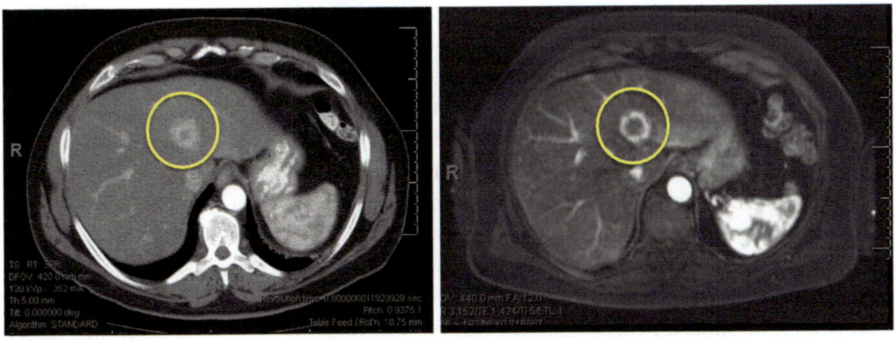

Fig. 38.1 Case #1: Stable liver metastases over 9 years demonstrated by high-resolution computerized tomography (left panel: August 2010) and magnetic resonance imaging (right panel: January 2020). Representative liver metastasis remains stable at 3.5 × 3.0 cm

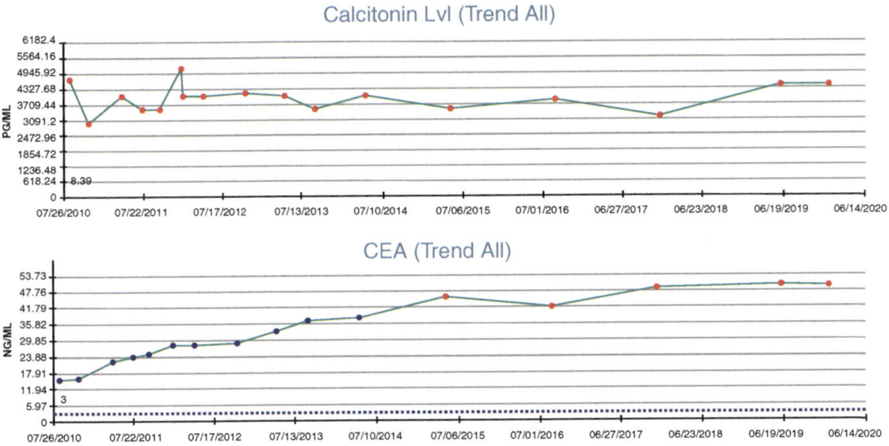

Fig. 38.2 Case #1: Stable calcitonin levels over 9 years with a doubling time of 10.6 years with indolent progression of carcinoembryonic antigen with a doubling time of 14.9 years

Active Surveillance for Progressive Disease

Evaluating serum tumor markers (Ctn and CEA) over time in conjunction with obtaining serial cross-sectional imaging is an effective and objective strategy for monitoring for progression of MTC. Serum Ctn is the primary biochemical marker used for postoperative surveillance and prediction of disease progression. CEA is a less specific biomarker for MTC but one whose magnitude can be useful in understanding the extent of disease and prognosis. Ctn and CEA doubling times correlate with rate of progression, recurrence, and survival [3]. Higher disease-specific survival and recurrence-free survival rates are associated with doubling times of over 1 year, with the CEA doubling time having a higher predictive value. Importantly, doubling times can be used to guide the frequency of imaging studies. In patients with prolonged doubling times of over 1 year, the time between imaging studies can be lengthened to every 6–12 months, thus lowering the cost of observation and reducing the radiation exposure risks associated with frequent imaging studies.

A broad spectrum of imaging modalities can be used to detect metastatic disease. Ultrasound of the neck is the most sensitive technique for detection of thyroid bed or nodal recurrence. Areas not easily imaged by ultrasound, such as the retropharyngeal region or superior mediastinum, can be best imaged by computed tomography (CT) with contrast or magnetic resonance imaging (MRI). Fine-section spiral CT or MRI of the chest or abdomen with liver protocol is useful for detection of pulmonary or hepatic metastasis. As case no. 1 clearly demonstrates, MTC has a predilection to metastasize to the bone. In a large retrospective study at a cancer institution, 19% of MTC patients had bone metastases with 25% of these patients demonstrating the bone metastases within 3 months of MTC diagnosis [4]. The spine and pelvis were the most commonly involved locations (92% and 69%, respectively). In patients with metastatic MTC, it is important to perform periodic bone scans or MRI examination of the spine; however, the presence of a spinal metastasis in the absence of concern about neurologic compressive symptoms is not an indication for therapeutic intervention and may be observed. Although ^{18}F-DOPA PET or a radiolabeled somatostatin analog may be useful in identifying areas of progression when standard imaging studies are unrevealing in the setting of rising tumor markers, their usefulness for routine surveillance of MTC is unproven.

Integration of Local Therapies into the Management of Progressive or Symptomatic Focal Metastases

Recurrent locoregional neck disease in the setting of distant metastases should be treated surgically if there is impending airway or other vital structural compromise. In selected cases, systemic therapy may be a consideration. For example, in a patient in whom the only surgical option for local airway involvement is total laryngectomy, it may be appropriate to delay surgery and initiate a MKI with the hope that surgery (and loss of voice) can be delayed or the procedure can be modified by reducing the size/extent of the metastatic lesion. Surgical wound healing is impaired by currently available MKIs with antiangiogenic effects; thus, such therapy must be stopped approximately 11 days (for cabozantinib: half-life, 55 hours) and 12 weeks (for vandetanib: half-life, 19 days) before a surgical procedure to allow for adequate clearance. The RET inhibitors have relatively little anti-VEGFR activity and a very low risk for bleeding.

It is unclear how targeted systemic therapy should be integrated with the use of external beam radiotherapy (EBRT). Prior to the availability of MKIs, EBRT was used postsurgically to control extensive nodal or soft tissue neck disease or bone metastases causing pain or neurologic deficit. Indeed, in a patient with localized but incurable disease, palliative EBRT may still be a useful adjuvant therapy, although there is no evidence for overall survival benefit. There is currently a bias (although there are no data supporting it) to defer EBRT to gross disease in the neck in the setting of other progressive, distant disease (and consequently, an indication for systemic therapy), given the risk of upper tracheoesophageal or tracheo-tumor fistula formation with antiangiogenic therapy [5]. In patients with brain metastases, where there is an inherent risk for bleeding into the brain lesions during treatment with MKIs, it is recommended that these lesions be irradiated (EBRT or stereotactic radiosurgery) prior to initiation of MKIs. For this reason, brain imaging should be performed prior to proceeding with systemic therapy. It is important to balance the risks and benefits of EBRT and MKI systemic therapy versus watchful waiting.

Distant metastases limited to the lung that are indolent and asymptomatic can usually be followed with serial imaging. Pulmonary metastases can occasionally cause symptoms such as dyspnea, obstructive pneumonia, and hemoptysis. In selected patients with isolated or localized pulmonary metastases, surgical resection or radiotherapy may offer palliation. For patients with liver metastases that are progressive or symptomatic, trans-arterial chemoembolization or radioembolization can be considered [6].

Skeletal metastases of MTC are often clinically silent. Skeletal-related events (SREs) are defined as pain, spinal cord compression, or pathological fracture necessitating external beam irradiation or surgery. It is extremely important to identify bone metastases and initiate palliative treatment modalities before SREs occur. EBRT, stereotactic radiotherapy, vertebroplasty, radiofrequency ablation, cryosurgery, and arterial embolization can be considered to palliate painful metastases or to prevent further progression that could lead to fracture or neurological compromise. Metastasectomy is sometimes performed if there is only one site of bone involvement. Agents that inhibit osteoclast activity, such as bisphosphonates or denosumab, are used in patients with osteolytic bone metastases from several neoplasms (lung, breast, prostate, kidney, and multiple myeloma), and anecdotal experience supports their use in MTC. Zoledronic acid (4 mg) or denosumab (120 mg) given at the approved monthly dosing schedule, in our experience, has been effective in reducing pain and progression of disease associated with bone metastases, although there have been no controlled trials of their use in patients with MTC. Although less frequent dosing of these antiresorptive agents has not been evaluated formally for efficacy in thyroid cancer patients, it is reasonable to surmise that less frequent dosing while maintaining suppression of bone turnover may be as effective in reducing SREs with less risk for side effects, such as osteonecrosis of the jaw. Little is known about the efficacy of MKIs or RET inhibitors in treating metastatic bone lesions. Bone lesions are not considered to be measurable targets; thus, bone metastases were not assessed in clinical trials of vandetanib, cabozantinib, or RET inhibitors although there are some reports of response with these agents [7]. Clinical trials in patients with MTC and bone metastases are needed to evaluate which agents are effective.

Case 2: Treating with a Systemic Agent and Management of Adverse Effects

A 32-year-old woman was diagnosed with sporadic medullary thyroid carcinoma at the age of 25 years. Prior to coming to our institution, she underwent total thyroidectomy, left central lymph neck dissection, and superior mediastinal lymph node dissection followed by external beam radiotherapy to the left lower neck. Her post-treatment Ctn was 81 pg/mL (preoperative >5000 pg/mL) and CEA was 2.2 ng/mL (preoperative 186 ng/mL). Serum Ctn and CEA levels progressed steadily over the next 3 years to 323 pg/mL and 59 ng/mL, respectively. Ultrasound of the neck identified a recurrent supraclavicular lymph node metastasis, and CT of the chest identified mediastinal adenopathy (2.4cm in right hilum, 2.9cm in subcarinal region) and subcentimeter lung metastases. CT of the abdomen with liver protocol was unremarkable. Given the lack of prior imaging of the chest to understand progressive rate, the recommendation was for short-term surveillance for progression. Mutational testing on a 50-gene NGS platform on the originally resected thyroidectomy specimen was positive for a somatic *RET* M918T mutation. Over the next 7 months, her Ctn rose to 468 pg/mL and CEA to 165 ng/mL, correlating with asymptomatic, progressive mediastinal lymph node metastases (4.3cm in right hilum, 3.5cm in subcarinal region) and pulmonary metastases and new bone metastases in C2 and C3 vertebral body [Fig. 38.3a]. Systemic chemotherapy with vandetanib was favored over cabozantinib due to the patient's history of neck irradiation, which led to a partial response after 9 months of therapy [Fig. 38.3b]. However, she developed progressive disease 26 months after being on vandetanib [Figs.. 38.3c and

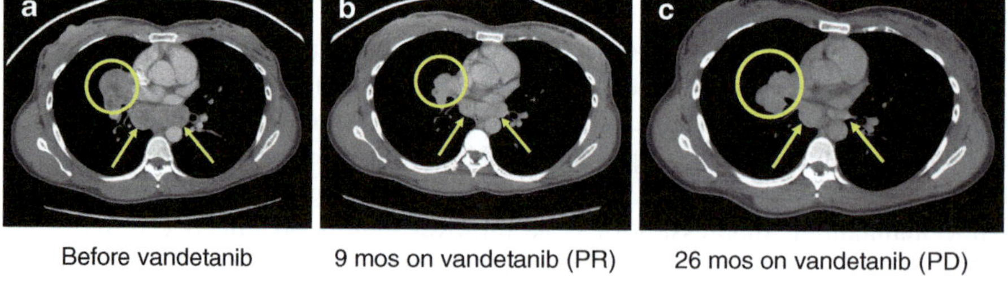

Fig. 38.3 Case #2: Right hilar (yellow circle) and subcarinal (yellow arrows) lymphadenopathy before vandetanib (panel A), on vandetanib for 9 months with partial response (PR) (panel B), and with progressive disease (PD) after 26 months on vandetanib (panel C)

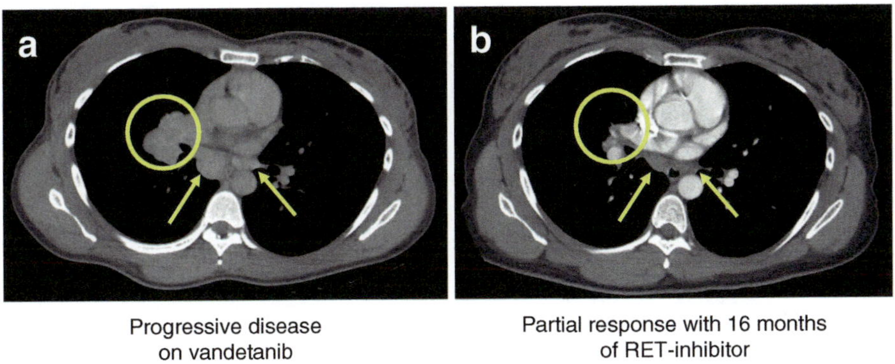

Fig. 38.4 Case #2: Right hilar (yellow circles) and subcarinal (yellow arrows) lymphadenopathy at progression on vandetanib (panel A) and with partial response after 16 months on a selective RET inhibitor (panel B)

38.4a]. She had no significant adverse effects other than grade 1 acneiform rash and taste change altering her appetite. Due to the fact that she has a somatic *RET* mutation, she was initiated on a phase I trial with a selective RET inhibitor and achieved a partial response of 41% reduction in target lesions after 12 months of therapy. She continues on treatment 27 months from initiation of the study drug [Fig. 38.4b]. She has not experienced any adverse effects with the RET inhibitor.

Approved Agents for MTC: Cabozantinib, Vandetanib, and Selpercatinib

On the basis of two randomized, placebo-controlled phase III trials that demonstrated efficacy (prolongation of progression-free survival), vandetanib and cabozantinib are approved in the USA and Europe for the treatment of symptomatic or progressive MTC in patients with unresectable, locally advanced, or metastatic disease [8, 9]. The cabozantinib (EXAM) and vandetanib (ZETA) trials had some important differences [Table 38.1]. The most notable differences are the requirement for progressive disease within 14 months in the cabozantinib trial and the presence of a crossover design in the vandetanib trial, making it impossible to compare outcomes in these two trials in any meaningful way.

Selpercatinib (LOXO-292) and pralsetinib (BLU-667) are potent, selective RET inhibitors that have been tested in phase I clinical trials since early 2016, both of which have additional activity against the gatekeeper *RET* V804 mutation. This gatekeeper mutation is known to lead to resistance to both cabozantinib and vandetanib in vitro [10–12]. Selpercatinib led to an objective response rate (ORR) of 56% (95% CI: 42, 70) in MTC patients previously treated with cabozantinib and/or

Table 38.1 Phase III trials for cabozantinib and vandetanib in patients with MTC

	Cabozantinib phase III (EXAM)		Vandetanib phase III (ZETA)	
Patients	Cabozantinib $N=219$	Placebo $N=111$	Vandetanib $N=231$	Placebo $N=100$
Inclusion criteria	Documented RECIST progression within 14 months of enrollment		Locally advanced or metastatic disease and serum Ct ≥ 500 pg/mL, with no requirement for progression	
Crossover design with progression during trial	Not allowed		Allowed	
Median PFS	11.2 months	4.0 months	Not reached (estimated 30.5 months)	19.3 months
OS	Immature analysis 44 % died at PFS cutoff		Immature analysis 15 % died at PFS cutoff	
Objective response rates	28 %	0 %	45 %	13 %[a]

[a]Twelve of the thirteen responses observed in patients randomized to the placebo group occurred while the patients were receiving open-label vandetanib

vandetanib and 59% (95% CI: 47, 70) in treatment-naïve patients [(13)]. Pralsetinib led to an ORR of 56% (95% CI: 38, 74) in MTC patient previously treated with cabozantinib and/or vandetanib and 63% (95% CI: 35, 85) in treatment-naïve patients [14]. Responses were long in duration and occurred regardless of specific germline and somatic *RET* mutation, even in patients with the gatekeeper *RET* V804 mutation. With these encouraging findings, selpercatinib received accelerated approval by the US FDA on May 8, 2020. Pralsetinib is undergoing evaluation by the FDA and will likely receive approval as well later in 2020. Notably, two additional RET inhibitors (TPX-0046 and BOS172738) are also currently in phase I clinical trials [15, 16]. TPX-0046, a RET and SRC inhibitor, has a potential added benefit in that it has activity against the solvent front mutation *RET* G810R, which has been associated with resistance to MKIs and other selective RET inhibitors under investigation [15] [17].

The timing to initiate therapy varies greatly among physicians and practices. However, the recommended indications for initiation of systemic chemotherapy include [18]:

1. Progressive (based on RECIST – Response Evaluation Criteria in Solid Tumors) [19] and clinically significant disease. Most clinical trials in thyroid cancer require progression within 12–14 months in order to qualify for enrollment in a trial, and therefore this is the standard most centers use for initiating systemic therapy in asymptomatic patients.
2. Symptomatic metastatic disease that cannot be treated with local or symptom-specific therapies such as surgery, radiotherapy, embolization, cryoablation, or diarrhea management.
3. Bulky disease that compromises organ function and cannot be managed with localized therapies.

In selected cases, additional consideration for systemic therapy includes:

1. Calcitonin doubling time of less than 6 months and structural evidence of clinically significant disease that cannot be treated with local therapies. Rising tumor markers alone are not sufficient to demonstrate progression and warrant initiating systemic therapy [1].
2. Severe, intractable MTC-related diarrhea or Cushing's syndrome and lack of efficacy of other medical treatments and presence of structural and clinically significant disease.

Adverse Events Associated with Approved Agents

Compared with cytotoxic chemotherapeutic agents, the adverse events (AEs) associated with MKIs are generally manageable in the setting of a clinical trial or in the hands of physicians familiar with the toxicity profile of each MKI. Some AEs are serious or can cause a worsening of a patient's quality of life; therefore, it is extremely important to apply an individualized, patient-centered approach concerning when to initiate a systemic therapeutic agent and which drug to use [18]. While patients with progressive metastatic disease may benefit from the treatment, potential serious AEs of these drugs may outweigh the benefits in patients with indolent or stable disease. The RET inhibitors have a more favorable and tolerable side effect profile due to the potent selectivity for the RET receptor with relatively low or no inhibition of VEGFR or other kinase receptors.

Before starting treatment with vandetanib, cabozantinib, or selpercatinib, all patients should sign an informed consent after describing the common and serious AEs, symptoms of serious AEs, and the expected efficacy with medical therapy. Baseline symptoms should be assessed prior to initiation of treatment with documentation of new and/or ongoing AEs throughout the treatment period [20]. The assessment and grading of each AE is performed at each visit using the Common Terminology Criteria for Adverse Events version 4.0 (CTCAE v4.0) [21]. Additionally, the Eastern Cooperative Oncology Group (ECOG) performance status (an assessment of general well-being) should be noted and be used as a basis for whether a patient can be safely treated with a proposed treatment or whether dose adjustment is necessary [22].

MKIs are associated with numerous side effects due to the variety of targeted kinase receptors, including skin effects (palmar-plantar erythrodysesthesia, photosensitivity, or acne), mucositis, taste alteration, hypertension, diarrhea, nausea, decreased appetite, weight loss, fatigue, and uncontrolled hypothyroidism. Vandetanib is associated with QTc prolongation in 14% of treated patients. Cabozantinib leads to a higher risk for hemorrhage, venous thrombosis, intestinal perforation, and fistula formation as it is a more potent inhibitor of VEGFR-2 than vandetanib. Patient quality of life, compliance, and optimal response to drug therapy can all be limited without implementation of preventative strategies and aggressive management of AEs. The management of AEs associated with MKIs used for metastatic thyroid cancer is complex and beyond the scope of this article; it has been well described elsewhere [23].

The RET inhibitors generally had low-grade and reversible AEs. Selpercatinib led to dry mouth, diarrhea, hypertension, and increased liver transaminases in ≥15% of patients, with most being grade 1 or 2 [13]. Only 1.7% of all cancer patients treated (n = 531) with selpercatinib discontinued therapy due to a treatment-related AE. Pralsetinib was associated with hypertension, neutropenia, constipation, and leukopenia in ≥15% of patients with no grade 4 or 5 AEs [14]. Across the entire study, 4% discontinued drug due to a treatment-related toxicity.

Choosing a Therapeutic Agent Based on Adverse Event Risk Rather than Efficacy

The MKIs and RET inhibitors have established efficacy in patients with extensive MTC. At present, there are no efficacy data favoring one over another agent. A great deal of clinical judgment needs to be applied when deciding which drug to initiate. However, it is certainly clear now that mutational testing for somatic mutations, if the germline testing is negative, is warranted in patients with metastatic disease to determine if there is a targetable *RET* mutation. The most recent NCCN guidelines for thyroid cancer has incorporated the recommendation for somatic mutation testing in appropriate MTC patients [1]. If the patient has a germline or somatic *RET* mutation and radiologic progressive disease, a selective RET inhibitor would be the favored choice due to the high efficacy seen in phase I trials and the lack of significant AEs. If there is no *RET* mutation, then one would choose from one of the MKIs available or referral to an appropriate clinical trial [Fig. 38.5].

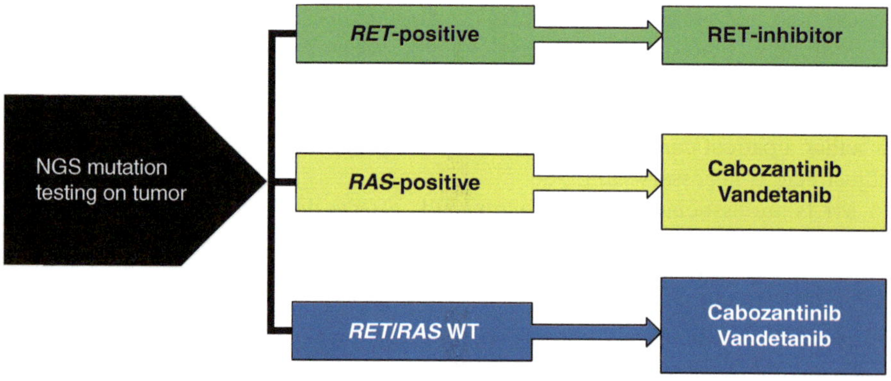

Fig. 38.5 Treatment algorithm based on mutation profile in advanced, progressive MTC. *NGS* next-generation sequencing; *WT* wild type

A systematic and patient-centered approach for deciding which MKI to choose first was recently developed by our group [18]. This takes into account multiple factors including patient medical history, physical examination findings, baseline laboratory data, electrocardiogram, concomitant medications, and extension of tumor to surrounding tissues. From this evaluation, it is possible to assess the impact of a particular drug-related side effect for the individual patient. For example, a patient with a history of long QT syndrome or treatment with medications known to prolong the QT interval would be best treated with cabozantinib. On the other hand, a patient with a history of peptic ulcer disease, diverticulitis, or tumoral encroachment or invasion into the trachea/esophagus/major vascular structures might be better treated with vandetanib.

Finally, if a patient develops progression on systemic treatment, it is recommended to biopsy a progressing lesion to evaluate for emergent mutations conveying resistance, such as a gatekeeper or solvent front *RET* mutation or a *RAS* bypass mutation [17] [24].

Clinical Pearls

- The majority of patients with residual MTC, after standard treatment with surgical resection, have indolent disease and can be actively monitored for objective progression on radiologic imaging performed at appropriate intervals.
- Systemic chemotherapy is not indicated in patients with indolent or structurally nonthreatening disease, even in the setting of distant metastases.
- In patients with progressive or symptomatic MTC without reasonable surgical or localized treatment options, testing for somatic mutations (if germline *RET* is negative) should be performed to identify if a targetable *RET* mutation exists.
- Selpercatinib, cabozantinib, or vandetanib should be considered to improve progression-free survival.
- A patient-centered approach must be used toward drug selection with diligent prevention and aggressive management strategies for adverse events.
- A patient with progressive MTC intolerant or unresponsive to the approved agents should be referred for a clinical trial.
- Although these agents have had a significant impact on the management of MTC, more effective treatment options for this small but difficult-to-treat population are needed.

References

1. NCCN. Clinical practice guidelines in oncology: thyroid carcinoma. J Natl Compr Canc Netw. 6(2020)
2. www.cancer.sanger.ac.uk/cosmic.

3. Meijer JA, le Cessie S, van den Hout WB, Kievit J, Schoones JW, Romijn JA, et al. Calcitonin and carcinoembryonic antigen doubling times as prognostic factors in medullary thyroid carcinoma: a structured meta-analysis. Clin Endocrinol (Oxf). 2010;72(4):534–42.
4. Xu JY, Murphy WA Jr, Milton DR, Jimenez C, Rao SN, Habra MA, et al. Bone metastases and skeletal-related events in medullary thyroid carcinoma. J Clin Endocrinol Metab. 2016;101(12):4871–7.
5. Blevins DP, Dadu R, Hu M, Baik C, Balachandran D, Ross W, et al. Aerodigestive fistula formation as a rare side effect of antiangiogenic tyrosine kinase inhibitor therapy for thyroid cancer. Thyroid. 2014;24(5):918–22.
6. Fromigue J, De Baere T, Baudin E, Dromain C, Leboulleux S, Schlumberger M. Chemoembolization for liver metastases from medullary thyroid carcinoma. J Clin Endocrinol Metab. 2006;91(7):2496–9.
7. Cabanillas ME, Brose MS, Holland J, Ferguson KC, Sherman SI. A phase I study of cabozantinib (XL184) in patients with differentiated thyroid cancer. Thyroid. 2014;24(10):1508–14.
8. Wells SA Jr, Robinson BG, Gagel RF, Dralle H, Fagin JA, Santoro M, et al. Vandetanib in patients with locally advanced or metastatic medullary thyroid cancer: a randomized, double-blind phase III trial. J Clin Oncol. 2012;30(2):134–41.
9. Elisei R, Schlumberger MJ, Muller SP, Schoffski P, Brose MS, Shah MH, et al. Cabozantinib in progressive medullary thyroid cancer. J Clin Oncol. 2013;31(29):3639–46.
10. Carlomagno F, Guida T, Anaganti S, Vecchio G, Fusco A, Ryan AJ, et al. Disease associated mutations at valine 804 in the RET receptor tyrosine kinase confer resistance to selective kinase inhibitors. Oncogene. 2004;23(36):6056–63.
11. Bentzien F, Zuzow M, Heald N, Gibson A, Shi Y, Goon L, et al. In vitro and in vivo activity of cabozantinib (XL184), an inhibitor of RET, MET, and VEGFR2, in a model of medullary thyroid cancer. Thyroid. 2013;23(12):1569–77.
12. Mologni L, Redaelli S, Morandi A, Plaza-Menacho I, Gambacorti-Passerini C. Ponatinib is a potent inhibitor of wild-type and drug-resistant gatekeeper mutant RET kinase. Mol Cell Endocrinol. 2013;377(1-2):1–6.
13. Wirth L, Sherman E, Drilon A, Solomon B, Robinson B, Lorch J, et al. Registrational results of LOXO-292 in patients with RET-altered thyroid cancers. Ann Oncol. 2019;30(suppl 5):LBA93.
14. Taylor MH, Gainor JF, Hu MI, Zhu VW, Lopes B, Leboulleux S, et al. Activity and tolerability of BLU-667, a highly potent and selective RET inhibitor, in patients with advanced RET-altered thyroid cancers. JCO. 2019;37(suppl 15):abstr 6018.
15. Drilon A, Rogers E, Zhai D, Deng W, Zhang X, Lee D, et al. TPX-0046 is a novel and potent RET/SRC inhibitor for RET-driven cancers. Ann Oncol. 2019;30(suppl 5):506P.
16. Schoffski P, Aftimos PG, Massard C, Italiano A, Jungels C, Andreas K, et al. A phase I study of BOS172738 in patients with advanced solid tumors with RET gene alterations including non-small cell lung cancer and medullary thyroid cancer. JCO. 2019;37(suppl 15):TPS3162.
17. Solomon BJ, Tan L, Lin JJ, Wong SQ, Hollizeck S, Ebata K, et al. RET solvent front mutations mediate acquired resistance to selective RET inhibition in RET-driven malignancies. J Thorac Oncol. 2020;15(4):541–9.
18. Cabanillas ME, Hu MI, Jimenez C. Medullary thyroid cancer in the era of tyrosine kinase inhibitors: to treat or not to treat–and with which drug--those are the questions. J Clin Endocrinol Metab. 2014;99(12):4390–6.
19. https://recist.eortc.org/
20. Carhill AA, Cabanillas ME, Jimenez C, Waguespack SG, Habra MA, Hu M, et al. The non-investigational use of tyrosine kinase inhibitors in thyroid cancer: establishing a standard for patient safety and monitoring. J Clin Endocrinol Metab. 2013;98(1):31–42.

21. https://evs.nci.nih.gov/ftp1/CTCAE/CTCAE_4.03/CTCAE_4.03_2010-06-14_QuickReference_5x7.pdf.
22. http://www.ecog.org/general/perf_stat.html
23. Cabanillas ME, Hu MI, Durand JB, Busaidy NL. Challenges associated with tyrosine kinase inhibitor therapy for metastatic thyroid cancer. J Thyroid Res. 2011;2011:985780.
24. Hu MI, Cote G, Hai T, Busaidy NL, Cabanillas ME, Dadu R, et al. Emergence of resistance-associated mutations of RET V804M and KRAS in medullary thyroid carcinoma (MTC) patients treated with tyrosine kinase inhibitors (TKI) cabozanitinib and vandetanib. Thyroid. 2019;29:A-13.

Chapter 39
Screening Leading to Diagnosis of C cell Hyperplasia

Giuseppe Costante

Introduction

The neoplastic proliferation of calcitonin (CT)-secreting thyroid parafollicular cells (C cells), broadly defined *C cell disease*, includes medullary thyroid carcinoma (MTC) and C cell hyperplasia (CCH) [1]. Both MTC and CCH are usually associated with increased circulating CT levels and may occur in sporadic or hereditary forms [2, 3].

MTCs represent approximately 4–10% of all thyroid malignancies [2–4]. Seventy-five percent of them are sporadic [2–4], while 25% are hereditary tumors [2–4], associated with specific germline mutations of the *REarranged during Transfection* (RET) proto-oncogene [2–4].

CCH with cytologic and/or nuclear features of atypia was initially described as a lesion associated with familial MTC and multiple endocrine neoplasia (MEN) type 2A and 2B [1–4] and is considered a C cell carcinoma in situ [3]. CCH histologically similar to that occurring in hereditary MTC may be observed in individual cases of chronic lymphocytic thyroiditis [3]. Moreover, up to 33% of thyroids from normal subjects (15% in women and 41% in men) may fulfill the histologic criteria of CCH [2, 4], but the exact significance of this sporadic form is unclear, and its progression to MTC has never been demonstrated.

CT determination in the washout fluid of the nodule could represent a promising preoperative ancillary procedure for MTC diagnosis, but the reference range and the appropriate international standards are not precisely defined.

G. Costante (✉)
Endocrinology Clinic, Medicine Department, Institut Jules Bordet, Comprehensive Cancer Center – Université Libre de Bruxelles, Brussels, Belgium
e-mail: giuseppe.costante@bordet.be

G. Grani et al. (eds.), *Thyroid Cancer*,
https://doi.org/10.1007/978-3-030-61919-0_39

Case Presentation

A 37-year-old woman presented an incidental (13.8×15.7×20.1 mm) ultrasonographically suspicious (solid, hypoechoic nodule with regular margins; classified as intermediate suspicion by the 2015 American Thyroid Association guidelines) nodule in the right thyroid lobe. Serum TSH was 1.2 mU/l, and anti-TPO antibodies were absent. US-guided fine-needle aspiration biopsy (FNAB) repeatedly yielded insufficient cytology (Class 1 of the Bethesda classification system). Basal calcitonin (CT) was 21 pg/ml (n.v. <10 pg/ml), with increased response to 84 pg/ml (n.v. <71 pg/ml) after Ca^{2+} stimulation.

Due to inconclusive cytology and CT provocative test indicating C cell disease, the patient was submitted to total thyroidectomy. Surgical pathology showed nodular thyroid hyperplasia, and immunohistochemistry showed low-power microscopic fields containing at least 50 C cells, consistent with CCH. L-thyroxine replacement therapy was immediately started. Three months after thyroidectomy, the patient was euthyroid, the serum TSH was 1.2 mU/l, and the basal CT levels were undetectable. The patient is presently in good health.

Case Discussion

Preoperative diagnosis of nonhereditary C cell disease is challenging. CCH, in fact, can only be diagnosed at surgical pathology. MTCs usually present as thyroid nodules [2–4], and cytology displays poor sensitivity (< 50%) for preoperative MTC diagnosis [2, 4, 5].

Being CT specifically secreted by C cells, its circulating levels usually rise to a limited extent in CCH and sharply increase in MTCs, paralleling disease progression [2, 4]. It is worth recalling, however, that interfering factors such as heterophilic antibodies or high-molecular-weight aggregates (*macrocalcitonin*) may determine falsely elevated circulating CT levels [4]. Several pathological conditions and pharmacological agents (Table 39.1) may also cause increased serum CT levels [2, 4]. The role of thyroid autoimmunity is controversial, with elevated or decreased [2, 4] serum CT concentrations, or even comparable to those found in control subjects [2, 4]. Greatly increased serum CT levels can occasionally be observed in patients with neuroendocrine tumors (Table 39.1), such as gastrointestinal, small and large cell lung cancers [2–4]. In all such instances, a confirmatory stimulation test can improve the diagnostic specificity of CT measurement [2, 4].

Classically, pentagastrin was the most used CT provocative test [2–4]. Due to PG unavailability, a short intravenous Ca^{2+} infusion nowadays represents an effective alternative [2, 3, 6], providing results comparable to pentagastrin stimulation, in both normal subjects and C cell disease patients [2, 3, 6]. The procedure consists in the injection of a 25 mg calcium gluconate [i.e., 2.3 mg or 0.12 mEq of elemental calcium/kg body weight during a minimum 3 minutes infusion time (5 ml/min)] and

Table 39.1 Causes of spurious elevations of serum calcitonin

Assay interference		
	Heterophilic antibodies	
	Macrocalcitonin	
Pathological conditions		
	Neoplastic	
		Small-cell lung carcinoma
		Breast cancer
		Neuroendocrine tumors of the lung or gastrointestinal tract
		Zollinger's syndrome
		Follicular thyroid tumors
		Papillary thyroid micro-carcinoma
	Nonneoplastic	
		Chronic renal failure
		Autoimmune thyroiditis (*debated*)
		Pernicious anemia
		Pancreatitis
		Hyperparathyroidism
		Nonneoplastic hypergastrinemia
		Mastocytosis
		Type 1A pseudohypoparathyroidism
		Sepsis
Pharmacological agents		
		Proton-pump inhibitors

determination of serum CT in basal conditions, 2, 5, and 10 minutes after stopping the infusion [6]. The stimulated CT peak is <10 pg/ml in approximately 80% of normal subjects, with a maximal response <30 pg/ml in 95% of normals [4]. Notably, more limited CT increase (0 to 2-fold rise) occurs in other neuroendocrine tumors [2–4]. The optimal reported CT cutoff values for considering thyroidectomy were >79 pg/ml for female and >544 pg/ml for male subjects [6].

Due to MTC poor prognosis in classical series, systematic CT measurement has been advocated in thyroid nodular disease patients, for early diagnosis and better outcome [2, 4]. Overall, the diagnostic sensitivity of circulating CT for C cell disease approximated 100% [2, 4], with an important proportion of false positives. Thus, the positive predictive value (PPV) was low (10–40%), even after excluding all known causes of spurious CT elevation [2, 4]. Additionally, the frequency of isolated CCH resulted high (30–75%) [2, 4]. Concerning MTC, the PPV was 100% only for CT values >100 pg/ml [7], leading the American Thyroid Association to recommend this cutoff as highly suspicious [8]. For basal CT increases <100 pg/ml, the PPV for MTC diagnosis dropped to approximately 10% [2, 4], and a stimulation test was necessary for improving sensitivity and specificity [2, 4], with a wide variation among studies in terms of both basal CT cutoff levels (5–20 pg/ml) for performing provocative tests and CT peaks (30–1,000 pg/ml) considered diagnostic for MTC [2, 4]. Indeed, the universal CT screening in thyroid nodular disease patients has not been endorsed by most scientific societies [9].

In the present case, the US findings were suspicious, FNAB was inconclusive, and both basal and Ca^{2+} stimulated CT levels were consistent with C cell disease. Thus, histological verification was advised, indicating benign thyroid nodule and sporadic CCH.

Should sporadic CCH be considered a false positive in the CT screening of thyroid nodules? Unless future studies will provide evidence that it actually represents a precancerous lesion evolving to MTC, surgery would not be required in such patients. Indeed, CCH frequency in screening studies was 0.12–1.56% [2], accounting for 30–75% of the cases with basal CT levels between 20 and 100 pg/ml and positive CT stimulation test [2, 4]. Thus, distinguishing preoperatively CCH from MTC could avoid unnecessary surgery. In this perspective, the amplitude of the CT peak at provocative testing could also help, with different cutoff values proposed by different reports [2, 4]. Particularly, one study found an 80% PPV for CCH in case of PG-stimulated CT peak 100–1000 pg/ml and a 100% PPV for MTC for response >1000 pg/ml [7]. Another study defined a cutoff of CT peak at 275 pg/ml, reporting a 100% PPV for MTC above this cutoff and an 89 % PPV for CCH in case of positive stimulated CT response <275 pg/ml [10].

Future studies should define the threshold windows of peak CT levels differentiating MTC from CCH, using Ca^{2+} stimulation. A promising preoperative ancillary procedure could be CT determination in the washout fluid of the nodule (FNAB-CT), with a reported sensitivity for MTC diagnosis of 80–100% [4]. Nonetheless, the exact reference range for FNAB-CT levels in relation to C cell density in normal thyroid tissue, as well as international standards for CT measurement in biological fluids other than serum, needs to be precisely defined.

Clinical Pearls

- Serum calcitonin is a highly sensitive biomarker for C cell disease.
- Increased circulating basal calcitonin levels are more frequently associated to CCH than to MTC.
- CCH does not represent a precancerous condition in the nonfamilial setting.
- Preoperative differentiation between MTC and CCH is often difficult, even after provocative testing (e.g., calcium stimulation).
- There is insufficient evidence supporting systematic calcitonin screening in the initial management of thyroid nodular disease patients.

References

1. LiVolsi VA. C cell hyperplasia/neoplasia. J Clin Endocrinol Metab. 1997;82:39–41.
2. Costante G, Durante C, Francis Z, Schlumberger M, Filetti S. Determination of calcitonin levels in C-cell disease: clinical interest and potential pitfalls. Nat Clin Pract Endocrinol Metab. 2009;5(1):35–44.
3. Leboulleux S, Baudin E, Travagli JP, Schlumberger M. Medullary thyroid carcinoma. Clin Endocrinol (Oxf). 2004;61:229–31.

4. Costante G., Meringolo D. Calcitonin as a biomarker of C cell disease: recent achievements and current challenges. Endocrine 2020;67:273–280. doi: https://doi.org/10.1007/s12020-019-02183-6.
5. Essig GF Jr, Porter K, Schneider D, Debora A, Lindsey SC, Busonero G, et al. Fine needle aspiration and medullary thyroid carcinoma: the risk of inadequate preoperative evaluation and initial surgery when relying upon FNAB cytology alone. Endocr Pract. 2013;19:920.
6. Mian C, Perrino M, Colombo C, Cavedon E, Pennelli G, Ferrero S, et al. Refining calcium test for the diagnosis of medullary thyroid cancer: cutoffs, procedures, and safety. J Clin Endocrinol Metab. 2014;99:1656–64.
7. Costante G, Meringolo D, Durante C, Bianchi D, Nocera M, Tumino S, et al. Predictive value of serum calcitonin levels for preoperative diagnosis of medullary thyroid carcinoma in a cohort of 5817 consecutive patients with thyroid nodules. J Clin Endocrinol Metab. 2007;92:450–5.
8. Haugen BR, Alexander EK, Bible KC, Doherty GM, Mandel SJ, Nikiforov YE, Pacini F, Randolph GW, Sawka AM, Schlumberger M, Schuff KG, Sherman SI, Sosa JA, Steward DL, Tuttle RM, Wartofsky L. 2015 American Thyroid Association Management Guidelines for Adult Patients with Thyroid Nodules and Differentiated Thyroid Cancer: The American Thyroid Association Guidelines Task Force on Thyroid Nodules and Differentiated Thyroid Cancer. Thyroid. 2016;26:1–133. https://doi.org/10.1089/thy.2015.0020.
9. Costante G, Filetti S. Early diagnosis of medullary thyroid carcinoma: is systematic calcitonin screening appropriate in patients with nodular thyroid disease? Oncologist. 2011;16:49–52. https://doi.org/10.1634/theoncologist.2010-0344.
10. Milone F, Ramundo V, Chiofalo MG, Severino R, Paciolla I, Pezzullo L, et al. Predictive value of pentagastrin test for preoperative differential diagnosis between C-cell hyperplasia and medullary thyroid carcinoma in patients with moderately elevated basal calcitonin levels. Clin Endocrinol (Oxf). 2010;73:85–8.

Chapter 40
Increased Basal Calcitonin in Nodular Goiter: Is It Micromedullary Thyroid Cancer?

Andreas Machens and Henning Dralle

Case Presentation

A 64-year-old woman with a 17-year history of thyroid nodules was referred with elevated basal calcitonin serum levels for a second opinion regarding the need for thyroidectomy.

Evaluation for Surgery

Eight years and eight months before referral, outside thyroid ultrasonography had identified a 22 × 13 mm hypoechoic nodule in the left lobe, for which the patient had been placed on a daily levothyroxine dose of 75 μg to suppress serum TSH.

Five months before referral, the left lobe hypoechoic nodule, measuring 28 × 12 mm, appeared hypofunctional on thyroid scintigraphy carried out elsewhere. Thyroid ultrasonography at that hospital disclosed two additional 3 and 5 mm nodules in an otherwise normal-appearing thyroid gland. The patient's basal

A. Machens (✉)
Department of Visceral, Vascular and Endocrine Surgery, University Hospital, Halle (Saale), Germany

Medical Faculty, University of Halle-Wittenberg, Halle (Saale), Germany

H. Dralle
Department of General, Visceral and Transplantation Surgery, Section of Endocrine Surgery, University Hospital, Essen, Germany

Medical Faculty, University of Duisburg-Essen, Essen, Germany

G. Grani et al. (eds.), *Thyroid Cancer*,
https://doi.org/10.1007/978-3-030-61919-0_40

calcitonin serum level was slightly elevated: 15.2 pg/mL (unspecified calcitonin assay; upper normal limit, 11.8 pg/mL).

One month before referral, high-resolution thyroid ultrasonography at the same facility uncovered, apart from the large left nodule (now measuring 26 × 16 mm), two hypoechoic nodules in the left lobe, measuring 10 × 6 mm and 7 × 4 mm, respectively, and a 3 × 1 mm hypoechoic, calcified nodule in the right lobe. Ultrasound-guided fine-needle aspiration of the large left nodule yielded a cytological diagnosis of follicular neoplasia (Bethesda class IV). Using a more sensitive calcitonin assay (IMMULITE 2000, Diagnostic Products Corporation, USA; normal upper limit <5 pg/mL), serum calcitonin was 25 pg/mL basally and peaking at 256 pg/mL 2 min after intravenous stimulation with 0.5 μg of pentagastrin per kilogram body weight. Carcinoembryonic antigen serum levels were normal (1.6 and 1.5 μg/L; upper normal limit <5.0 μg/L).

Upon first presentation to our institution, calcitonin serum level was 16.5 pg/mL basally and peaked at 194 pg/mL 5 min (IMMULITE 2000, Diagnostic Products Corporation, USA; normal upper limit <5 pg/mL) after intravenous stimulation at 10 mL/min with 2.5 mg of calcium gluconate per kg body weight. Repeat ultrasonography confirmed the cytologically indeterminate left hypoechoic nodule at 25 × 16 mm (Fig. 40.1) and the small right calcified nodule measuring 4.8 mm (Fig. 40.2).

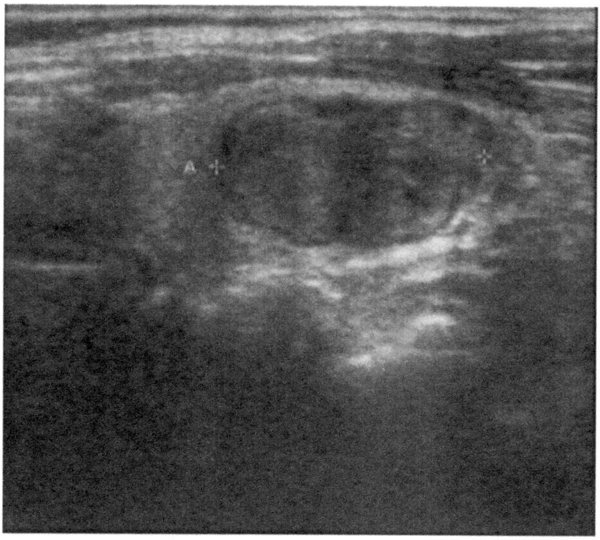

Fig. 40.1 Ultrasound of the left thyroid lobe showing a hypoechoic nodule 25 × 16 mm in size

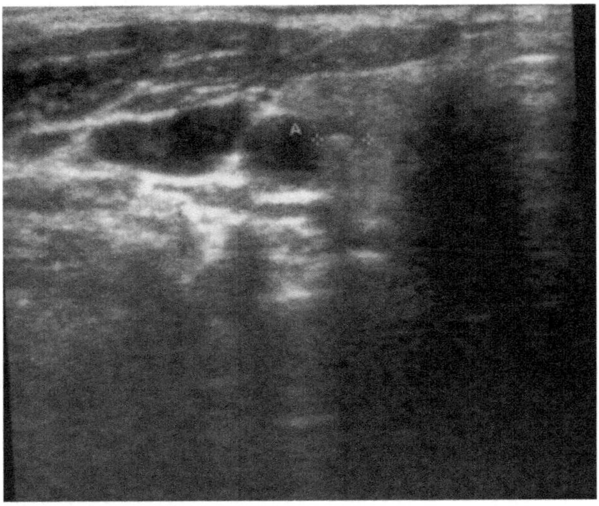

Fig. 40.2 Ultrasound of the right thyroid lobe showing a small calcified nodule 4.8 mm in size

Assessment and Literature Review

Is It Medullary Thyroid Cancer?

Calcitonin is an important predictive biomarker useful for diagnosis and follow-up of medullary thyroid cancer, which affects 0.3–1.4% of patients with thyroid nodules [1–4]. Medullary thyroid cancer, also called C cell cancer, synthesizes and secretes calcitonin proportional to overall tumor mass into the bloodstream. In the setting of nodular thyroid disease, an elevated basal calcitonin ≤ 100 pg/mL can pose a diagnostic dilemma that becomes more problematic as the serum calcitonin levels move lower and lower. In fact, calcitonin secretion is moderately influenced by cigarette smoking, proton-pump inhibitors, chronic renal failure, pernicious anemia, Zollinger-Ellison syndrome, and pancreatitis. Because male thyroid glands contain larger numbers of parafollicular C cells than female thyroids, men have higher serum calcitonin levels. Thus, there are gender-specific basal calcitonin thresholds for thyroidectomy: 20 pg/mL for women (positive predictive value, PPV 88%) and 80–100 pg/mL for men (PPV 100%) [5]. Corresponding absolute calcitonin thresholds after stimulation with pentagastrin are 250 pg/mL for women and 500 pg/mL for men (PPV 100% each) [5]. Interestingly, our patient's calcitonin serum levels, ranging from 15.2 pg/mL to 25 pg/mL basally depending on the assay and reaching 256 pg/mL after stimulation with pentagastrin, crossed the absolute calcitonin thresholds for women of 20 pg/mL basally and 250 pg/mL after stimulation with pentagastrin by a narrow margin. Although it may be a more suitable provocative agent than calcium, pentagastrin has been unavailable since 2005 in many countries, including the USA. In the era of more sensitive immunochemiluminometric calcitonin assays, the need for provocative testing is dwindling. Although calcium stimulation tests have been used for differential diagnosis in patients with moderately elevated serum calcitonin levels [6], cutoffs are less well defined, which can make interpretation of tests results challenging. It is noteworthy that our patient required thyroid surgery for the cytological diagnosis of follicular neoplasia from the indeterminate left nodule, which is what prompted calcitonin screening in the first place.

If It Is Medullary Thyroid Cancer, Will It Be Confined to the Thyroid Gland?

The diagnosis of sporadic medullary thyroid cancer raises the question of whether the tumor is limited to the thyroid gland or has already spread beyond the thyroid capsule. On preoperative neck ultrasonography, more than one-third of patients with MTC have false-negative findings [7]. This is why basal calcitonin serum levels provide important clues as to the presence of occult lymph node metastases [8].

The overall risk of lymph node metastases is estimated at:

- 0%—when basal calcitonin is ≤20 pg/mL
- 11%—when basal calcitonin is 20.1–50 pg/mL
- 17%—when basal calcitonin is 50.1–100 pg/mL
- 35%—when basal calcitonin is 100.1–200 pg/mL

Lymph node metastases begin to appear in the:

- Ipsilateral central and lateral neck—when basal calcitonin exceeds 20 pg/mL
- Contralateral central neck—when basal calcitonin exceeds 50 pg/mL
- Contralateral lateral neck—when basal calcitonin exceeds 200 pg/mL

Absent clinical and ultrasonographic evidence of suspicious lymph nodes, the patient's most recent basal calcitonin of 16.5 pg/mL argued against the presence of lymph node metastases.

If Basal Calcitonin Fails to Normalize, Will Reoperation Be Worthwhile for Minimal Disease?

Calcitonin levels typically normalize within 1 week and within a fortnight in those with node-positive MTC and preoperative calcitonin levels of 500.1–1000 pg/ml. With node-positive MTC and preoperative calcitonin levels exceeding 1000 pg/ml, and with more than ten nodal metastases, calcitonin normalization takes longer [9].

The prospect of biochemical cure after a second neck operation is contingent on the residual basal calcitonin level, as long as no more than five lymph node metastases were removed at the initial operation [10]:

- 75–77% for a residual basal calcitonin <10 pg/mL
- 35–36% for a residual basal calcitonin of 10.1–100 pg/mL

The pros and cons of reoperation in a scarred neck (high chance of definitive cure versus expectant observation of minimal residual disease) need to be detailed to the patient. Reoperations in a scarred neck, as a matter of principle, should not be embarked on outside specialist centers to keep surgical morbidity to a minimum. The one-time cost of reaching a definitive cure and the cost of daily levothyroxine supplementation may be smaller from a societal perspective than the need for continual biochemical follow-up and imaging studies, some of which may prompt additional operations at incremental costs [5].

Management of the Case

After informed consent, the patient opted for thyroidectomy under intraoperative nerve monitoring as a minimum procedure, with possible lymph node dissection depending on intraoperative evidence of nodal disease. Inside the dorsal portion of the right lobe, a small firm nodule was noted. The central neck was explored for suspicious nodes but none were found, as to be expected with a basal calcitonin level ≤ 20 pg/mL, so that no neck dissection was performed.

Histopathological examination revealed a 15 mm follicular adenoma in the left lobe and a 5 mm medullary thyroid cancer surrounded by normal thyroid parenchyma in the absence of C cell hyperplasia.

The patient made an uneventful recovery. Video laryngoscopy confirmed normal vocal cord function after the operation. On the second postoperative day, basal and calcium gluconate-stimulated calcitonin levels were below the assay detection limit (<2 pg/mL; IMMULITE 2000, Diagnostic Products Corporation, USA) reflecting biochemical cure. Follow-up examinations 4 weeks later showed normal parathyroid hormone serum levels, whereas serum calcitonin remained below the assay detection limit.

RET (rearranged during transfection) screening (exons 5, 8, 10, 11, 13, 14, 15, and 16) was negative, excluding hereditary medullary thyroid cancer with a probability of 99%.

Importance of Identifying Occult Medullary Thyroid Cancer

For any medical intervention, there is a continuum of benefit vs. harm. The net benefit of surgical intervention for medullary thyroid microcarcinoma is a continuous function of the following:

- Risk of morbidity if left untreated (the risk of which is unknown)
- The relative risk reduction of treatment (surgical cure, likely to be high)
- The risk of harm from the treatment (surgical morbidity, likely to be low in expert hands)

Sporadic micromedullary thyroid cancer is found pathologically in 0.3–0.4% of patients with nodular thyroid disease [2]. In the absence of good natural history data, it is important to note the close relationships between primary tumor diameter [11] and the following:

- Preoperative basal calcitonin serum levels: means of 136.5 pg/mL (≤2 mm) to 926.0 pg/mL (9–10 mm)
- The rates of lymph node metastases: from 13% (≤2 mm) to 43% (9–10 mm)
- The biochemical cure rate: from 85% (≤2 mm) to 77% (9–10 mm)

Although cancer-specific death is extremely uncommon, as many as 24% of patients harboring micromedullary thyroid cancer are not biochemically cured, perhaps reflecting locally metastatic or systemic disease [11].

Owing to the lack of long-term follow-up data, the same body of scientific evidence has led to different conclusions. In Europe, the Thyroid Section of the German Society for Endocrinology in 2004 [12] and the European Thyroid Association in 2006 [13] started supporting calcitonin screening in patients with nodular thyroid disease. In a decision model developed for a hypothetical group of adult patients presenting for evaluation of thyroid nodules in the USA, serum calcitonin screening, which is sensitive to age and gender, appeared to be cost-effective in patients undergoing evaluation for thyroid nodules [14]. The American Thyroid Association, raising concerns of cost-effectiveness and unproven benefit, advises neither for nor against calcitonin screening [4, 15].

Despite these professional disagreements, a strong consensus exists to actively detect and, in most cases, to resect involved nodes [2].

Clinical Pearls/Pitfalls

- Gender-specific basal calcitonin thresholds for sporadic medullary thyroid cancer are 20 pg/mL for women and 80–100 pg/mL for men.
- Lymph node metastases begin to appear in the ipsilateral central and lateral neck when basal calcitonin exceeds 20 pg/mL, in the contralateral central neck when basal calcitonin exceeds 50 pg/mL, and in the contralateral lateral neck when basal calcitonin exceeds 200 pg/mL.
- In sporadic micromedullary thyroid cancer, there are significant relationships between primary tumor diameter and (1) preoperative basal calcitonin serum levels (means of 136.5–926.0 pg/mL), (2) the rates of lymph node metastases (from 13 to 43%), and (3) biochemical cure rates (85–77%).

References

1. Costante G, Meringolo D, Durante C, Bianchi D, Nocera M, Tumino S, Crocetti U, Attard M, Maranghi M, Torlontano M, Filetti S. Predictive value of serum calcitonin levels for preoperative diagnosis of medullary thyroid carcinoma in a cohort of 5817 consecutive patients with thyroid nodules. J Clin Endocrinol Metab. 2007;92:450–5.
2. Ahmed SR, Ball WC. Incidentally discovered medullary thyroid cancer: diagnostic strategies and treatment. J Clin Endocrinol Metab. 2011;96:1237–45.
3. Chambon G, Alovisetti C, Idoux-Louche C, Reynaud C, Rodier M, Guedj AM, Chapuis H, Lallemant JG, Lallemant B. The use of preoperative routine measurement of basal serum thyrocalcitonin in candidates for thyroidectomy due to nodular thyroid disorders: results from 2733 consecutive patients. J Clin Endocrinol Metab. 2011;96:75–81.
4. Wells SA Jr, Asa SL, Dralle H, Elisei R, Evans DB, Gagel RF, Lee NY, Machens A, Moley JF, Pacini F, Raue F, Frank-Raue K, Robinson B, Rosenthal MS, Santoro M, Schlumberger M, Shah MH, Waguespack SG. The American Thyroid Association Guidelines Task Force on Medullary Thyroid Carcinoma Revised American Thyroid Association guidelines for the management of medullary thyroid cancer. Thyroid. 2015;25:567–610.
5. Machens A, Hoffmann F, Sekulla C, Dralle H. Importance of gender-specific calcitonin thresholds in screening for occult medullary thyroid cancer. Endocr Relat Cancer. 2009;16:1291–8.
6. Mian C, Perrino M, Colombo C, Cavedon E, Pennelli G, Ferrero S, De Leo S, Sarais C, Cacciatore C, Manfredi GI, Verga U, Iacobone M, De Pasquale L, Pelizzo MR, Vicentini L, Persani L, Fugazzola L. Refining calcium test for the diagnosis of medullary thyroid cancer: cutoffs, procedures, and safety. J Clin Endocrinol Metab. 2014;99:1656–64.
7. Kouvaraki MA, Shapiro SE, Fornage BD, Edeiken-Monro BS, Sherman SI, Vassilopoulou-Sellin R, Lee JE, Evans DB. Role of preoperative ultrasonography in the surgical management of patients with thyroid cancer. Surgery. 2003;134:946–55.
8. Machens A, Dralle H. Biomarker-based risk stratification for previously untreated medullary thyroid cancer. J Clin Endocrinol Metab. 2010;95:2655–63.
9. Machens A, Lorenz K, Dralle H. Time to calcitonin normalization after surgery for node-negative and node-positive medullary thyroid cancer. Br J Surg. 2019;106:412–8.
10. Machens A, Dralle H. Benefit-risk balance of reoperation for persistent medullary thyroid cancer. Ann Surg. 2013;257:751–7.
11. Machens A, Dralle H. Biological relevance of medullary thyroid microcarcinoma. J Clin Endocrinol Metab. 2012;97:1547–53.
12. Karges W, Dralle H, Raue F, Mann K, Reiners C, Grussendorf M, Hüfner M, Niederle B, Brabant G, German Society for Endocrinology (DGE). Thyroid section. Calcitonin measurement to detect medullary thyroid carcinoma in nodular goiter: German evidence-based consensus recommendations. Exp Clin Endocrinol Diabetes. 2004;112:52–8.
13. Pacini F, Schlumberger M, Dralle H, Elisei R, Smit JW, Wiersinga W, European Thyroid Cancer Taskforce. European consensus for the management of patients with differentiated thyroid carcinoma of the follicular epithelium. Eur J Endocrinol. 2006;154:787–803.
14. Cheung K, Roman SA, Wang TS, Walker HD, Sosa JA. Calcitonin measurements in the evaluation of thyroid nodules in the United States: a cost-effectiveness and decision analysis. J Clin Endocrinol Metab. 2008;93:2173–80.
15. Haugen BR, Alexander EK, Bible KC, Doherty GM, Mandel SJ, Nikiforov YE, Pacini F, Randolph GW, Sawka AM, Schlumberger M, Schuff KG, Sherman SI, Sosa JA, Steward DL, Tuttle RM, Wartofsky L. 2015 American Thyroid Association management guidelines for adult patients with thyroid nodules and differentiated thyroid cancer: The American Thyroid Association Guidelines Task Force on thyroid nodules and differentiated thyroid cancer. Thyroid. 2016;26:1–133.

Chapter 41
Timing and Extent of Surgery for a Pediatric Patient with Hereditary MTC and Positive Screening for the p.S891A *RET* Mutation

Henning Dralle and Andreas Machens

Case Presentation

A 17-year-old male non-index patient (patient 3.1.2; Table 41.1, Fig. 41.1) was referred for surgical intervention with positive screening for the p.S891A *RET* mutation, which had been prompted by a positive *RET* gene test in his father (index patient 2.1; Fig. 41.1) after outside surgery for medullary thyroid cancer (MTC). Familial screening uncovered eight additional gene carriers.

Evaluation for Surgery

On stimulation with pentagastrin, the adolescent carrier's calcitonin serum levels rose from 24 pg/mL basally (upper normal limit <8.4 pg/mL; Immulite 2000 assay, Diagnostic Products Corp., Los Angeles, CA) to a peak level of 510 pg/mL after 5 min (patient 3.1.2; Table 41.1, Fig. 41.1). Physical examination of the thyroid gland and high-resolution neck ultrasonography were negative. Thyroid examination of the other eight non-index patients, including ultrasonography, identified multinodular goiter disease without evidence of lymph node metastases in the

H. Dralle (✉)
Department of General, Visceral and Transplantation Surgery, Section of Endocrine Surgery, University Hospital, Essen, Germany

Medical Faculty, University of Duisburg-Essen, Essen, Germany
e-mail: henning.dralle@uk-essen.de

A. Machens
Department of Visceral, Vascular and Endocrine Surgery, University Hospital, Halle (Saale), Germany

Medical Faculty, University of Halle-Wittenberg, Halle (Saale), Germany

G. Grani et al. (eds.), *Thyroid Cancer*,
https://doi.org/10.1007/978-3-030-61919-0_41

Table 41.1 Clinical histopathological characteristics of all eight non-index patients carrying the p.S891A *RET* mutation

Patient no., gender, age (years)	Preoperative calcitonin (pg/mL)		Extent of surgery	Histopathology; pTNM	Postoperative calcitonin (pg/mL)	
	Basal	Peak			Basal	Peak
1.1; f; 78	312	2634	TT, LND central and lateral	Bilateral MTC (10 mm, 11 mm); 1/45 LNM; pT1bpN1aM0	7	48
2.3; m; 46	60	nd	TT, LND central and lateral	Bilateral MTC (3 mm, 5 mm), unilateral PTC (1 mm); 0/31 LNM; pT1apN0M0	<2	<2
3.1.2; m; 17	24	510	TT, LND central	Bilateral MTC (3 mm, 3 mm), 0/7 LNM; pT1apN0M0	<2	<2
3.2.4; f; 10	9	27	TT	Bilateral CCH, no MTC, 0/1 LNM	<2	<2
3.1.3; m; 8	4	79	TT	No CCH, no MTC; 0/1 LNM	<2	<2
3.2.3; m; 8	9	nd	TT	Bilateral CCH, no MTC	<2	<2
3.2.2; m; 6	9	57	TT	Bilateral CCH, no MTC, 0/1 LNM	<2	<2
3.2.1; f; 5	3	nd	TT	Bilateral CCH, no MTC, 0/1 LNM	<2	<2

Patient numbers are the same as in Fig. 41.1. The calcitonin assay's upper normal limit was <5.0 pg/mL for women and <8.4 for men (Immulite 2000 assay, Diagnostic Products Corp., Los Angeles, CA)
pTNM according to Amin et al. [13]
TT total thyroidectomy, *LND* lymph node dissection, *CCH* C cell hyperplasia, *f* female, *m* male, *MTC* medullary thyroid cancer, *LNM* lymph node metastasis, *nd* not determined

78-year-old grandmother (patient 1.1) and a suspicious small hypoechoic lesion in her 46-year-old son (patient 2.3) (Fig. 41.2). With the exception of two 5- and 8-year-old children (patients 3.2.1 and 3.1.3), all non-index patients exhibited elevated basal calcitonin levels. All family members who had a pentagastrin stimulation test performed showed peak calcitonin levels markedly increased over baseline (Table 41.1). None of the eight non-index patients had biochemical or imaging evidence for adrenal medullary or parathyroid disease.

Assessment and Literature Review

The *RET* proto-oncogene encodes a single-pass transmembrane receptor of the tyrosine kinase family. *RET* germline mutations cause hereditary MTC, pheochromocytoma, and primary hyperparathyroidism to different degrees. They have an autosomal dominant transmission: over 100 mutations, duplications, insertions, or deletions

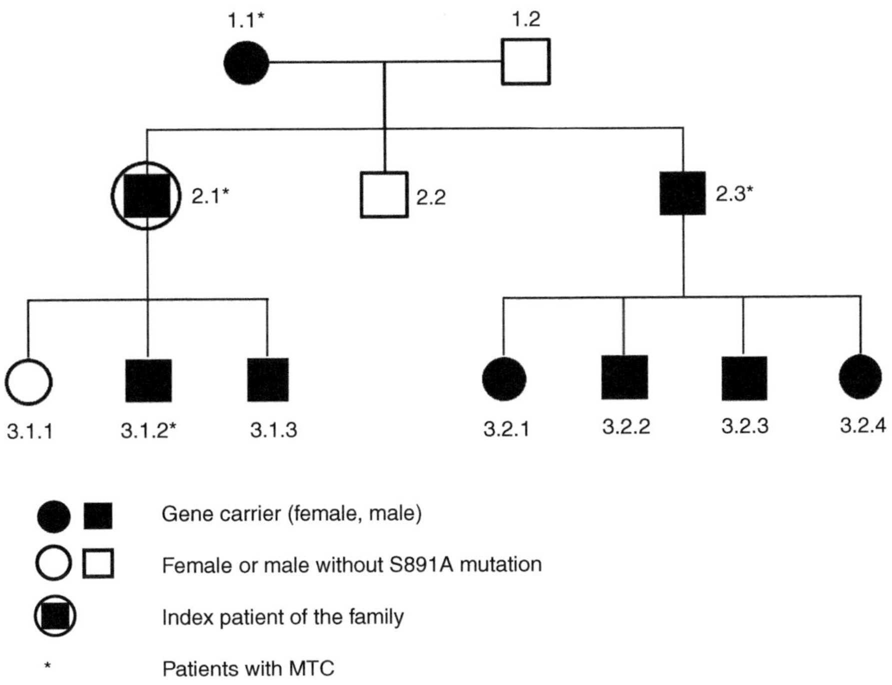

Fig. 41.1 Pedigree of the three-generational family carrying the heterozygous p.S891A *RET* mutation. *Filled circle, filled square* Gene carrier (female, male). *Open circle, open square* Kindred (female, male) without p.S891A mutation. *Open circle with filled square* Male index patient of the family. *Asterisk* Patients with MTC

involving RET have been described. Patients with presumed sporadic MTC should have genetic testing to detect a germline *RET* mutation. If a *RET* mutation is confirmed, the patient should have genetic counseling, and the same should be offered to all first-degree relatives of patients with proven hereditary MTC.

The c.2671T>G (p.S891A) *RET* missense mutation affects 2.9–9.8 % of all *RET* gene carriers across geographic boundaries [1, 2], depending on the intensity of national screening programs (every patient diagnosed with MTC as opposed to no more than family screening for confirmation of clinically manifest disease) and the presence of founder effects [3]. Within the spectrum of hereditary C cell disease, the S891A mutation is part of a group of intracellular *RET* mutations (tyrosine kinase sub-domain 2) and carries a low-moderate risk for aggressive MTC [American Thyroid Association (ATA) risk level MOD] [4, 5]. Carriers of the p.S891A mutation have a <10 % risk of pheochromocytoma or hyperparathyroidism [6].

Because of the weaker genotype-phenotype relationship and the C cells' need to acquire additional mutations (dubbed "second hits") for malignant transformation, there is more variability in the onset of MTC (range 13–48 years) among carriers of

Fig. 41.2 Ultrasound of the left thyroid lobe visualizing a medullary thyroid microcarcinoma of 5 mm in size (patient 2.3)

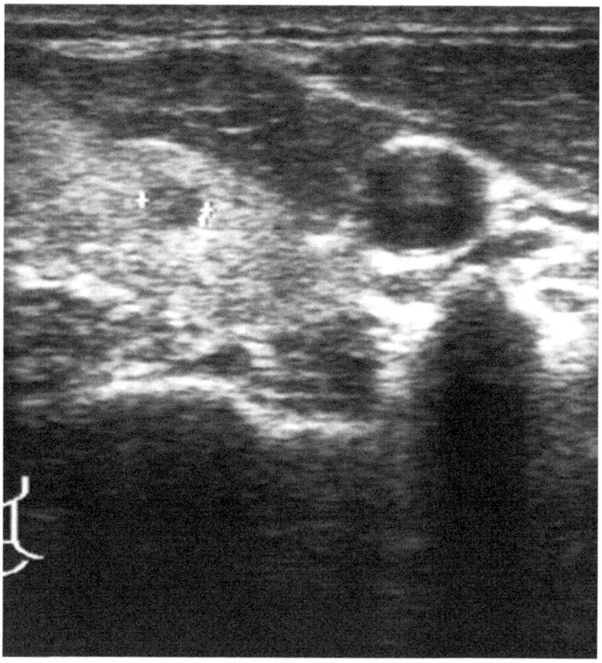

the p.S891A mutation [1, 2, 5, 7], reflecting the play of chance. This variability hampers predictions regarding the age by which tumors will have developed. This is why a carrier's age is less useful than his or her calcitonin levels to determine the optimum time for prophylactic thyroidectomy [8, 9]. Basal calcitonin levels within the upper normal range of the assay can reliably distinguish between C cell diseases limited to, or spreading beyond, the confines of the thyroid capsule so that these patients can safely forego central lymph node dissection, sparing them incremental surgical morbidity [2, 7–9]. For an individual patient with p.S891A ATA MOD low-moderate-risk mutation as in the presented family, prophylactic parathyroid preserving thyroidectomy without node dissection should be performed before basal calcitonin levels are exceeding the upper normal limit. Lymph node metastases have only been observed in patients with calcitonin levels beyond the upper normal limit (2, 4, 7–9). It is important to note that basal calcitonin levels as high as 33.8 pg/mL in 1-month-old newborns, 14.1 pg/mL in 1-year-old children, and 8.5 pg/mL in 2-year-old children can be normal [10]. Because it is less sensitive than calcitonin to spot MTC in hereditary C cell disease, ultrasonography is only of limited use for the clinical workup of pediatric *RET* mutation carriers [11].

Management of the Cases

After informed consent, balancing the pros and cons, all eight non-index patients (including those children who had normal or slightly elevated basal calcitonin levels only) opted for surgical treatment. As detailed in Table 41.1 and Fig. 41.1, MTC or CCH was present in seven of eight patients and in all three generations, including the 17-year-old adolescent gene carrier (patient 3.1.2; Table 41.1 and Fig. 41.1). No lymph node metastases were seen up to a basal calcitonin serum level of 60 pg/mL. One carrier (patient 2.3) also harbored a 1 mm papillary thyroid microcarcinoma in addition to bilateral MTC, in all likelihood a chance occurrence [12]. Intriguingly, it was the 78-year-old grandmother, displaying high basal calcitonin serum levels, who had node-positive MTC (patient 1.1), and not the index patient who was operated on elsewhere.

Outcome

All non-index patients with node-negative C cell disease were biochemically cured, as shown in Table 41.1, and made an uneventful recovery without recurrent laryngeal nerve palsy or postoperative hypoparathyroidism. As long as basal calcitonin serum levels did not exceed the upper limit of the assay reference range, total thyroidectomy alone was adequate to reach biochemical cure.

Clinical Pearls/Pitfalls

- The p.S891A *RET* mutation carries a low-moderate risk for aggressive MTC. Manifestation of MTC has not been described before age 17.
- Owing to the considerable variation in the time of malignant transformation from C cell hyperplasia to MTC and tumor spread to lymph nodes, preoperative calcitonin levels, being more sensitive than ultrasonography in detecting pediatric MTC, should be considered for the timing of prophylactic thyroidectomy.
- As long as calcitonin serum levels are within the normal range, prophylactic parathyroid preserving thyroidectomy alone is adequate, sparing gene carriers the incremental surgical morbidity attendant to lymph node dissection.
- Elevated basal calcitonin levels in excess of 60 pg/mL are associated with an increased risk of lymph node metastases, warranting compartment -oriented lymph node dissection.

References

1. Machens A, Niccoli-Sire P, Hoegel J, Frank-Raue K, van Vroonhoven TJ, Roeher HD, Wahl RA, Lamesch P, Raue F, Conte-Devolx B, Dralle H, European Multiple Endocrine Neoplasia (EUROMEN) Study Group. Early malignant progression of hereditary medullary thyroid cancer. N Engl J Med. 2003;349:1517–25.
2. Machens A, Dralle H. Long-term outcome after DNA-based prophylactic neck surgery in children at risk of hereditary medullary thyroid cancer. Best Pract Res Clin Endocrinol Metab. 2019;33:101274.
3. Giacché M, Panarotto A, Tacchetti MC, Tosini R, Campana F, Mori L, Cappelli C, Pirola I, Lombardi D, Pezzola DC, Casella C, Castellano M. p.Ser891Ala RET gene mutations in medullary thyroid cancer: Phenotypical and genealogical characterization of 28 apparently unrelated kindreds and founder effect uncovering in Northern Italy. Hum Mutat. 2019;40:926–37.
4. Wells SA Jr, Asa SL, Dralle H, Elisei R, Evans DB, Gagel RF, Lee N, Machens A, Moley JF, Pacini F, Raue F, Frank-Raue K, Robinson B, Rosenthal MS, Santoro M, Schlumberger M, Shah M, Waguespack SG. American Thyroid Association Guidelines Task Force on Medullary Thyroid Carcinoma. Revised American Thyroid Association guidelines for the management of medullary thyroid carcinoma. Thyroid. 2015;25:567–610.
5. Machens A, Lorenz K, Weber F, Dralle H. Genotype-specific progression of hereditary medullary thyroid cancer. Hum Mutat. 2018;39:860–9.
6. Schulte KM, Machens A, Fugazzola L, McGregor A, Diaz-Cano S, Izatt L, Aylwin S, Talat N, Beck-Peccoz P, Dralle H. The clinical spectrum of multiple endocrine neoplasia type 2a caused by the rare intracellular RET mutation S891A. J Clin Endocrinol Metab. 2010;95:E92–7.
7. Machens A, Elwerr M, Lorenz K, Weber F, Dralle H. Long-term outcome of prophylactic thyroidectomy in children carrying RET germline mutations. Br J Surg. 2018;105:e150–7.
8. Machens A, Lorenz K, Dralle H. Individualization of lymph node dissection in RET (rearranged during transfection) carriers at risk for medullary thyroid cancer. Ann Surg. 2009;250:305–10.
9. Elisei R, Romei C, Renzini G, Bottici V, Cosci B, Molinaro E, Agate L, Cappagli V, Miccoli P, Berti P, Faviana P, Ugolini C, Basolo F, Vitti P, Pinchera A. The timing of total thyroidectomy in RET gene mutation carriers could be personalized and safely planned on the basis of serum calcitonin: 18 years experience at one single center. J Clin Endocrinol Metab. 2012;97:426–35.
10. Castagna MG, Fugazzola L, Maino F, Covelli D, Memmo S, Sestini F, Fioravanti C, Ferraris Fusarini C, Scapellato C, Macchini F, Cevenini G, Pacini F. Reference range of serum calcitonin in pediatric population. J Clin Endocrinol Metab. 2015;100:1780–4.
11. Morris LF, Waguespack SG, Edeiken-Monroe BS, Lee JE, Rich TA, Ying AK, Warneke CL, Evans DB, Perrier ND, Grubbs EG. Ultrasonography should not guide the timing of thyroidectomy in pediatric patients diagnosed with multiple endocrine neoplasia syndrome 2A through genetic screening. Ann Surg Oncol. 2013;20:53–9.
12. Machens A, Dralle H. Simultaneous medullary and papillary thyroid cancer: a novel entity? Ann Surg Oncol. 2012;19:37–44.
13. Amin MB, Edge S, Greene F, Byrd DR, Brookland RK, Washington MK, Gershenwald JE, Compton CC, Hess KR, Sullivan DC, Jessup JM, Brierley JD, Gaspar LE, Schilsky RL, Balch CM, Winchester DP, Asare EA, Mandera M, Gress DM, Meyer LR (eds.), American Joint Commission on Cancer: AJCC Cancer Staging Manual (8th edition). Springer International Publishing 2017.

Part VII
Anaplastic Thyroid Cancer

Chapter 42
Anaplastic Thyroid Cancer: Surgery or Not in Locally Advanced Disease

Ashish V. Chintakuntlawar, Keith C. Bible, and Robert C. Smallridge

Introduction

Anaplastic thyroid carcinoma (ATC) is one of the most aggressive and lethal of all malignancies, accounting for approximately 1.7 % of all thyroid cancers in the USA and a median of 3.6 % (range, 1.3–9.8 %) worldwide [1]. According to the American Joint Committee on Cancer (AJCC) TNM classification, ATC is always stage IV at presentation; stage IVA tumors are intrathyroidal, IVB tumors have extrathyroidal extension and may involve locoregional lymph nodes, and IVC tumors are distantly metastatic.

Survival generally correlates inversely with TNM stage and correlates directly/positively with extent of surgery, administration of high-dose radiotherapy, and absence of distant metastases. The American Thyroid Association management guidelines for ATC recommends initial surgery in potentially grossly resectable (R0, negative surgical margins; R1, microscopically involved margins) stage IVA or IVB disease in patients who are in reasonably good health and who elect aggressive treatment [1]. The role of R2 (gross residual disease)/debulking/resection is uncertain. In this chapter, we will discuss the role of surgery in the treatment of ATC.

A. V. Chintakuntlawar (✉) · K. C. Bible
Division of Medical Oncology, Mayo Clinic, Rochester, MN, USA
e-mail: Chintakuntlawar.ashish@mayo.edu

R. C. Smallridge
Division of Endocrinology, Mayo Clinic, Jacksonville, FL, USA

G. Grani et al. (eds.), *Thyroid Cancer*,
https://doi.org/10.1007/978-3-030-61919-0_42

Case Report

A 60-year-old Caucasian gentleman noticed a left-sided neck swelling that grew rapidly over 2–3 weeks, seeking medical care locally. He denied symptoms of local invasion such as dysphagia, stridor, hoarseness, or pain. He underwent neck ultrasound that demonstrated a large neck mass likely arising from the thyroid gland. Fine needle aspiration demonstrated high-grade carcinoma, likely undifferentiated/anaplastic thyroid carcinoma, but other high-grade carcinomas including medullary or insular carcinoma could not be excluded. Tissue was insufficient for further classification. The patient had no significant medical comorbidities but had a long history of smoking tobacco.

He was referred to our institution and underwent further testing including CT of the neck and positron emission tomography-CT (PET-CT) from the skull to thigh. PET-CT scan demonstrated a large mass in the left neck that resulted in deviation of the trachea (Fig. 42.1a and b) but showed no evidence of any distant metastatic disease. After a thorough multidisciplinary evaluation that included radiation oncology, medical oncology, endocrinology, and head and neck surgery, surgical resection was recommended. The patient underwent near-total thyroidectomy and left modified neck dissection with recurrent laryngeal nerve monitoring. Surgical pathology demonstrated high-grade carcinoma most compatible with anaplastic

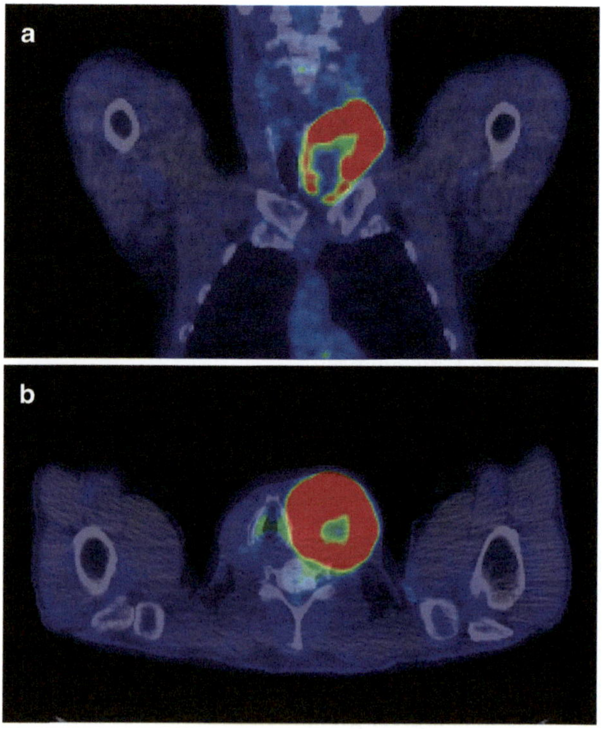

Fig. 42.1 Positron emission tomography-CT scan with coronal (**a**) and axial (**b**) images of large left thyroid mass with central necrosis. Mass results in deviation of the trachea. The glottic opening is preserved

(undifferentiated) thyroid carcinoma measuring 14.0 x 9.8 x 7.5 cm. Margins were negative but close at less than 1 mm. Tumor cells were negative for S100, TTF-1, and thyroglobulin but positive for cytokeratins.

Postoperative course was complicated by infection and development of seroma (drained and treated with amoxicillin-clavulanic acid complicated by antibiotic-associated diarrhea). Ultimately, 4 weeks after his operation, the patient initiated adjuvant chemoradiotherapy with weekly docetaxel and doxorubicin, 20 milligram/meter square each administered intravenously. His treatments were complicated with mucositis, oral candidiasis, malnutrition, and need for percutaneous gastric feeding tube. He received a total dose of 60 Gy external beam radiotherapy and four out of his six planned doses of chemotherapy.

Five months later, the patient developed a left lower lobe lesion in the medial lung, measuring 2.5 cm. This was treated with stereotactic radiotherapy, 48 Gy in four fractions.

Literature Review

A PubMed search for "anaplastic thyroid cancer" and "surgical resection" was performed for publications from January 2000 to November 2019. We intended to include studies that explored the role of surgery in the treatment of ATC. One hundred and eleven publications were found. Expert reviews and case reports were excluded. Studies from single institutions with large cohorts (>50 patients), systematic reviews/meta-analysis, and population-based studies were reviewed. References from these studies were reviewed so as to also capture additional studies. One recent study exploring the role of neoadjuvant BRAF-MEK inhibitor therapy was also included considering the novelty of the approach in the treatment of ATC [2–36].

Most of these examined studies, including the population-based studies and systematic reviews, demonstrated that surgical treatment was independently prognostic of better survival, especially when combined with postoperative radiotherapy or chemoradiotherapy [3–5, 8, 9, 15, 22, 25, 26]. For example, from the Korean multicenter nationwide study (2000–2012), the patients who underwent curative resection followed by adjuvant radiotherapy or chemoradiotherapy showed the best 1-year overall survival rate of 50.2%. Most patients with stage IVA (80.6%) and IVB (73.6%) disease were treated with curative surgical resection followed by adjuvant therapy and led to significant survival benefit. This survival benefit was, however, not seen in stage IVC patients [4]. Similar results were also obtained with aggressive multimodality therapy at the authors' institution in this same time period [6]. On the other hand, patients from the National Cancer Database (1998–2012) who were treated without any upfront surgery but received >60 Gy radiotherapy dose had 1-year overall survival of 31% [3].

There were very few studies that demonstrated no benefit of surgery. For example, Besic et al. examined outcomes in 26 patients in the primary surgery group and 53 in the nonsurgical group. Patients with distant metastases at presentation were excluded. Patients in the nonsurgical group had larger tumors and were older. When directly compared, there was no difference in the overall survival of these two groups [37]. Kim et al. demonstrated in a multicenter study that multimodality therapies including surgical resection were not associated with overall survival on a multivariable analysis [32].

It is also clear from the reviewed studies that locoregional control is improved with multimodality therapy that includes surgery. A general exclusion criterion for offering surgery has been presenting with stage IVC disease, as reflected in the ATA guidelines which recommend radiotherapy and chemotherapy for those desiring aggressive treatment [1]. However, Brignardello et al. [14] observed that surgery may have a role in patients presenting with distant metastases. They examined 55 patients (31 with stage IVC disease) who underwent either "maximal debulking" (R0, R1, or R2 resection with only minimal residual macroscopic tumor) or "partial debulking." Maximal debulking was associated with improved median survival in both stage IVB (10.9 vs. 3.0 months) and IVC (6.5 vs. 3.2 months) patients. The improvement in overall survival was attributed to fewer deaths from locoregional tumor progression. However, most studies demonstrated no overall survival benefit in stage IVC patients [4, 6] as locoregional control could also be alternatively obtained from chemoradiotherapy [25]. Therefore, surgery likely has a less important role in stage IVC ATC patients for locoregional control.

All of the examples presented above, however, reflect retrospective analyses. There were no prospective studies except for two older studies from Europe – which also showed that surgical resection is an important prognostic factor [35, 38]. The recently completed RTOG 0912 trial also included patients with or without surgery, and hence a post hoc analysis of this cohort could also inform us about the role of surgery in a prospective fashion. There are no studies with randomized prospective comparison of a surgical versus nonsurgical approach. Therefore, it is not possible to conclude definitively, and conclusions presented here are best considered hypothesis generating. However, in the authors' opinion, surgical treatment should be preferred whenever feasible commensurate with the guidelines from the American Thyroid Association.

Presurgical evaluation should be completed expeditiously by an expert multidisciplinary team so as not to delay therapy for this rapidly growing malignancy. Surgery is not recommended if there is overt involvement of the pharynx, larynx, trachea, or esophagus, if mediastinal vessels are involved, or if prevertebral fascia and paraspinous muscles are involved.

The approach to surgical therapy for ATC could be categorized into three separate pathways (Fig. 42.2). The most common approach is to proceed with upfront surgical resection followed by adjuvant therapy [6, 11]. Several studies from Europe have alternatively utilized an approach where neoadjuvant chemoradiotherapy is utilized with an intention to proceed with surgical resection thereafter [7, 35]. As previously mentioned, up to half of ATCs carry the *BRAFV600E* somatic mutation, thereby providing an opportunity for initial/neoadjuvant targeted systemic therapy [39, 40]. Capitalizing on this genetic aberration, a recent study investigated the use

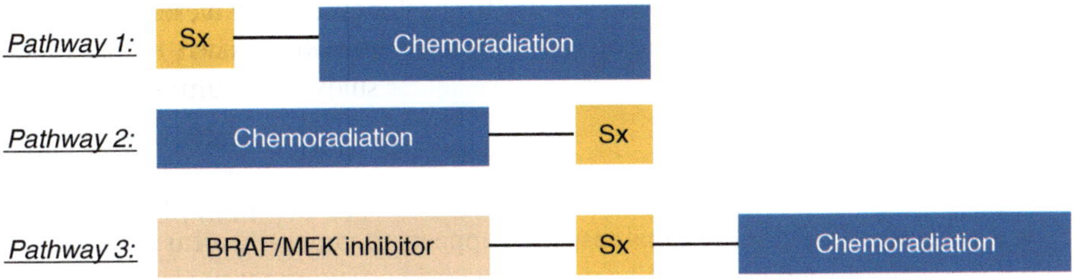

Fig. 42.2 Three distinct treatment pathways wherein surgery (Sx) could be employed in the treatment of anaplastic thyroid carcinoma. The most common program involves upfront surgical resection with adjuvant chemoradiotherapy (top). Less commonly, chemoradiotherapy could also be employed in neoadjuvant fashion followed by surgical resection where feasible (middle). Recently, in BRAF-mutated anaplastic thyroid carcinoma, systemic therapy with a BRAF/MEK inhibitor combination was used as initial therapy followed by surgical resection of anaplastic thyroid carcinoma. Adjuvant therapy was delivered in select patients (bottom). *Sx* surgery

of targeted therapy in *BRAF*-mutated ATC as a neoadjuvant therapy, with the goal to proceed to surgical resection as feasible depending upon therapeutic response [2]. This is an exciting development that needs further careful study in larger populations to confirm the feasibility and efficacy.

Summary

The preponderance of the literature supports the notion that patients with ATC incur longer survival if they undertake complete or near-complete surgical resection (R1). However, no studies to date have been randomized. It is quite possible therefore that available studies are biased, with elderly and/or more debilitated patients and/or those who have extensive unresectable locoregional disease or widespread distant metastases less likely to be offered surgery. Given severe molecular dysregulation in ATC [39, 41], the recognition that almost all patients eventually die from their disease (suggesting micrometastases upon presentation), and the observation that some patients may respond to targeted therapy exquisitely with durable responses [2, 40], the exact role of surgery in each individual patient is best determined by an experienced multidisciplinary team. Multicenter prospective studies can be designed to better characterize and optimize the individual contributions of surgery, external radiation, and systemic therapies (both cytotoxic and targeted).

Back to the Patient

Returning to our patient, he remains alive and active with a good quality of life, with no evidence of disease 5.5 years after his diagnosis. We propose that aggressive multimodal therapy directed at both locoregional control and control of systemic disease currently offers the best opportunity for prolonging survival, but with considerable side effect and complication risks. We have, however, much to learn about this horrific tumor.

Pearls

In most series, maximal surgical resection appears to improve 1-year survival, but resectability depends on the extent of the primary tumor at presentation.

- Aggressive multimodal therapy presently offers the most successful approach to attempt to prolong survival in patients with ATC but imposes risks of considerable side effects and of complications.
- *BRAFV600E*-mutated ATCs can show excellent response to targeted therapy in the metastatic setting, and its role in neoadjuvant therapy is currently being defined.

References

1. Smallridge RC, Ain KB, Asa SL, Bible KC, Brierley JD, Burman KD, Kebebew E, Lee NY, Nikiforov YE, Rosenthal MS, Shah MH, Shaha AR, Tuttle RM. American Thyroid Association guidelines for management of patients with anaplastic thyroid cancer. Thyroid. 2012;22:1104–39.
2. Wang JR, Zafereo ME, Dadu R, Ferrarotto R, Busaidy NL, Lu C, Ahmed S, Gule-Monroe MK, Williams MD, Sturgis EM, Goepfert RP, Gross ND, Lai SY, Gunn GB, Phan J, Rosenthal DI, Fuller CD, Morrison WH, Iyer P, Cabanillas ME. Complete surgical resection following neoadjuvant dabrafenib plus trametinib in BRAF(V600E)-mutated anaplastic thyroid carcinoma. Thyroid. 2019;29:1036–43.
3. Pezzi TA, Mohamed ASR, Sheu T, Blanchard P, Sandulache VC, Lai SY, Cabanillas ME, Williams MD, Pezzi CM, Lu C, Garden AS, Morrison WH, Rosenthal DI, Fuller CD, Gunn GB. Radiation therapy dose is associated with improved survival for unresected anaplastic thyroid carcinoma: outcomes from the National Cancer Data Base. Cancer. 2017;123:1653–61.
4. Baek SK, Lee MC, Hah JH, Ahn SH, Son YI, Rho YS, Chung PS, Lee YS, Koo BS, Jung KY, Lee BJ. Role of surgery in the management of anaplastic thyroid carcinoma: Korean nationwide multicenter study of 329 patients with anaplastic thyroid carcinoma, 2000 to 2012. Head Neck. 2017;39:133–9.
5. Hu S, Helman SN, Hanly E, Likhterov I. The role of surgery in anaplastic thyroid cancer: A systematic review. Am J Otolaryngol. 2017;38:337–50.
6. Prasongsook N, Kumar A, Chintakuntlawar AV, Foote RL, Kasperbauer J, Molina J, Garces Y, Ma D, Neben Wittich MA, Rubin J, Richardson R, Morris J, Hay I, Fatourechi V, McIver B, Ryder M, Thompson G, Grant C, Richards M, Sebo TJ, Rivera M, Suman V, Jenkins SM, Smallridge RC, Bible KC. Survival in response to multimodal therapy in anaplastic thyroid cancer. J Clin Endocrinol Metab. 2017.
7. Jacobsen AB, Groholt KK, Lorntzsen B, Osnes TA, Falk RS, Sigstad E. Anaplastic thyroid cancer and hyperfractionated accelerated radiotherapy (HART) with and without surgery. Eur Arch Otorhinolaryngol. 2017;274:4203–9.
8. Kwon J, Kim BH, Jung HW, Besic N, Sugitani I, Wu HG. The prognostic impacts of postoperative radiotherapy in the patients with resected anaplastic thyroid carcinoma: A systematic review and meta-analysis. Eur J Cancer. 2016;59:34–45.

9. Goffredo P, Thomas SM, Adam MA, Sosa JA, Roman SA. Impact of timeliness of resection and thyroidectomy margin status on survival for patients with anaplastic thyroid cancer: an analysis of 335 cases. Ann Surg Oncol. 2015;22:4166–74.
10. Paunovic IR, Sipetic SB, Zoric GV, Diklic AD, Savic DV, Marinkovic J, Zivaljevic VR. Survival and prognostic factors of anaplastic thyroid carcinoma. Acta Chir Belg. 2015;115:62–7.
11. Mohebati A, Dilorenzo M, Palmer F, Patel SG, Pfister D, Lee N, Tuttle RM, Shaha AR, Shah JP, Ganly I. Anaplastic thyroid carcinoma: a 25-year single-institution experience. Ann Surg Oncol. 2014;21:1665–70.
12. Sugitani I, Hasegawa Y, Sugasawa M, Tori M, Higashiyama T, Miyazaki M, Hosoi H, Orita Y, Kitano H. Super-radical surgery for anaplastic thyroid carcinoma: a large cohort study using the Anaplastic Thyroid Carcinoma Research Consortium of Japan database. Head Neck. 2014;36:328–33.
13. Aslan ZA, Granados-Garcia M, Luna-Ortiz K, Guerrero-Huerta FJ, Gomez-Pedraza A, Namendys-Silva SA, Meneses-Garcia A, Ordonez-Mosquera JM. Anaplastic thyroid cancer: multimodal treatment results. Ecancermedicalscience. 2014;8:449.
14. Brignardello E, Palestini N, Felicetti F, Castiglione A, Piovesan A, Gallo M, Freddi M, Ricardi U, Gasparri G, Ciccone G, Arvat E, Boccuzzi G. Early surgery and survival of patients with anaplastic thyroid carcinoma: analysis of a case series referred to a single institution between 1999 and 2012. Thyroid. 2014;24:1600–6.
15. Sugitani I, Miyauchi A, Sugino K, Okamoto T, Yoshida A, Suzuki S. Prognostic factors and treatment outcomes for anaplastic thyroid carcinoma: ATC Research Consortium of Japan cohort study of 677 patients. World J Surg. 2012;36:1247–54.
16. Ito K, Hanamura T, Murayama K, Okada T, Watanabe T, Harada M, Ito T, Koyama H, Kanai T, Maeno K, Mochizuki Y, Amano J. Multimodality therapeutic outcomes in anaplastic thyroid carcinoma: improved survival in subgroups of patients with localized primary tumors. Head Neck. 2012;34:230–7.
17. Segerhammar I, Larsson C, Nilsson IL, Backdahl M, Hoog A, Wallin G, Foukakis T, Zedenius J. Anaplastic carcinoma of the thyroid gland: treatment and outcome over 13 years at one institution. J Surg Oncol. 2012;106:981–6.
18. Akaishi J, Sugino K, Kitagawa W, Nagahama M, Kameyama K, Shimizu K, Ito K. Prognostic factors and treatment outcomes of 100 cases of anaplastic thyroid carcinoma. Thyroid. 2011;21:1183–9.
19. Sherman EJ, Lim SH, Ho AL, Ghossein RA, Fury MG, Shaha AR, Rivera M, Lin O, Wolden S, Lee NY, Pfister DG. Concurrent doxorubicin and radiotherapy for anaplastic thyroid cancer: a critical re-evaluation including uniform pathologic review. Radiother Oncol. 2011;101:425–30.
20. Swaak-Kragten AT, de Wilt JH, Schmitz PI, Bontenbal M, Levendag PC. Multimodality treatment for anaplastic thyroid carcinoma--treatment outcome in 75 patients. Radiother Oncol. 2009;92:100–4.
21. Yau T, Lo CY, Epstein RJ, Lam AK, Wan KY, Lang BH. Treatment outcomes in anaplastic thyroid carcinoma: survival improvement in young patients with localized disease treated by combination of surgery and radiotherapy. Ann Surg Oncol. 2008;15:2500–5.
22. Kebebew E, Greenspan FS, Clark OH, Woeber KA, McMillan A. Anaplastic thyroid carcinoma. Treatment outcome and prognostic factors. Cancer. 2005;103:1330–5.
23. Pierie JP, Muzikansky A, Gaz RD, Faquin WC, Ott MJ. The effect of surgery and radiotherapy on outcome of anaplastic thyroid carcinoma. Ann Surg Oncol. 2002;9:57–64.
24. McIver B, Hay ID, Giuffrida DF, Dvorak CE, Grant CS, Thompson GB, van Heerden JA, Goellner JR. Anaplastic thyroid carcinoma: a 50-year experience at a single institution. Surgery. 2001;130:1028–34.
25. Wendler J, Kroiss M, Gast K, Kreissl MC, Allelein S, Lichtenauer U, Blaser R, Spitzweg C, Fassnacht M, Schott M, Fuhrer D, Tiedje V. Clinical presentation, treatment and outcome of anaplastic thyroid carcinoma: results of a multicenter study in Germany. Eur J Endocrinol. 2016;175:521–9.

26. Chen J, Tward JD, Shrieve DC, Hitchcock YJ. Surgery and radiotherapy improves survival in patients with anaplastic thyroid carcinoma: analysis of the surveillance, epidemiology, and end results 1983-2002. Am J Clin Oncol. 2008;31:460–4.
27. Bhatia A, Rao A, Ang KK, Garden AS, Morrison WH, Rosenthal DI, Evans DB, Clayman G, Sherman SI, Schwartz DL. Anaplastic thyroid cancer: Clinical outcomes with conformal radiotherapy. Head Neck. 2010;32:829–36.
28. Sun XS, Sun SR, Guevara N, Fakhry N, Marcy PY, Lassalle S, Peyrottes I, Bensadoun RJ, Lacout A, Santini J, Cals L, Bosset JF, Garden AS, Thariat J. Chemoradiation in anaplastic thyroid carcinomas. Crit Rev Oncol Hematol. 2013;86:290–301.
29. Besic N, Hocevar M, Zgajnar J, Pogacnik A, Grazio-Frkovic S, Auersperg M. Prognostic factors in anaplastic carcinoma of the thyroid-a multivariate survival analysis of 188 patients. Langenbecks Arch Surg. 2005;390:203–8.
30. Goutsouliak V, Hay JH. Anaplastic thyroid cancer in British Columbia 1985-1999: a population-based study. Clin Oncol (R Coll Radiol). 2005;17:75–8.
31. Lee DY, Won JK, Choi HS, Park do J, Jung KC, Sung MW, Kim KH, Hah JH, Park YJ. Recurrence and survival after gross total removal of resectable undifferentiated or poorly differentiated thyroid carcinoma. Thyroid. 2016;26:1259–68.
32. Kim TY, Kim KW, Jung TS, Kim JM, Kim SW, Chung KW, Kim EY, Gong G, Oh YL, Cho SY, Yi KH, Kim WB, Park DJ, Chung JH, Cho BY, Shong YK. Prognostic factors for Korean patients with anaplastic thyroid carcinoma. Head Neck. 2007;29:765–72.
33. Steggink LC, van Dijk BA, Links TP, Plukker JT. Survival in anaplastic thyroid cancer in relation to pre-existing goiter: a population-based study. Am J Surg. 2015;209:1013–9.
34. Sun C, Li Q, Hu Z, He J, Li C, Li G, Tao X, Yang A. Treatment and prognosis of anaplastic thyroid carcinoma: experience from a single institution in China. PLoS One. 2013;8:e80011.
35. Tennvall J, Lundell G, Wahlberg P, Bergenfelz A, Grimelius L, Akerman M, Hjelm Skog AL, Wallin G. Anaplastic thyroid carcinoma: three protocols combining doxorubicin, hyperfractionated radiotherapy and surgery. Br J Cancer. 2002;86:1848–53.
36. Zivaljevic V, Tausanovic K, Paunovic I, Diklic A, Kalezic N, Zoric G, Sabljak V, Vekic B, Zivic R, Marinkovic J, Sipetic S. Age as a prognostic factor in anaplastic thyroid cancer. Int J Endocrinol. 2014;2014:240513.
37. Besic N, Auersperg M, Us-Krasovec M, Golouh R, Frkovic-Grazio S, Vodnik A. Effect of primary treatment on survival in anaplastic thyroid carcinoma. Eur J Surg Oncol. 2001;27:260–4.
38. De Crevoisier R, Baudin E, Bachelot A, Leboulleux S, Travagli JP, Caillou B, Schlumberger M. Combined treatment of anaplastic thyroid carcinoma with surgery, chemotherapy, and hyperfractionated accelerated external radiotherapy. Int J Radiat Oncol Biol Phys. 2004;60:1137–43.
39. Landa I, Ibrahimpasic T, Boucai L, Sinha R, Knauf JA, Shah RH, Dogan S, Ricarte-Filho JC, Krishnamoorthy GP, Xu B, Schultz N, Berger MF, Sander C, Taylor BS, Ghossein R, Ganly I, Fagin JA. Genomic and transcriptomic hallmarks of poorly differentiated and anaplastic thyroid cancers. J Clin Invest. 2016;126:1052–66.
40. Subbiah V, Kreitman RJ, Wainberg ZA, Cho JY, Schellens JHM, Soria JC, Wen PY, Zielinski C, Cabanillas ME, Urbanowitz G, Mookerjee B, Wang D, Rangwala F, Keam B. Dabrafenib and trametinib treatment in patients with locally advanced or metastatic BRAF V600-mutant anaplastic thyroid cancer. J Clin Oncol. JCO2017736785. 2017.
41. Smallridge RC, Copland JA. Anaplastic thyroid carcinoma: pathogenesis and emerging therapies. Clin Oncol (R Coll Radiol). 2010;22:486–97.

Chapter 43
A Patient with *BRAF*V600E-Mutated Anaplastic Thyroid Cancer with Metastatic Disease

Maria E. Cabanillas and Jennifer R. Wang

Anaplastic thyroid cancer (ATC) is a deadly disease, and, until recently, little progress had been made to change the outcomes of these patients. In 2018, the US Food and Drug Administration (FDA) approved a BRAF/MEK inhibitor combination, dabrafenib/trametinib, for *BRAF*V600E-mutated ATC. These drugs are highly efficacious in this ATC subtype, and therefore, *BRAF*V600E status is now part of the initial evaluation for all ATC patients. Dabrafenib/trametinib is now the standard of care for BRAFV600E-mutated ATC patients in the USA.

Case Presentation

A 72-year-old woman presented to the local emergency room with dyspnea and palpitations. She was found to have a right-sided neck mass, a pulmonary embolism, and a large pleural effusion. Thoracentesis was performed, revealing metastatic adenocarcinoma, positive for PAX8 (diffuse) and TTF-1 (weak) and negative for thyroglobulin and estrogen receptor, compatible with a thyroid primary. Ultrasound of the neck revealed a 5.5 cm partially cystic mass in the right supraclavicular region and multiple thyroid nodules. CT scan of the neck and chest revealed

M. E. Cabanillas (✉)
Department of Endocrine Neoplasia and Hormonal Disorders, The University of Texas MD Anderson Cancer Center, Houston, TX, USA
e-mail: mcabani@mdanderson.org

J. R. Wang
Department of Head and Neck Surgery, The University of Texas MD Anderson Cancer Center, Houston, TX, USA

G. Grani et al. (eds.), *Thyroid Cancer*,
https://doi.org/10.1007/978-3-030-61919-0_43

similar findings as well as mediastinal adenopathy. Taken together, the clinical picture was consistent with stage IVC ATC. The patient subsequently underwent biopsy of the supraclavicular mass, which showed poorly differentiated carcinoma. The patient was referred to an academic cancer center.

On initial staging FDG-PET/CT, shown in Fig. 43.1, (panel a), a large right necrotic mass adjacent to right thyroid hypermetabolic nodule was identified. Additional sites of disease included bilateral cervical lymph nodes, bilateral pulmonary nodules, a left sternal bone metastasis, and paracaval lymph nodes. An MRI of the brain showed no evidence of metastatic disease.

Fine-needle aspiration with cell block preparation of the supraclavicular lesion was performed in order to obtain immunohistochemistry staining for *BRAF*V600E. The biopsy showed high-grade, poorly differentiated carcinoma with squamoid features, positive for PAX-8, TTF-1, and *BRAF*V600E. She was started on dabrafenib 150mg twice a day and trametinib 2mg once daily by mouth. The patient noticed a rapid reduction in her neck mass. Restaging FDG-PET scan performed 2 months after starting dabrafenib/trametinib (Fig. 43.1, panel b) showed significant reductions in size and FDG avidity within the right supraclavicular mass, right thyroid nodule, sternal metastasis, bilateral lung, pleural, and nodal disease in the chest and abdomen. The patient's disease has remained stable on dabrafenib/trametinib.

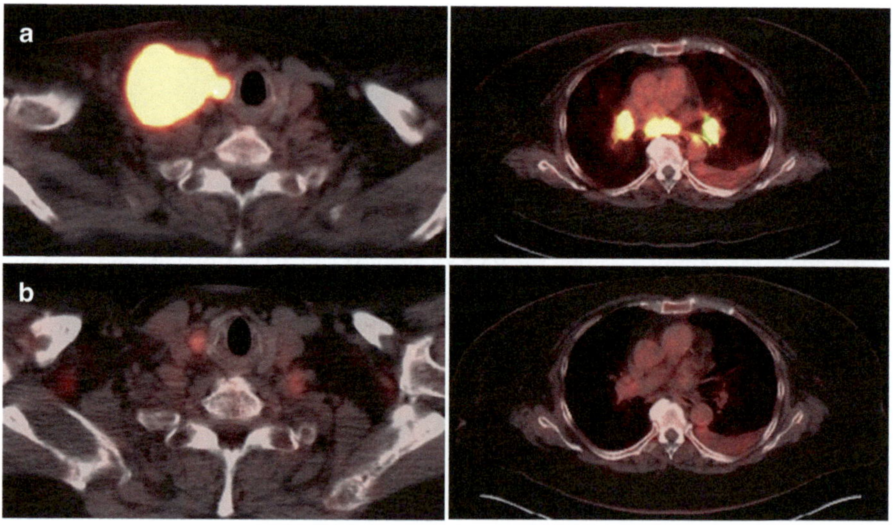

Fig. 43.1 Pre- and post-treatment FDG-PET/CT imaging. (**a**) Baseline FDG-PET/CT imaging showing a right supraclavicular mass with an SUV of 32, a small right-sided thyroid nodule in the neck (left panel), and multiple mediastinal adenopathy and left pleural effusion (right panel). (**b**) FDG-PET/CT was performed after treatment with dabrafenib/trametinib for 2 months, showing near resolution of metastatic lymphadenopathy in the neck and lungs. The right thyroid nodule shows significantly less metabolic activity

Assessment and Literature Review

ATC is a rare form of thyroid cancer and the most aggressive. The clinical picture is of a rapidly growing neck mass causing dyspnea, stridor, hoarseness, and/or dysphagia. Because ATC is often derived from well-differentiated thyroid cancer ("anaplastic transformation"), patients may report a history of prior thyroid cancer. The diagnosis of ATC can be made via fine-needle (FNA), core, or incisional biopsy. Core biopsy or FNA with a cell block preparation is preferred, to allow for immunohistochemical staining for BRAFV600E and molecular testing. Image guidance is helpful to avoid tumor areas with significant necrosis to increase diagnostic yield.

*BRAF*V600*E* is the most common actionable mutation in ATC and influences initial treatment. Thus it must be assessed at diagnosis in all ATC patients. Although next-generation sequencing (NGS) of tumor is the gold standard for molecular testing, results can take several weeks to obtain. Therefore, rapid methods are used as an adjunct to NGS. The most rapid method is immunohistochemistry (IHC) staining for BRAFV600E protein [1]. This test should only be performed on FNA cell blocks or core/surgical specimens to maximize accuracy. The second test is cell-free DNA (cfDNA) on peripheral blood specimens [2, 3]. The pathologic diagnosis is at times difficult to make, as this is a rare tumor and there are many pathologic morphologies, some of which can mimic other cancers. For example, the squamous morphology is often confused with squamous cell carcinoma of the head and neck or lung.

Assessment of the airway, staging, and *BRAF*V600E status should be performed quickly and in tandem, in order to initiate treatment as soon as possible. The first step is to ensure that the airway is secure. The airway may be threatened by vocal cord paralysis, laryngeal edema, external compression, and/or direct invasion by disease. Laryngoscopy should be performed on all patients with a new diagnosis of ATC. Tracheostomy may be necessary to secure the airway in patients presenting with significant respiratory distress. Patients without respiratory distress or concerning physical exam findings may not require upfront prophylactic tracheostomy. Imaging of the neck and chest with contrast is necessary for staging and determination of resectability. Cross-sectional imaging with CT or MRI of the body and brain is also necessary to determine the extent of disease at other sites, as 50% of patients have distant metastases at diagnosis. FDG-PET/CT is very helpful with identifying areas of metastasis that may be difficult to evaluate with cross-sectional imaging alone.

Once staging is complete and *BRAF*V600E status has been determined, further treatment planning can start. Surgery can be considered as the primary treatment for stage IVA patients who are fit for surgery and can undergo resection without significant morbidity. Stage IVB patients (nodal metastasis or disease extending outside the thyroid without distant metastasis) with resectable disease may also be considered for upfront surgery on a case-by-case basis with goals of achieving complete resection. Surgery that leaves behind gross disease (R2) is not beneficial to patients and should not be performed. Furthermore, radical surgery such as laryngectomy and/or esophagectomy is not recommended in ATC patients. Stage IVB patients who do not have a *BRAF*V600E mutation and cannot be treated with surgical resection should receive external beam radiation to the neck with concomitant chemotherapy. Those who do have *BRAF*V600E-mutated stage IVB ATC may also undergo upfront chemoradiation. However, a newer approach to these patients is to start neoadjuvant dabrafenib plus trametinib and later undergo surgical resection followed by chemoradiation [4]. Ongoing clinical trials are evaluating whether this approach leads to improved survival.

Until recently, there were no effective systemic therapies for patients with stage IVC disease (distant metastasis). Targeted therapy against *BRAF*V600E with dabrafenib plus trametinib has shown high response rates (69%) and improved survival [5]. The median progression-free and overall survival were 14 and 20 months in clinical trial, respectively [6]. The BRAF/MEK inhibitor combination, dabrafenib/trametinib, is now approved in the USA and considered the standard of care for patients with tumors harboring a *BRAF*V600E mutation. It should be recognized, however, that the clinical trial that led to the approval enrolled only patients able to swallow whole pills. This likely biased the patient population. Others have reported shorter median overall survival [7, 8] and treatment resistance [9]. Thus, newer approaches to deter resistance, such as the addition of immunotherapy to the BRAF/MEK inhibitor combination [10], are being studied at this time.

In addition to *BRAF*V600E, gene fusions, particularly *NTRK* and *RET* fusions, are also potentially actionable in patients with ATC. There are currently selective NTRK and RET inhibitors approved for solid tumors harboring these fusions [11–14]. However, these alterations are rare in ATC, and response rates have not been established in a larger population of ATC patients.

Patients without an actionable mutation or fusion still lack effective therapies. Thus, patients with stage IVC without a *BRAF*V600E mutation should be referred for clinical trials. Emerging research suggests that the anti-PD1 checkpoint inhibitor, spartalizumab, may have efficacy in ATC patients with high PD-L1 expression and in those without a *BRAF*V600E mutation [15]. Combinations of checkpoint inhibitors [16] or checkpoint inhibitors plus targeted therapy [10] have also been studied in ATC and appear promising.

Clinical Pearls/Pitfalls

- *BRAF*V600E mutation status is now part of the initial evaluation of ATC patients.
- Rapid BRAF testing should be performed by immunohistochemistry on tumor biopsy specimens and/or assessment of cell-free DNA in peripheral blood.
- Dabrafenib (BRAF inhibitor) and trametinib (MEK inhibitor) are effective for ATC patients with *BRAF*V600E mutation and now the standard of care.
- Stage IVC ATC patients without a *BRAF*V600E mutation should be treated within the context of a clinical trial, as there are still no effective therapies for these patients.

References

1. Smith AL, Williams MD, Stewart J, Wang WL, Krishnamurthy S, Cabanillas ME, Roy-Chowdhuri S. Utility of the BRAF p.V600E immunoperoxidase stain in FNA direct smears and cell block preparations from patients with thyroid carcinoma. Cancer Cytopathol. 2018;126:406–13.
2. Iyer PC, Cote GJ, Hai T, Gule-Monroe M, Bui-Griffith J, Williams MD, Hess K, Hofmann M-C, Dadu R, Zafereo M, Busaidy NL, Ferrarotto R, Subbiah V, Gross N, Gunn BG, Skinner HD, Garden AS, Cabanillas ME. Circulating BRAF V600E cell-free DNA as a biomarker in the management of anaplastic thyroid carcinoma. JCO Precis Oncol. 2018;2:1–11.
3. Sandulache VC, Williams MD, Lai SY, Lu C, William WN, Busaidy NL, Cote GJ, Singh RR, Luthra R, Cabanillas ME. Real-time genomic characterization utilizing circulating cell-free DNA in patients with anaplastic thyroid carcinoma. Thyroid. 2017;27:81–7.
4. Wang JR, Zafereo ME, Dadu R, Ferrarotto R, Busaidy NL, Lu C, Ahmed S, Gule-Monroe MK, Williams MD, Sturgis EM, Goepfert RP, Gross ND, Lai SY, Gunn GB, Phan J, Rosenthal DI, Fuller CD, Morrison WH, Iyer P, Cabanillas ME. Complete surgical resection following neoadjuvant dabrafenib plus trametinib in BRAF(V600E)-mutated anaplastic thyroid carcinoma. Thyroid. 2019;29:1036–43.
5. Subbiah V, Kreitman RJ, Wainberg ZA, Cho JY, Schellens JHM, Soria JC, Wen PY, Zielinski C, Cabanillas ME, Urbanowitz G, Mookerjee B, Wang D, Rangwala F, Keam B. Dabrafenib and trametinib treatment in patients with locally advanced or metastatic BRAF V600-mutant anaplastic thyroid cancer. J Clin Oncol. 2017:JCO2017736785.
6. Keam B, Kreitman RJ, Wainberg ZA, Cabanillas ME, Cho DC, Italiano A, Stein A, Cho JY, Schellens JHM, Wen PY, Zielinski CC, Boran AD, Mookerjee B, Burgess P, Rangwala F, Subbiah V. Updated efficacy and safety data of dabrafenib (D) and trametinib (T) in patients (pts) with BRAF V600E–mutated anaplastic thyroid cancer (ATC). Ann Oncol. 2018;29(suppl_8):viii645–6.
7. Iyer P, Dadu R, Ferrarotto R, Busaidy N, Habra MA, Zafereo M, Gross ND, Hess K, Gule-Monroe M, Williams MD, Cabanillas M. Real world experience with targeted therapy for the treatment of anaplastic thyroid carcinoma. Thyroid. 2017;28:79–87.
8. Iyer PC, Dadu R, Gule-Monroe M, Busaidy NL, Ferrarotto R, Habra MA, Zafereo M, Williams MD, Gunn GB, Grosu H, Skinner HD, Sturgis EM, Gross N, Cabanillas ME. Salvage pembrolizumab added to kinase inhibitor therapy for the treatment of anaplastic thyroid carcinoma. J Immunother Cancer. 2018;6:68. https://doi.org/10.1186/s40425-018-0378-y.
9. Cabanillas ME, Dadu R, Iyer P, Wanland KB, Busaidy NL, Ying A, Gule-Monroe M, Wang JR, Zafereo M, Hofmann MC. Acquired secondary RAS mutation in BRAF(V600E)-mutated thyroid cancer patients treated with BRAF inhibitors. Thyroid. 2020;30(9):1288–96. https://doi.org/10.1089/thy.2019.0514.
10. Cabanillas ME, Dadu R, Ferrarotto R, Liu S, Fellman BM, Gross ND, Gule-Monroe M, Lu C, Grosu H, Williams MD, Duose D, Mallampati S, Dervin S, McKenna EF, Wang JR, Zafereo M, Busaidy N. Atezolizumab combinations with targeted therapy for anaplastic thyroid carcinoma (ATC). J Clin Oncol. 2020;38(Suppl):abstr 6514.
11. Bayer HeathCare Pharmaceuticals. Vitrakvi (larotrectinib) [package insert]. U.S. Food and Drug Administration website. https://www.accessdata.fda.gov/drugsatfda_docs/label/2018/211710s000lbl.pdf. Accessed 2 Jun 2020.
12. Roche Pharmaceutical. Rozlytrek (entrectinib) [package insert]. U.S. Food and Drug Adminstration website. https://www.accessdata.fda.gov/drugsatfda_docs/label/2019/212725s000lbl.pdf. Accessed 2 Jun 2020.
13. Eli Lilly and Company. Retevmo (selpercatinib) [package insert]. U.S. Food and Drug Administration website. https://www.accessdata.fda.gov/drugsatfda_docs/label/2020/213246s000lbl.pdf. Accessed 2 Jun 2020.
14. Wirth LJ, Sherman E, Robinson B, Solomon B, Kang H, Lorch J, Worden F, Brose M, Patel J, Leboulleux S, Godbert Y, Barlesi F, Morris JC, Owonikoko TK, Tan DSW, Gautschi O, Weiss

J, de la Fouchardiere C, Burkard ME, Laskin J, Taylor MH, Kroiss M, Medioni J, Goldman JW, Bauer TM, Levy B, Zhu VW, Lakhani N, Moreno V, Ebata K, Nguyen M, Heirich D, Zhu EY, Huang X, Yang L, Kherani J, Rothenberg SM, Drilon A, Subbiah V, Shah MH, Cabanillas ME. Efficacy of Selpercatinib in RET-Altered Thyroid Cancers. N Engl J Med. 2020;383:825–35.

15. Capdevila J, Wirth LJ, Ernst T, Ponce Aix S, Lin CC, Ramlau R, Butler MO, Delord JP, Gelderblom H, Ascierto PA, Fasolo A, Fuhrer D, Hutter-Kronke ML, Forde PM, Wrona A, Santoro A, Sadow PM, Szpakowski S, Wu H, Bostel G, Faris J, Cameron S, Varga A, Taylor M. PD-1 Blockade in Anaplastic Thyroid Carcinoma. J Clin Oncol. 2020:JCO1902727.
16. Lorch JH, Barletta JA, Nehs M, Uppaluri R, Alexander EK, Haddad R, Hanna GJ, Margalit DN, Tishler RB, Schoenfeld JD, Goguen LA, Jabiev A, Sorensen MJ, Ahmadi S, Marqusee E, Kim MI, Stanizzi D, Harris E, Kacew A. Barbie DA. A phase II study of nivolumab (N) plus ipilimumab (I) in radioidine refractory differentiated thyroid cancer (RAIR DTC) with exploratory cohorts in anaplastic (ATC) and medullary thyroid cancer (MTC). J Clin Oncol. 2020;38(Suppl):abstr 6513.

Index

G. Grani et al. (eds.), *Thyroid Cancer*,
https://doi.org/10.1007/978-3-030-61919-0

Q

R

GPSR Compliance

The European Union's (EU) General Product Safety Regulation (GPSR) is a set of rules that requires consumer products to be safe and our obligations to ensure this.

If you have any concerns about our products, you can contact us on ProductSafety@springernature.com

In case Publisher is established outside the EU, the EU authorized representative is:

Springer Nature Customer Service Center GmbH
Europaplatz 3
69115 Heidelberg, Germany

Batch number: 10732076

Printed by Printforce, the Netherlands